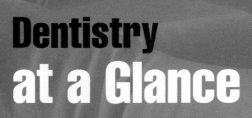

Dentistry
at a Glance

This title is also available as an e-book.
For more details, please see
www.wiley.com/buy/9781118629529
or scan this QR code:

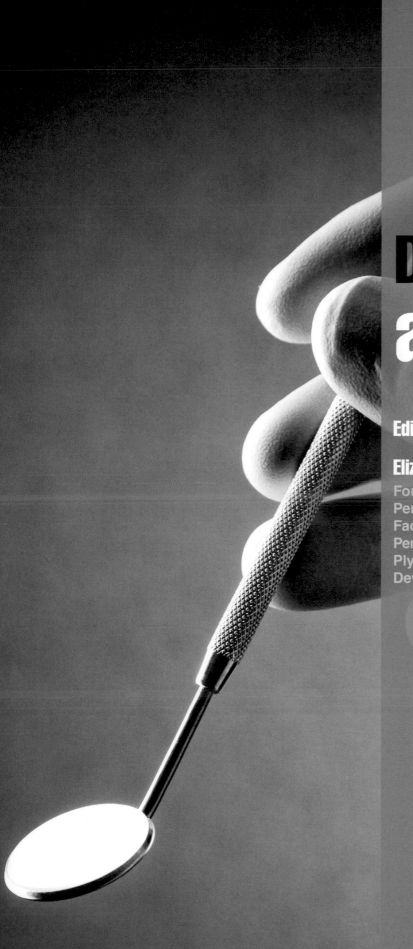

Dentistry
at a Glance

Edited by

Elizabeth Kay
Foundation Dean
Peninsula Dental School;
Faculty Associate Dean
Peninsula Schools of Medicine and Dentistry
Plymouth University
Devon, UK

WILEY Blackwell

This edition first published 2016 © 2016 by John Wiley & Sons Ltd.

Registered office:	John Wiley & Sons, Ltd, The Atrium, Southern Gate, Chichester, West Sussex, PO19 8SQ, UK
Editorial offices:	9600 Garsington Road, Oxford, OX4 2DQ, UK
	The Atrium, Southern Gate, Chichester, West Sussex, PO19 8SQ, UK
	1606 Golden Aspen Drive, Suites 103 and 104, Ames, Iowa 50010, USA

For details of our global editorial offices, for customer services and for information about how to apply for permission to reuse the copyright material in this book please see our website at www.wiley.com/wiley-blackwell

The right of the author to be identified as the author of this work has been asserted in accordance with the UK Copyright, Designs and Patents Act 1988.

Library of Congress Cataloging-in-Publication Data

Names: Kay, Elizabeth J., editor.
Title: Dentistry at a glance / edited by Elizabeth Kay.
Other titles: At a glance series (Oxford, England)
Description: Chichester, West Sussex ; Hoboken, NJ : John Wiley & Sons Inc.,
  2016. | Series: At a glance series | Includes index.
Identifiers: LCCN 2015033705 (print) | LCCN 2015035022 (ebook) | ISBN
  9781118629529 (pbk.) | ISBN 9781118629499 (ePub) | ISBN 9781118629512
  (Adobe PDF)
Subjects: | MESH: Dentistry—methods. | Tooth Diseases.
Classification: LCC RK56 (print) | LCC RK56 (ebook) | NLM WU 100 | DDC
  617.6—dc23
LC record available at http://lccn.loc.gov/2015033705

A catalogue record for this book is available from the British Library.

Wiley also publishes its books in a variety of electronic formats. Some content that appears in print may not be available in electronic books.

Cover image: ©iStockphoto/Casarsa

Set in Minion Pro 9.5/11.5 by Aptara, India
Printed and bound in Singapore by Markono Print Media Pte Ltd

1   2016

Contents

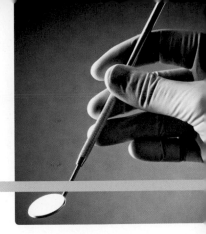

Part 1 — Introduction   1

Part 2 — Clinical presentations   37

Medical emergencies

Prevention of dental diseases

Teeth and disease of tooth hard tissue

The medically compromised patient   199

Orthodontics   219

Contributors

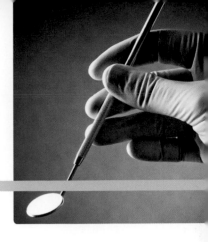

Kamran Ali
Associate Professor / Clinical Lead in Oral Surgery, Peninsula Schools of Medicine and Dentistry, Plymouth University, Devon, UK

Finbarr Allen
Consultant in Prosthodontics and Oral Rehabilitation, Cork Dental School and Hospital, Cork, Ireland

Rupert Austin
Clinical Lecturer in Prosthodontics, King's College London Dental Institute, King's College London, London, UK

Toni Batty
Practice Manager, Torrington Dental Practice, Devon, UK

Igor R. Blum
Consultant and Hon. Senior Lecturer in Restorative Dentistry, The Dental Institute, King's College Hospital, King's College London, London, UK

Tatiana M. Botero
Clinical Associate Professor, Cariology Restorative Sciences and Endodontics School of Dentistry, University of Michigan, Michigan, USA

Andrew Bridgman
Barrister, St Johns Buildings, St John Street, Manchester, UK

Malcolm Bruce
Year 2 Lead and Clinical Dentistry Module Lead, Peninsula Schools of Medicine and Dentistry, Plymouth University, Devon, UK

Martyn Cobourne
Professor of Orthodontics, King's College London Dental Institute, London, UK;
Hon Consultant in Orthodontics, Guy's and St Thomas' NHS Foundation Trust, London, UK

Jennifer Collins
General Dental Practitioner, UK

StJohn Crean
Dean, School of Medicine and Dentistry, University of Central Lancashire, Lancashire, UK

Martin Fulford
Professional Lead - Dentistry, Bristol, N. Somerset, Somerset and S. Gloucester Area Team, NHS England, Somerset, UK

Sue Greening
Consultant in Special Care Dentistry and Clinical Director of the Community Dental Service - Aneurin Bevan Health Board, Wales, UK

Nick Grey
Faculty Associate Dean for Teaching and Learning, The University of Manchester, Manchester, UK

Duncan Parker-Groves
Dental Officer, Defence Dental Service, RAFC Cranwell, Royal Air Force, Lincolnshire, UK

Stephen Hancocks OBE
Editor-in-Chief, British Dental Journal, London, UK

G. R. Holland
Professor, School of Dentistry, University of Michigan, Michigan, USA

Ian Holloway
Associate Dean Df1, NHS South West, UK

Matthew Jerreat
Consultant in Restorative Dentistry, Peninsula Schools of Medicine and Dentistry, Plymouth University, Devon, UK

Elizabeth Kay
Foundation Dean, Peninsula Dental School; Faculty Associate Dean, Peninsula Schools of Medicine and Dentistry, Plymouth University, Devon, UK

Nigel M. King
Winthrop Professor of Paediatric Dentistry, University of Western Australia, Australia

Russ Ladwa
Private Practitioner, London, UK

Kevin Lewis
Dental Director, Dental Protection Limited, London, UK

Michael A. O. Lewis
Professor of Oral Medicine and Dean, School of Dentistry, Cardiff University, Cardiff, UK

Gerry Linden
Professor of Periodontology, School of Medicine, Dentistry and Biomedical Sciences, Queen's University of Belfast, Belfast, UK

Fraser McCord
Emeritus Professor, University of Glasgow, Glasgow, UK

Colman McGrath
Clinical Professor, Faculty of Dentistry, The University of Hong Kong, Hong Kong, China

James Mehta
General Dental Practitioner, Creffield Lodge Dental Practice, Colchester, UK

Alasdair G. Miller
Dental Postgraduate Dean, NHS South West, UK

Ian Mills
Partner, Torrington Dental Practice, Torrington, Devon & Academic Clinical Fellow, Peninsula Schools of Medicine and Dentistry, Plymouth University, Devon, UK

David R. Moles
Director of Postgraduate Education and Research, Peninsula Schools of Medicine and Dentistry, Plymouth University, Devon, UK

Tim Newton
Professor of Psychology as Applied to Dentistry, King's College London Dental Institute, King's College London, London, UK

A. Robert Prashanth
School of Dentistry, University of Western Australia, Australia

Nigel D. Robb
Reader / Honorary Consultant in Restorative Dentistry, Specialist in Special Care Dentistry, School of Oral and Dental Sciences, University of Bristol, Bristol, UK

Anthony Roberts
Professor of Restorative Dentistry (Periodontology), Cork University Dental School and Hospital/University College Cork, Cork, Ireland

Douglas Robertson
Clinical Lecturer/Honorary Specialist Registrar in Restorative Dentistry, Glasgow Dental School, University of Glasgow, Glasgow, UK

Helen Rogers
Clinical Lecturer/Honorary SpR in Oral Medicine, School of Dentistry, Cardiff University, Cardiff, UK

Reza Vahid Roudsari
Clinical Lecturer and Honorary StR in Restorative Dentistry, School of Dentistry, The University of Manchester, Manchester, UK

Fleur R. Stoops
LDFT in Glasgow, NHS Education Scotland, UK

Carly L. Taylor
Clinical Lecturer / Honorary StR in Restorative Dentistry, Manchester Dental School, University of Manchester, Manchester, UK

S. R. Tinsley
Freelance photographer and illustrator, Cornwall, UK

Angus Walls
Director Edinburgh Dental Institute, University of Edinburgh, Edinburgh, UK

Robert Witton
Director of Social Engagement & Community-Based Dentistry, Peninsula Schools of Medicine and Dentistry, Plymouth University, Devon, UK

Hai Ming Wong
Clinical Assistant Professor in Paediatric Dentistry, The University of Hong Kong, Hong Kong, China

Graeme Wright
Specialist and Honorary Clinical Teacher in Paediatric Dentistry, Glasgow Dental Hospital and School, Glasgow, UK

Natasha Wright
Consultant in Orthodontics, Guy's and St Thomas' NHS Foundation Trust, London, UK

Cynthia Yiu
The University of Hong Kong, Hong Kong, China

Preface

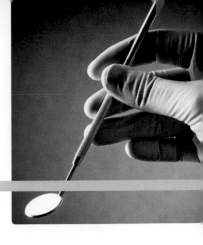

I was immensely honoured and flattered when, based on the reputation of Peninsula Dental School, of which I am Foundation Dean, John Wiley and Sons Publishers approached me to ask me to lead the production of a comprehensive dental textbook. They asked me if I felt that everything a dental undergraduate student needed to know about could be put into one book, and whether I could produce such a tome.

I agreed to the project because, in today's world, where information can be sourced so easily, what is important to students is that someone provides, not so much the detail of the information, but the signposts to show them what they need to look at, and think about, and what is important. A single text containing all that there is to know about dentistry would be a never ending task. However a book which has the intention of simply indicating and highlighting the essentials, whilst stimulating interest and a desire to learn, was a task I was delighted to take on.

I, and the colleagues who wrote this book, hope that this is how it will be seen – as a launchpad for the wonderful experience of a life of learning in dentistry. Every person who has contributed to this book has passion for their subject, and more importantly, and wonderfully, a will to spend their time giving a future generation of dentists the benefit of their knowledge and experience.

The authors are drawn from experts and enthusiasts all over the world and I am deeply grateful to all of my colleagues who have given of their expertise so willingly and so assiduously. Whilst *everyone* involved has done a fantastic job, I would like to thank a few people particularly. My profound gratitude goes to Dr Kamran Ali who contributed all of the oral pathology and oral surgery chapters. His substantial presence in this book is testament to his huge commitment to teaching and learning and perhaps explains the very high regard in which all of his students and staff hold him.

I also need to particularly mention Professor Mike Lewis, who not only contributed chapters, but also gave cheery moral support and was unfailingly and unremittingly generous with images for the book. Likewise Dr Ian Mills, whose expert general practitioner view is an essential component of this text. He also did a fantastic job with the provision of images to illustrate his, and other people's, texts.

My most grateful thanks and eternal gratitude go to Jane Newman. Without her this book would unquestionably never have seen the light of day! This book owes its very existence to her patient persistence, her unbelievable organisational skills and her charm and determination. Organising over forty busy academics to deliver pieces of work to set deadlines is no mean feat! Jane has contributed in many ways to the book, and co-ordinated and provided administrative support to the whole of this enormous project. *And* she remained calm, and buoyed my confidence that we would succeed and did so throughout the entire process. So, I hope everyone who uses the book, or answers the MCQs, or benefits in any way from this publication will remember that *Jane* made it all happen.

Finally, both Jane and I would like to thank our publishers, John Wiley and Sons, and their Associate Commissioning Editor, Sara Crowley-Vigneau and Editorial Assistant Jessica Evans. Their encouragement and support were invaluable and we hope that they are pleased with the end result.

I so hope you enjoy, as well as benefit from, this book. We would value any feedback you can give us. Good luck with your studies, and look forward to your lives. Dentistry is a wonderful profession. This book holds the foundations on which you will build the rest of your careers.

Professor Liz Kay
Foundation Dean Peninsula Dental School

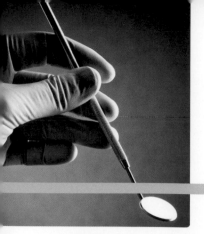

Acknowledgements

With very grateful thanks to the following people and organisations:

- Dentsply
- Pensilva Village Stores
- Tepe Oral Hygiene Products Ltd
- Carestream Dental Ltd
- Journal of the Canadian Dental Association
- The General Dental Council
- The Dental Trauma Guide
- Dr Nikolaos Silikas
- Mrs Margaret Newman
- Sue Greening

- iADH
- Department of Health
- RCSEng Photo Archives with permission from Royal College of Surgeons of England
- Royal Society of Medicine
- British Dental Association
- Torrington Dental Practice
- A-dec Dental UK Ltd
- UK Interprofessional Group

David Moles thanks Jenny Collins for help with producing figures.

About the companion website

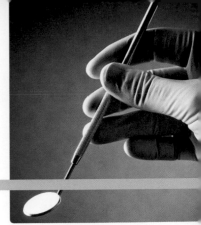

Don't forget to visit the companion website for this book:

**www.ataglanceseries.com/
dentistryseries/dentistry**

There you will find valuable material designed to enhance
your learning, including:

- Interactive multiple choice questions
- Further reading suggestions

Scan this QR code to visit the companion website

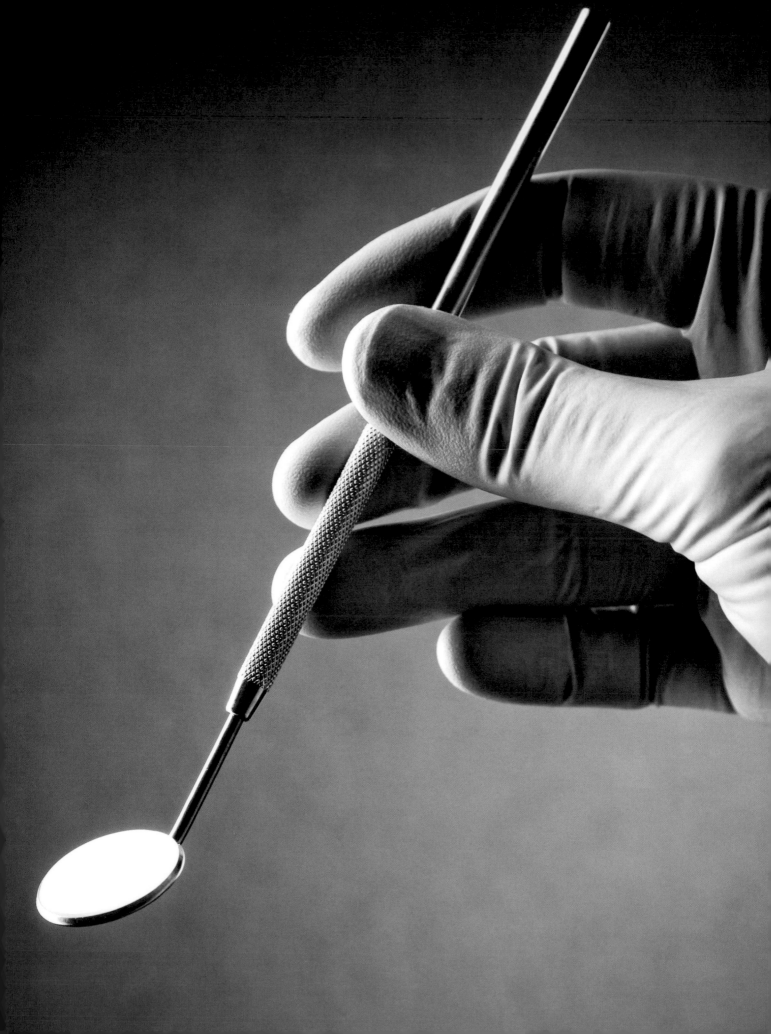

Introduction

Part 1

Chapters

1 Principles of dental practice

Dental practice has been carried out for over 7000 years, and there is evidence of dentistry being practised around the River Indus at that time. From 2600 BC, there are records of the Egyptians practising dentistry, making prostheses and carrying out oral surgery. The purpose of dental practice has, since its inception, been very similar. What has changed over time is the equipment, techniques and materials available to practitioners, and patients' desires and expectations.

The key principles

The key GDC principles are given in Box 1.1.

Box 1.1 The principles of practice in dentistry

As a dental professional, you are responsible for doing the following.
1 Put patients' interests first
2 Communicate effectively with patients
3 Obtain valid consent
4 Maintain and protect patients' information
5 Have a clear and effective complaints procedure
6 Work with colleagues in a way that is in patients' best interests
7 Maintain, develop and work within your professional knowledge and skills
8 Raise concerns if patients are at risk
9 Make sure your personal behaviour maintains patients' confidence in you and the dental profession

Source: General Dental Council (2015). Available at: http://standards.gdc-uk.org/. Information correct at the time of going to press. Please visit the General Dental Council website to check for any changes since publication. Reproduced with the permission of the General Dental Council.

The ethics of a profession is a complex area as it encompasses the views of the profession and those of the society which it serves. These may change over time. Some professional ethics are very obvious, for example the relief of a patient's dental pain should be the first objective for dentists treating patients. However, other issues, which have an ethical dimension, may change based on society's views. For example, there is a dilemma over the ethics of the provision of treatments simply to improve the appearance of teeth. Another major challenge to general practitioners is how to earn a living by providing care to patients whilst maintaining ethical professional standards. Dentists could provide treatments because the patient requests it, so long as it is feasible. The dentist could charge a higher fee, rather than offer a patient a simpler lower-cost procedure. Such decisions are not a simple matter of right or wrong. Ethics and professional standards are important as they provide a 'litmus test' to assist a practitioner decide what they should do. Asking the question 'can the proposed treatment be supported?', if reviewed against the GDC's key standards, is critical to providing appropriate care.

The purpose of dental practice in more detail

1 **Relief of pain to patients** – types of pain in the mouth in order of prevalence is:
- Sensitivity to cold and sweet, which is often due to loss of dentine around the cervical margin of teeth
- Pain from within a tooth – inflamed dental pulp tissues – which is reversible or irreversible
- Pain from the bone around and under a tooth with an abscess
- Pain from unhealthy gums or infection of the gums, gingivitis, periodontitis, e.g. acute ulcerative gingivitis
- Pain from ulcers of the soft tissues of the mouth
- Pain arising within the nervous system of the mouth, e.g. trigeminal neuralgia, psychogenic pain
- Pain from oral cancer
- Pain referred to the jaws, e.g. angina.

2 **Restore function of the oral tissues** so that patients can eat, drink and socialise as they require. Options are:
- Remove the painful or mobile tooth – extraction
- Restore the tooth with fillings or crowns, with or without root fillings
- Replace missing teeth with removable prostheses (e.g. dentures) or fixed prosthesis (e.g. bridges and dental implant retained crowns)
- Provision of orthodontics to straighten teeth to improve the function and appearance
- Provision of tooth whitening and other procedures to improve the aesthetics of the teeth.

3 **Provide advice and treatments to prevent further dental disease:**
- Advice on diet and frequency of consumption of sugar and acid drinks
- Advice on tooth pastes, mouth washes and cleaning of teeth, including interdentally, gum margins and the tongue
- Advice on lifestyle issues – smoking, alcohol consumption
- Procedures to reduce the chance of dental decay, e.g. the application of high-concentration fluoride varnishes, gels and fissure sealants

The object of these interventions is the promotion and maintenance of dental and oral health.

4 **Promotion of the oral health of the community** – dentists may be involved in dental health promotion in their community. This might be talks to schools and other groups, encouragement of local authorities to add fluoride to water, education of staff who care for patients (e.g. in residential and nursing homes), oral cancer awareness months, etc.

The key points

- Dentistry can – relieve pain, restore function, improve appearance, give individual and societal advice on promoting oral and general health
- The delivery of care is defined by professional clinical standards and professional standards which are in turn based on professional ethics and the wishes of the society it serves. These are determined by society in consultation with the profession.

Dentistry at a Glance. First Edition. Edited by Elizabeth Kay. © 2016 John Wiley & Sons, Ltd. Published 2016 by John Wiley & Sons, Ltd.
Companion website: www.ataglanceseries.com/dentistryseries/dentistry

Patient confidentiality

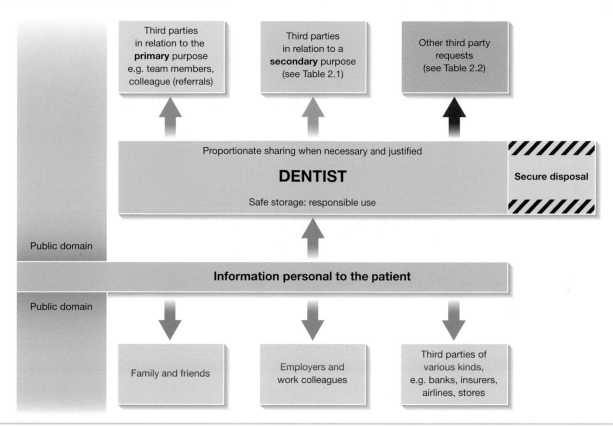

Figure 2.1 Diagram illustrating the flow of information and the escalating level of controls required (green>amber>red). The patient must agree to the onward sharing of information at each point represented by the three coloured arrows. Specific consents may be required in certain situations (refer to text and Tables 2.1 and 2.2)

Any information that a patient has entrusted to you in your professional capacity remains the property of the patient. Failing to keep that information safe and secure, or passing it on to others without the patient's knowledge and agreement, is a breach of the professional trust that the patient has vested in you. Not only would this violate a fundamental ethical principle, but many forms of inappropriate disclosure would also be a criminal offence, under Data Protection legislation.

Patients disclose many different kinds of information to us in the course of our professional relationship with them – some of it being of a sensitive personal nature. Additionally, they will often allow us to capture less obvious forms of information about them, such as study models, X-rays and clinical photographs. In all these cases, they do so in the trust and expectation that we will keep this information safe, and only hold and use it in association with their own dental care and treatment unless they specifically agree otherwise.

Some of the information we hold regarding a patient may already be in the public domain, for example their name, address and phone number may appear in a public directory. But if we have been given this information by the patient within the confidentiality of our professional relationship with them, the fact that it may also be in the public domain for other reasons does not diminish our own ethical obligations in relation to that same information. The underlying principle is that it will always remain the patient's information, not ours (Figure 2.1).

Secondary information

We hold other forms of information, such as the fact that the patient attended (or is due to attend) the practice at a particular date and time. We may know what job the patient does or which company they work for. We may know the names of other people in the patient's family. Even the simple fact that the patient is under your care is information that you have no right to pass on without the patient's agreement.

Permission

The patient may give us permission (consent) to pass on to a third party some or all of the information that they have

Dentistry at a Glance. First Edition. Edited by Elizabeth Kay. © 2016 John Wiley & Sons, Ltd. Published 2016 by John Wiley & Sons, Ltd.
Companion website: www.ataglanceseries.com/dentistryseries/dentistry

disclosed to us, for a purpose directly related to their dental care, for example when being referred to a hygienist or a professional colleague elsewhere. They may also allow us to use some of this information for a purpose unrelated to, or secondary to, their own dental care (Table 2.1). In all these cases the patient must be fully aware of the purpose for which the information will be used, the context in which it will appear, who will have access to it, for how long/ how often, etc.

Table 2.1 Secondary uses of confidential patient information, unrelated to their own care and treatment

Research	Supplying information about the patient and their dental/oral status for the purpose of a bona fide research project (e.g. one which has been approved by a recognised research ethics committee) may be justified in appropriate circumstances.
Lectures and publications	Patient information and images of a patient might be used within professional/ academic circles for the purposes of education through discussion of case studies, published articles, seminars, and lectures at courses and conferences.
Practice promotion/ marketing	The use of images of a patient (especially but not limited to those from which they might readily be identified) for advertisements, printed marketing material, websites etc. This would include any quotes from the patient used for the same purposes.
Mailing/ communications	A mailing house might be provided with the names and addresses of a group of patients (and/or their email address) for the purposes of a direct mailing of paper communication or email campaign.
Audit and investigation	Third-party payment agencies and health insurers may wish to be provided with patient records in order to satisfy themselves as to the treatment provided, details of any payments made by the patient etc. The patient may have provided a qualified or absolute consent to this when applying for treatment and details of this should be sought before releasing any information.

The specific agreement of the patient is needed for any of the above, for each occasion when the information is used. If the intention is to use the information on more than the one occasion for which their permission was originally sought, the patient must have agreed to this at the outset.

If the patient consents to (for example) an image of their mouth and teeth being used in a professional/ academic setting for the specific purposes of one or more lectures to be given by a specific dentist, it is not then acceptable for that dentist to use the same image for an entirely different purpose such as 'before' and 'after' images placed on a practice website. It is even less acceptable for the image to be passed on to anyone else, and used for any other purpose, if the patient did not give their agreement in the expectation that this would happen.

Exceptions

Most of the time, the principles and duties of confidentiality will be clear and obvious. There are, however, some other instances where it is not possible, or perhaps not always necessary, for the specific agreement of the patient to be obtained before passing on confidential information about them. A common example arises when disclosing information about a minor (child) to their parent or someone else with a legal right to be provided with the information. Some other rare exceptions are listed in Table 2.2.

Privacy and security

In any healthcare environment, there needs to be a shared understanding on the part of the entire team that the information that patients have given to us is precious, important and needs to be protected. The fact that the patient trusts us enough to have given us this information about them, and believes that we will keep it safe, is one of the many privileges of being a healthcare professional.

For as long as we hold this information, and whether held in paper form or electronically, we need to take appropriate measures to ensure that the information is only ever accessible to people who need to have it. The same principle extends to any situation where we might be discussing some aspect of the care of one patient within the hearing of another.

There should be adequate safeguards for the secure protection of patient information within the practice/ healthcare environment, and also if any information is ever taken off the premises where it is usually kept. The security of the patient's private information needs to be seamless.

In the case of any document or image from which the identity of the patient could be discovered, one should ask whether the information could be redacted in some way to de-identify the patient. Where information is held electronically, screensaver defaults, password protection and encryption are all examples of how one can prevent information becoming accessible to others unintentionally.

To manage the risks of holding, using and storing confidential information, any disclosure should always be limited to the minimum necessary to serve the required purpose. Similarly, information should be retained no longer than is absolutely necessary to serve the purpose for which it was collected. When, eventually, the information about a patient is no longer required, it is necessary to destroy that information in a safe and secure fashion.

Responsibility and accountability

Many different people have different kinds of responsibility in relation to information about a patient. In addition to the treating dentist, other members of the dental team will have access to information about the patient, some of it of a very sensitive personal nature. It should be a condition of every employment agreement that patient confidentiality is respected not only during the currency of the employment, but also thereafter.

Under Data Protection legislation, a named person within every work setting where health care is provided needs to be identified as the Data Controller, and must register as such with the Information Commissioner's Office. But every dental health profession registered with the General Dental Council is personally accountable to the General Dental Council for any breaches of confidentiality.

Table 2.2 Examples of situations where disclosure of confidential information about a patient to third parties may be acceptable in specific circumstances (advice should be sought from your indemnity provider regarding particular situations)

Disclosure to whom?	In what circumstances?	Safeguards
Tax authorities (HMRC)	To verify the date, amount and method of payments made to a dentist, and to corroborate a dentist's tax claims. HMRC may wish to see a range of information including clinical and financial records, laboratory and supplier invoices which identify the patient.	Establish whether or not the same information can be provided without disclosing any records that might contain other sensitive personal information about the patient, unrelated to the tax investigation. HMRC should be asked to provide a formal notice under Section 19A of the Taxes Management Act 1970, citing the reason why the information is required.
Police officers	This may be: (1) for the purpose of corroborating an alibi given by one of your patients who is suspected of having been involved in committing a criminal offence; (2) to facilitate police enquiries into the whereabouts of a missing person; (3) to assist in the identification of a body.	(a) Here the patient's right of confidentiality needs to be balanced against a legitimate public interest. The seriousness of the offence may be a consideration but there should normally be no objection to seeking the patient's consent in writing to the disclosure. (b, c) In both of these cases you should ask for formal documentation to confirm the nature and scope of the police enquiry, and generally co-operate in the public interest.
Solicitors instructed to act on behalf of a patient (including children under your care)	Usually, when they are making or investigating a potential claim against you or somebody else who has previously treated the patient. But occasionally the request may be in connection with intimated divorce or child custody proceedings.	No information should be supplied without a full explanation of the circumstance in which the requested information is needed. The solicitors should also be asked to supply a specific written authority signed by the patient.
Teachers (in the case of child patients)	For example, to verify details of a child's dental appointment(s) or the time when they arrived/left the surgery. This can occur where a child is citing their attendance at a dental appointment as the reason for them being absent from school.	In general this information should not be provided without the written authority of the parent(s) or person who has legal responsibility for the child. You should also ask for formal confirmation in writing that the enquiry is being made with the school's knowledge and authority.
Employers and work colleagues	For a similar purpose to that in the case of teachers (above).	No information should be provided unless and until the patient has given their consent.

3 Record keeping

Keeping proper records of the care and treatment we provide for our patients is an essential aspect of our overall duty of care. It is one of the basic principles that we are all taught at dental school, and this message is continually reinforced throughout our practising careers through lectures, publications and personal clinical experience. But even though the complexity of dental care and the context in which it is being provided has evolved over the years, this has not been reflected in a commensurate improvement in the quality and completeness of the records that are being kept.

There are many reasons why it is important to keep clear, full and contemporaneous notes of the care and treatment provided. The irony of record keeping and paperwork generally is that it is the part of dentistry that most dentists actively dislike. Consequently, many dentists spend as little time as possible on it, perhaps because it is often seen as a distraction from (and less important than) the main 'task', that is the clinical work itself. This can leave the dentist exposed and vulnerable to problems on all fronts.

Every member of the dental team can play a valuable part in ensuring that the practice's record keeping is of a high standard. This is the key to high-quality care as well as patient safety. Poor record keeping can make it difficult or impossible to defend allegations of clinical negligence, poor clinical performance or professional misconduct. It can also lead to disputes over money, can cause mistrust and confusion, and can lead directly to complaints. Endless hours of 'fire-fighting' can be wasted in trying to resolve problems caused by poor record keeping, and it can even lead to the most serious (and fatal) consequences. On some occasions, the records we make can change the entire course of our professional career.

Why keep records?

It is a common misconception that records are simply an *aide memoire* for the personal use of the clinician. Here in the UK, patients have a legal right of access to their records, and can obtain copies of them upon request. If and when any problems arise, other bodies such as NHS commissioners and independent premises and facilities inspectorates, such as the Care Quality Commission (CQC) and equivalent bodies elsewhere in the UK, the NHS Counter Fraud Service, the General Dental Council, experts and forensic odontologists or coroners acting on behalf of the courts will all examine dental records. In Denplan and similar capitation systems, they may be inspected by officers of these agencies, or by insurance companies. If litigation or disciplinary action is being contemplated against a dentist, then the records will usually need to be disclosed to patients' legal or other representatives.

The UK has become increasingly litigious in recent years and good record keeping can provide vital evidence of the proper level of skill, care and attention that a patient has received. Sometimes there will be a conflict of evidence between the versions of events given by the patient and the dentist, respectively. In such situations, the patient's version is often preferred unless

the records can provide clear evidence to support the dentist's account of events. It is often argued that the patient is much more likely to recall the events of a single dental appointment, with a single dentist on a specific occasion, than the dentist for whom this will have been one of many patients seen on that particular day, and with many more patients having been seen in the weeks, months and years since the events in question. Our memories are much more fallible than we might wish to imagine.

Adequate records will allow a clinician to reconstruct the details of a patient's dental care, without having to rely upon memory alone. Excellent records go further than this, because they provide evidence of the thought processes, which lie behind the decisions that were made. They will also provide a lot more useful detail and, because of this, they can anticipate and answer all the key questions that might be asked in the future, arising from the treatment provided (or sometimes not provided).

Think record, not record card

It will be clear from Box 3.1 that the totality of the available records of the care and treatment that you have provided for a particular patient is a lot wider than the clinical records alone. In some situations, these secondary records of various kinds will provide and corroborate crucial details that may not be available or obvious from the clinical records alone.

Box 3.1 Different kinds of records

The totality of the record of a patient's dental care could include many (or all) of the following:
- The treatment notes
- The current and historical medical history
- Radiographs (and any associated tracings), prints from magnetic resonance imaging (MRI), head and neck tomography and other imaging
- Results of other investigations (pathology or radiology reports, pulse oximeter printouts, blood tests etc.)
- Study models/casts
- Diagnostic records (bite registrations, stents, diagnostic wax-ups etc.)
- Photographs (including intraoral camera images)
- Correspondence
- Notes of meetings (e.g. joint consultations or case management conferences between different clinicians involved in the patient's treatment)
- Practice documentation of various kinds (perhaps including consent forms, although their relevance is considered separately in the Chapter Consent)
- Other sources of information, some of which might refer to the patient:
  - Laboratory tickets and invoices
  - Other invoices (e.g. for implant fixtures)
  - Financial records
  - Appointment diaries/ daylists

Many of these records may be held on paper, others in computerised/digital form. Either way, the records are only helpful if they have been preserved and remain available at the time they are subsequently required. Original documents are obviously preferable but scanned copies are better than nothing at all.

Dentistry at a Glance. First Edition. Edited by Elizabeth Kay. © 2016 John Wiley & Sons, Ltd. Published 2016 by John Wiley & Sons, Ltd.
Companion website: www.ataglanceseries.com/dentistryseries/dentistry

Communication

Dentists tend to be more diligent in recording the treatment that they provided than the details of the conversations that they have had with the patients. Yet these conversations often lie at the heart of disputes about what patient were and were not told about treatment recommended for them, or warnings and advice given in association with it. Box 3.2 summarises some of the detail that we need to be capturing. Training and involving a dental nurse to assist in ensuring that all key elements of these discussions have been properly recorded will make the best use of everyone's time and help to ensure that no important details are overlooked.

Box 3.2 What should the clinical record (treatment notes) contain?

- **The patient's name and contact details** (address, preferred phone/ fax/ e-mail or other contact details): it is important to keep this information up to date as it may be needed in an emergency situation.
- **An up to date medical history**: a full medical history (including a note of any prescribed or self-administered medication) should be taken at the initial examination and updated and checked for any changes at each subsequent visit. It is also helpful to have a note of the patient's medical practitioner. Everybody realises the importance of taking a full, written medical history at the time of the first examination of a new patient. The problem often arises, however, that at subsequent recall examinations (checkups) the medical history is not formally updated, and no written entry is made in the notes to the effect that the clinician has confirmed that the medical history is unchanged.
- **Evidence of a thorough case assessment**: it should be possible for a third party, long after the event, to understand from the records you have kept each detail of the examination, diagnosis and treatment planning process. A detailed baseline charting of the dentition, showing the location, type and extent of any restorations, is an invaluable starting point. The attention to detail shown in the clinician's approach to the patient's personal, social/employment, medical and dental history, and to other aspects of the case assessment, help to create a picture of a thorough, caring and competent professional. The reverse is equally true.
  An accurate record of positive findings and signs (what you can discover for yourself) and symptoms (what the patient tells you about the problem) are important, so also is the absence of them (tooth *not* tender to percussion, lymph nodes *not* enlarged, *no* swelling, *not* painful, *not* loose or mobile, *no* change in medical history, etc.).
- **Risk factors**: it should be clear that any relevant risk factors have been screened for, identified and appropriately managed. The records should confirm that the patient has been made aware of the risk factors, their relevance to the prognosis and any action on the part of the patient that will be necessary to mitigate and/or manage them.
- **Investigations**: a summary of each investigation carried out with a note of both positive and negative findings. This should include monitoring information such as Basic Periodontal Examination (BPE) scores, periodontal probing depths and other indices, tracking of oral pathology and other conditions.
- **Treatment information**: the date, diagnosis and treatment notes every time a patient is seen, with full details of the treatment carried out. This should specify the teeth treated, materials used and clinical findings as the treatment proceeds.
  These notes should include a summary of any particular incidents, episodes or discussions (e.g. if a patient declines a referral or other treatment recommended for them).
- **Appointment attendance record**: the date and details of any appointment offered to a patient but declined, or which a patient fails to attend, or cancels or when the patient arrives late and/or needs to be re-booked.
- **Phone contacts**: dates and details of any telephone conversations with the patient, whether this involves the dentist or other dental team members. Similarly, any fax or e-mail contact should be retained within the records.
- **Financial records**: although it is sensible to keep these separate from the clinical notes themselves, records should be kept of all fees quoted and charged and payments made by the patient. Tax authorities may request financial data from the dentist and issues of confidentiality can be avoided if the financial transactions are kept as a separate element within the record, rather than being mixed up within clinical records. Processes in which any unpaid fees are pursued should also be meticulously recorded.
- **Correspondence**: all correspondence to and from the patient or any third party (including specialists, medical practitioners, other dentists, etc.).
- **Consents** obtained, information provided about the nature and extent of any procedures proposed, and specific warnings given of possible adverse outcomes: the necessary elements of the consent process are covered in more detail in the Chapter Consent.
- **Advice**: notes of advice (including oral hygiene, dietary and/or general health advice such as the discontinuation of smoking or attention to other risk factors).
- **Instructions**: given pre- and postoperatively to the patient (or parents).
- **Drugs given**: including not only the identity of the drug, but also the route of administration, dosages, frequency and quantity ordered. Any adverse reaction to any such medication should be recorded.
- **Anything else that you consider relevant**: here, the patient's *dental history* can be particularly relevant. For example, a record should contain the reason why the patient has requested a consultation or examination, and (unless a regular patient) a note of when the patient last received dental care. This is extremely important, especially in the case of a new patient, because it is always helpful to be able to refer back to notes made at the initial examination to recall what signs and symptoms the patient was actually exhibiting when he or she was first seen.
  It is equally important to have a record of what treatment the patient initially requested or required, and of any constraints placed by the patient upon the treatment approach. A relevant part of the records in this connection might be a summary of the patient's past experience of various kinds of restoration (e.g. a denture with palatal coverage).

Authenticity

There is a particular value and integrity in records made at the time of the events that are being described. This is often described as a 'contemporaneous' record. There is nothing wrong with making a later addition to a previous record if you realise that something important has been overlooked, providing that it is clear who made the additional entry and when. No such amendment should be made in a way that is designed to suggest that this record was contemporaneous. The worst scenario is when it later comes to light that the additional entry was made only after the dentist became aware that a challenge was imminent, in a foolhardy attempt to strengthen their defence to any potential allegations.

In fact, such actions do precisely the opposite because they create doubt regarding the honesty of the clinician concerned. Never be tempted to destroy and rewrite records or embellish them and attempt to pass them off as the original, contemporaneous record. Many dentists over the years have fallen into the trap of being panicked into altering their records of a patient's treatment. Even the most deficient original, contemporaneous records have a greater value in their support of a dentist than the most immaculate and comprehensive records that later prove to be something other than what they purported to represent.

Consent

Figure 4.1 Staying on track through a valid consent process

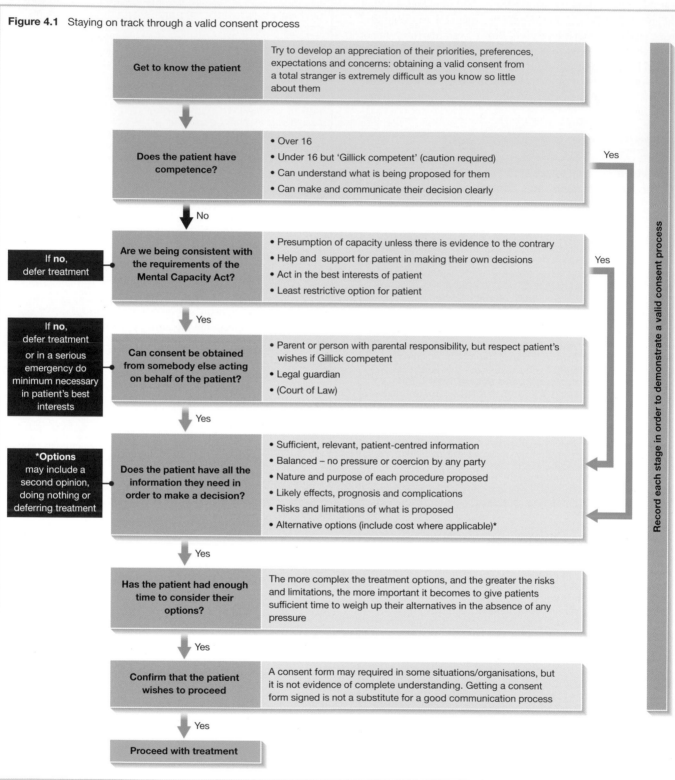

Dentistry at a Glance. First Edition. Edited by Elizabeth Kay. © 2016 John Wiley & Sons, Ltd. Published 2016 by John Wiley & Sons, Ltd.
Companion website: www.ataglanceseries.com/dentistryseries/dentistry

Respecting our patients and their personal autonomy – that is, their right to make decisions for themselves regarding what (if any) treatment they are willing to undertake, when and from whom – is one of the most important aspects of modern health care. It is an extension of the right of every human being to 'self-determination', which is essentially the right to decide, without compulsion or undue influence by others, what will happen to them. In the era of so-called 'medical paternalism', there was a wide gulf in knowledge and understanding of medical matters between patients and the healthcare professionals treating them. As a result, doctors were often trusted by patients to do whatever they believed to be in their best interests.

This so-called 'Doctor knows best' approach started to change in the 1980s and this trend has accelerated rapidly since the internet empowered many more people with information about health care. Now, the patient should be at the centre of all decisions regarding their care and treatment.

Three dimensions

It may be helpful to view consent as having three dimensions:
• **An ethical dimension** – what patients have a right to expect from us as healthcare professionals in whom they have placed their trust
• **A legal dimension** – what the law expects of us (in practical terms, failures in this regard generally take the form of an allegation of negligence although in very rare instances a charge of assault or battery may be possible)
• **A human dimension** – treating our patients in the same way that we would want ourselves or a close friend or family member to be treated in the same circumstances.

While all three are important, and they share several key principles in common, pausing to reflect upon the human dimension will often take us towards the right decisions when approaching questions relating to patient consent.

Preliminary considerations
Competence

In order to understand information given to them about their condition and treatment options, and to give a valid consent on their own behalf, a first prerequisite is that the patient is 'competent'. Such a patient has the 'capacity' to understand the nature and purpose of a particular procedure, its likely effects and risks, what other treatment options are available and their relative advantages and disadvantages. They must also be able to ask relevant questions and to communicate their decision clearly at the time it needs to be made – this is a key consideration when assessing capacity. A young child may lack the intellectual capacity to assimilate and objectively consider this kind of information, and is deemed to be incompetent. But an older child may be competent because they have the capacity to understand the same information and make rational decisions for themselves – this is referred to as 'Gillick competence' where it involves a patient who has not yet reached the age of consent, this term originating from a landmark test case of the same name.

On the other hand, a normally competent adult patient may lack competence at a specific moment in time (e.g. when unconscious or under the influence of substances affecting their mental capacity). Some patients suffer from chronic mental incapacity and may never be able to give a valid consent for themselves. For these situations, a Code of Practice has been established under the Mental Capacity Act 2005, at the heart of

which is a '**presumption of capacity**', which places the onus on healthcare practitioners to demonstrate that the patient is not competent, rather than the reverse.

Authority

Competent adults aged 16 years or more have the authority to give or withhold consent for any treatment proposed for them. The question of who has the legal authority to give consent on behalf of a minor (child) is complex and varies form one part of the UK to another, and to some extent depends upon what is being proposed and the circumstances.

The consent process
Information

Choice in the absence of sufficient, balanced information, communicated in terms that the patient can understand and relate to, is not really a meaningful choice at all. But much more important than the information itself, is the extent to which the patient can understand it, consider it, reflect upon it and come to a decision. This is why many eminent authorities believe that the widely used term 'informed consent' is actually unhelpful because it places too much emphasis on the transfer of information, and insufficient emphasis on the patient's understanding and internalisation of the information.

Far preferable to a long and text-heavy 'universal' consent form that comprehensively describes every risk and adverse outcome ever known to be associated with a given procedure, is evidence of a two-way discussion in which the patient was helped to understand what was likely to happen in their own individual case, and where any areas of uncertainty existed. Information should be particularised (i.e. using specific rather than vague terms), and personalised – too much irrelevant information can actually obscure the key facts and obstruct the patient's understanding.

Voluntariness

The patient needs to make their decision freely, with no pressure, manipulation or coercion from the healthcare provider or any other person (such as a relative or carer). Healthcare professionals must be careful not to abuse their position of great influence in terms of the treatment options that they do and do not discuss, or how they explain them to patients, or the words used, the timing of the discussion, their body language etc.

Documentation

Every stage of the consent process, and especially the details of any discussions, explanations and warnings of risks and any uncertain prognosis, needs to be meticulously documented. Consent forms are one way to show that some information was given to the patient, but they do not provide evidence of any real understanding. They should never be seen as an effective substitute for a thorough communication process.

Summary

This information, coupled with the flowchart in Figure 4.1, is necessarily a very brief overview of what is an important and, in some respects, complex area of clinical practice in the UK. The law in Scotland is subtly different, and a more detailed advice booklet for each jurisdiction of the UK is available at: www.dentalprotection.org.

5 Communication with patients

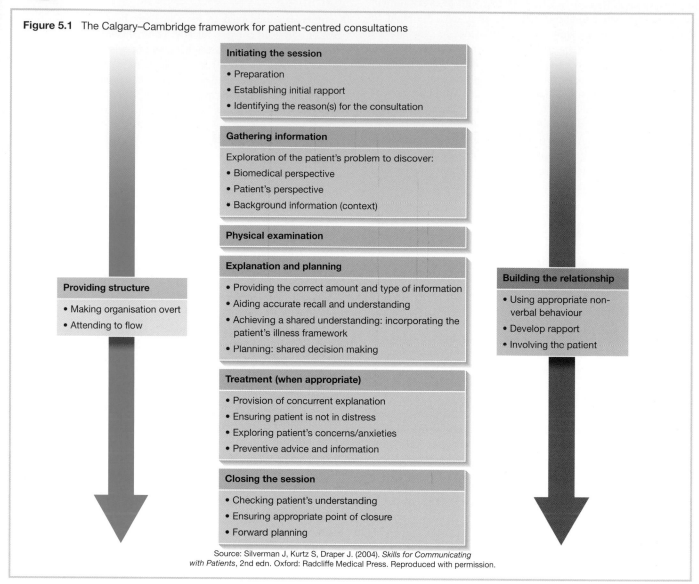

Figure 5.1 The Calgary–Cambridge framework for patient-centred consultations

Initiating the session

- Preparation
- Establishing initial rapport
- Identifying the reason(s) for the consultation

Gathering information

Exploration of the patient's problem to discover:
- Biomedical perspective
- Patient's perspective
- Background information (context)

Physical examination

Providing structure

- Making organisation overt
- Attending to flow

Explanation and planning

- Providing the correct amount and type of information
- Aiding accurate recall and understanding
- Achieving a shared understanding: incorporating the patient's illness framework
- Planning: shared decision making

Building the relationship

- Using appropriate non-verbal behaviour
- Develop rapport
- Involving the patient

Treatment (when appropriate)

- Provision of concurrent explanation
- Ensuring patient is not in distress
- Exploring patient's concerns/anxieties
- Preventive advice and information

Closing the session

- Checking patient's understanding
- Ensuring appropriate point of closure
- Forward planning

Source: Silverman J, Kurtz S, Draper J. (2004). *Skills for Communicating with Patients*, 2nd edn. Oxford: Radcliffe Medical Press. Reproduced with permission.

Effective communication lies at the heart of healthcare and dental practice. The benefits of improved communication are numerous and include increased patient satisfaction, improvements in adherence to health-related advice, better patient outcomes and a decreased risk of litigation.

Interpersonal communication is founded on three channels of communication through which we transfer information. These are: the verbal channel – the actual words we use; the paralinguistic channel – essentially our tone of voice; and the non-verbal channel, which includes a whole range of behaviours that we interpret without consciousness but which convey a great deal of information, for example facial expressions, gestures and eye contact. Communication is most effective if all three channels (verbal, tone of voice and non-verbal communication) are congruent, that is they all give the same message. It is not enough to say the right words, if your tone of voice and non-verbal communication belie the importance of your message. For example when giving oral hygiene advice, does your body language and tone of voice tell the patient the importance of this topic?

The Calgary–Cambridge framework provides an overview of the key tasks that a dentist needs to achieve when communicating with their patients (Figure 5.1). This can be summarised as a central description of the process together with two themes running throughout the consultation.

Providing structure

The dentist needs to be conscious of the structure of the consultation and make clear to the patient what is happening. For instance, 'Today I will make some notes on your medical history, we can discuss how your teeth have been and then I will take a look and perhaps get some X-rays. Once we have all that information we can decide on the next steps'. The dentist also needs to ensure that the stages progress satisfactorily.

Building the relationship

A relationship of trust and mutual respect will enable the dentist and their patient to work towards joint decisions about the most effective pathway of care. Three key skills help to build such relationships, that is developing rapport through showing an interest in the patient and a willingness to help, as well as appropriate empathic responses. Involving the patient in decision making is simple and helps them feel positive towards the decisions made. Such involvement need not be complex, for example asking the patient whether they would like upper or lower impressions first, or their opinion of the priorities for treatment. Throughout, the dentist's non-verbal communication should be warm and welcoming.

The consultation

The dental consultation has an overall structure that is similar to nearly all healthcare encounters, but varies in the emphasis given to each phase. The Calgary–Cambridge framework gives the detail of this. It identifies tasks to achieve at each stage of the consultation. The specific communication skills that you will need to achieve these tasks are:

- Active listening
- Empathic responses
- Open and closed questions
- Summarizing
- Clarification and negotiation
- Clear explanations.

Active listening

Though we generally believe that we are listening to somebody, we recall less than 25% of the information that we have been told. Active listening refers to a process where the individual listens and, at the same time, attempts to discern, interpret and summarise what the speaker is saying. This necessarily requires a great deal of attention on the part of the listener. This attention will be reflected in the body language and non-verbal communication of the listener. Active listening involves trying to understand a speaker's viewpoint and requires a degree of empathy on the part of the listener.

One way of thinking about active listening is to imagine that at the end of the initial discussion you will be asked to give a summary of the patient's concerns and expectations. The summary should be concise and precise. Making such a summary is good communication practice, and if recorded in patient notes is a useful statement of the agreed goals at the start of treatment.

Empathy

Empathy refers to the feeling that the listener is making an effort to understand the situation from the speaker's point of view. Empathy is an attempt to understand how the other person is feeling – it is not the same as sympathy, which is an emotional reaction to someone's emotion. Empathy may be conveyed in body language and tone of voice, and also in the way that the dental healthcare professional talks about the patient's problems.

Use of open and closed questions

The quality and amount of information acquired in a consultation is related to the appropriate use of open-ended questions, frequent summaries, clarification and negotiation. Open questions allow the patient a free possibility of response, rather than limiting the replies to a number of options. 'How are you?' is an open question; 'Do you have a toothache?' is a closed question. Using open questions allows the patient to discuss all their concerns. If questioning is inappropriately restricted to closed questions (about their desire for change etc.) important concerns for the patient (such as their anxiety) may be missed.

In general, open questions should be used to initiate consultations, closed questions to focus down on the issues that are raised. Closed questions may inappropriately restrict choice but they are essential in getting accurate information on specific issues.

Summarising

As the consultation progresses, the use of frequent summaries allows the dentist to check that he or she has understood the patient. It may also help the patient to clarify in their own mind what they are trying to express. A simple technique is the use of 'chunk and check' – group information into meaningful chunks and then check after every 'chunk' that the patient has clearly understood and remembered that bit of information before moving on to the next.

Clarification and negotiation

Clarification aims to demonstrate to the patient that the dentist is seeking a shared understanding of the patient's problem. Offering patients simple choices in their treatment is a good way to introduce the notion of negotiation and to demonstrate that the opinion of the patient is important.

Clear explanations

Patients who are given clear explanations also feel more satisfied with their interactions. Consider rehearsing a clear explanation for the advice you commonly give. Remember that though you may give the same message several times a day it is important that your tone of voice and non-verbal behaviour suggest that you are interested in helping the patient.

Summary

Communication is central to being a good dentist. Communication occurs through the words we use, the tone of voice we say them in and the actions that accompany our communication. It is best if all three of these channels give the same message. Through the use of key communication skills such as active listening, empathy, summarizing and question techniques, the dentist seeks to establish rapport with their patient, and steer the patient through the consultation, achieving the best possible care.

6 History taking

Figure 6.1 Talk to patient with chair upright and make eye contact

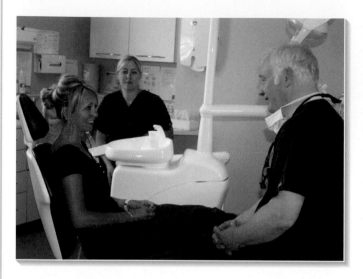

Figure 6.2 Adopting a compassionate manner includes careful explanation

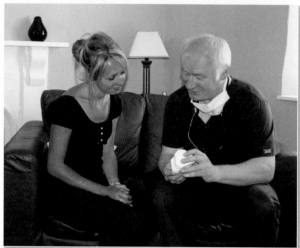

Table 6.1 Common causes of dental pain

Pain	Character	Duration	Aggravating/relieving factors
Dentine hypersensitivity	Sharp pain on response to thermal or tactile stimulus	Seconds	Stimulus evokes response
Reversible pulpitis	Sharp Pain not easy to locate	As long as the stimulus – seconds	Cold/ hot/ sweet Removing stimulus relieves symptoms
Irreversible pulpitis	Dull Spontaneous Throbbing Maybe worse at night Not easy to locate	Minutes/ hours	Remove stimulus Analgesics
Apical periodontitis	Dull ache on biting Easy to associate with a specific tooth	Minutes/ hours	Biting
Cracked tooth	Sharp pain on biting	Seconds	Biting hard foods

Table 6.2 Common causes of non-dental pain

Pain	Character	Duration	Aggravating/relieving factors
Muscular	Dull Aching Difficult to pinpoint	Constant	Clenching Grinding Habits – nail/pen biting Analgesics may help
Migraine	Moderate Associated nausea/ visual disturbance	Hours	Alcohol Foods (cheese/ chocolate) Light
Cluster headaches	Severe	Hours	
Atypical dental pain	Atypical by definition but not easily falling in to any other category No obvious dental cause	Variable	Relived by medication
Trigeminal neuralgia	Excruciating pain Unusual to be at night	Very short – not more than seconds	'Trigger' points Diagnostic use of carbamazepine may confirm diagnosis

Dentistry at a Glance. First Edition. Edited by Elizabeth Kay. © 2016 John Wiley & Sons, Ltd. Published 2016 by John Wiley & Sons, Ltd.
Companion website: www.ataglanceseries.com/dentistryseries/dentistry

Sir William Osler is well known for supposedly saying 'Listen to your patient, he is telling you the diagnosis'. His words are as true now as they were in the 19th century.

Greeting the patient

Taking an accurate and thorough history and examination for a patient is essential if the patient is to be managed safely and effectively. As first impressions do count, it is important that the first encounter with a patient goes well. As not all patients are the same, it is difficult to have a style that suits all but there are some general points worthy of consideration.

Run on time: There can be few patients who will be happy about not being seen on time. The nature of dentistry is such that running late does occasionally occur and where it does, there should be mechanisms in place to inform the patient. When the patient is eventually seen, it is sensible to apologise for running late with an explanation if appropriate.

The environment: A pleasant and relaxing environment can only assist a more effective consultation with the patient. A cluttered surgery with the noise of instruments from a previous patient being cleared away is hardly likely to relax the patient.

Communication skills

Introduce yourself: Saying 'good morning, how are you today?' with a smile is polite and will most often get a response 'fine'. Where it does not, it allows a conversation about what might not be going well and personalises the attention you are giving the patient very quickly.

Making eye contact and body language: Writing up patient notes is essential but not at the same time as having a conversation with them as it prevents the dentist from making eye contact. Talking with the patient sitting upright and at the same level as them is more natural than with the patient laid back in the dental chair (Figure 6.1).

Addressing the patient: Times change but common courtesy is probably still such that a person's title should be used. There are some who would never think to call a patient by their first name, thinking this would be overfamiliar, and those who feel that using patients first names encourages a more relaxed atmosphere. Either way, it is a good idea to ask the patient how they wish to be addressed and make a note of that for the next time the patient attends. If the patient wishes to bring someone in with them, it is polite to acknowledge their presence and ask the patient 'who have you come in with today?' rather than make any assumptions.

Adopting a compassionate manner: There are many factors that contribute to being compassionate; including listening, responding, explaining in a form of language the patient can understand (Figure 6.2).

Presenting complaint

This is straightforward, with the aim of recording the reason the patient is being seen.

It can therefore be 'none' if the patient is in for a regular check up, or note that the patient is in pain, dislikes the appearance of their teeth, cannot eat, has bleeding gums, or has difficulty opening their mouth or other such problems.

It is important to record what the patient reports in their own words.

History of presenting complaint

The art of listening is key to establishing the course of events leading to the patient attending the surgery. Some patients are expert at relaying on signs and symptoms that make diagnosis straightforward, while others struggle. For those that do struggle, questions can be tailored to glean more information but without resorting to asking leading questions.

Common complaints fall into one the following:

Pain: More detail is needed to aid reaching a diagnosis – site (and spread), onset, duration, character, aggravating and relieving factors, and it is sometimes also helpful to ask the patient what they think may be related to the pain. See Table 6.1 for common causes of dental pain and Table 6.2 for common causes of non-dental pain. A General Medical Practitioner or a specialist in Oral Medicine is better placed to investigate atypical dental or facial pain with a suspected psychological cause.

Appearance: Complaints relating to appearance are personal to the patient, with some patients being more particular than others. There are many factors relating to the mouth that may affect appearance – position, colour and contour of teeth, symmetry and proportion, soft tissue contour.

Function: There is sufficient literature indicating that a shortened dental arch is viable for the majority of patients and most seem reassured when told that not every space needs to be restored. Some patients, however, do mourn the loss of a tooth or teeth despite still being able to function.

Bleeding gums/ bad breath: Halitosis is a common complaint and one that merits further questioning, which should focus on oral hygiene procedures.

Speech: The number of patients reporting problems with speech is fortunately very rare as speech is the end result of a very complex neuromuscular mechanism. The history may reveal an association between speech difficulties and a dental procedure, which may help identify changes that are potentially needed.

Trauma: The dentist may be the first port of call for a patient who has suffered trauma to the teeth. The first fact to ascertain is whether the patient has been rendered unconscious or shows any sign of head injury, in which case they need to be seen in hospital immediately.

Other (a good catch all for the unusual): Patients occasionally present with complaints that do not fit with any obvious dental cause and their management depends on the nature of the complaint.

7 Past medical history

Figure 7.1 The medical history is taken at the beginning of each course of treatment and checked at each subsequent visit

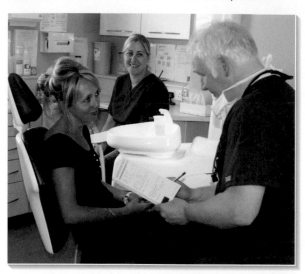

Figure 7.2 Comfortable surroundings promote accurate history taking

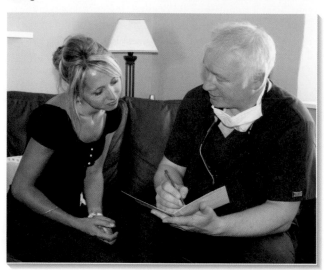

The importance of the medical history

An accurate and up to date medical history is essential if safe care is to be delivered to patients. The General Dental Council (GDC) states 'Make and keep accurate and complete records including a medical history, at the time that you treat them' (Standards for Dental Professionals, GDC, 2005. Available at: www.gdc-uk.org). Local Trusts often have additional guidance and it is the responsibility of the dentist to make sure they are adhered to. In the locality of the author (Central Manchester NHS Foundation Trust, 2010), it is suggested that:

• A detailed record of the medical history must be obtained at the beginning of each course of treatment (Figure 7.1).
• The patient registration booklet must be signed and dated by the patient.
• At each subsequent visit, the medical history should be verbally checked and that must be recorded in the notes.
• A detailed record of the medical history must be repeated annually if the course of treatment lasts longer than 12 months.

The medical history taking may be taken verbally by the dentist (writing in the answers on a proforma) or by asking the patient to fill in a proforma before the appointment to be discussed with the dentist in the surgery (Figure 7.2). The Dental Protection Society's article *Exercise In Risk Management: The Medical History* states: 'Dentists and other members of the practice team should resist the temptation to complete the "yes" and "no" answers on the patient's behalf, to avoid the suggestion that they might have incorrectly recorded the patient's actual responses. Wherever possible, the patient (or parent) should complete the questionnaire personally.' With respect to computers, the Dental Protection Society also notes that 'computerised practices strenuously avoid the creation and storage of any paper documents, and so a clinician will often take a medical history verbally, perhaps using screen-based prompts

and entering the patient's responses on screen. This again invites the suggestion that the patient's responses were incorrectly recorded. It is more sensible to take a written medical history, this being signed and dated by the patient. This document could either be retained in its original form, or alternatively could be scanned into the patient's electronically held file.'

Whatever method is used, the dentist needs to be assured that the medical history is accurate and, if any doubt exists, the dentist should seek to clarify any areas of doubt with the patients general medical practitioner (GMP). If the doubt arises from a language barrier, an interpreter can be booked.

With easy access to the internet, finding out the relevance of the more unusual medical conditions to dental treatment is to be encouraged. This section therefore covers the more common issues that need managing on a regular basis.

Cardiovascular problems

Most patients with cardiovascular disease need no special care but there are some exceptions.
• In the past, antibiotic prophylaxis was routinely used if a dental procedure was likely going to cause a bacteraemia for a patient with a history of rheumatic fever. However, since the publication of NICE guidance this has changed significantly and reference should be made to the guidance for current advice (see NICE Guideline CG64 *Prophylaxis Against Infective Endocarditis*, 2008. Available at: www.nice.org.uk/guidance/cg64).
• Patients with hypertension should have the dental chair raised more slowly.
• If a patient has had a myocardial infarction, it is wise to avoid dental treatment within a 6-month period following the episode. If treatment is essential prior to this period having elapsed, a referral should be considered so that they can be managed safely.

Dentistry at a Glance. First Edition. Edited by Elizabeth Kay. © 2016 John Wiley & Sons, Ltd. Published 2016 by John Wiley & Sons, Ltd.
Companion website: www.ataglanceseries.com/dentistryseries/dentistry

Diabetes

There are two main types of diabetes:
• Type 1, which is due to the inability of the body to produce insulin
• Type 2 where the body's cells do not produce enough insulin or are unable to use it effectively.

The patient should be asked if their diabetes is well controlled and to follow their normal routine. Easy access to a glucose drink and the emergency drug kit is wise to deal with any hypoglycaemic attack.

Bleeding disorders

Common bleeding disorders can be categorised as:
• Coagulation deficiencies – haemophilia A/B, von Willibrand disease
• Platelet disorders – quantitative, qualitative
• Vascular disorders – scurvy, purpura, hereditary haemorrhagic telangiectasia
• Fibrinolytic defects – streptokinase therapy, disseminated intravascular coagulation

For any of the above, consultation with the patient's GMP is advised so that the patient can be managed appropriately.

The most common situation the dentist has to manage is for those patients taking warfarin. Guidance varies but a consensus view appears to be that if the international normalised ratio (INR) is below 4.0, primary care dental procedures can be carried out and bleeding managed locally by pressure, suturing or packing with a haemostatic dressing.

Fainting, blackouts and epilepsy

Patients with a history of fainting, fits or blackouts should have been investigated and treatment initiated and therefore hopefully the condition will be well controlled. If it is unclear how severe the patient's condition is, the GMP should be consulted.

Allergies

It is important to establish if the patient has any relevant allergies; the most common one is latex allergy with respect to the use of gloves, rubber dam and anaesthetic cartridges with a latex bung. Once known, an allergy to latex can easily be managed by use of alternatives and it might be prudent to consider the use latex-free gloves as standard, as prices have now come down considerably.

Occasionally, patients report being 'allergic' to local anaesthetic. This is fortunately rarely the case but the possibility cannot be ignored. Any hypersensitivity is often due to the use of ester-based solutions; therefore, local anaesthetics containing amides should be used. If the patient gives an obvious history of allergy, a referral can be made for testing where an anaphylactic reaction could be managed safely.

Allergy to dental materials is also rare but the most common one is allergy to nickel; use of nickel-free alloys by dental laboratories should be considered as standard.

For any other reported allergies, a referral to a dermatologist is advisable to confirm the status.

Hospitalisation and operations

It is advisable to check with the patient as to whether they have recently been in hospital, either for treatment or an operation. This quite often gives us more information about their medical history as patients sometimes do not appreciate the relevance of their GDP having a complete medical history.

Current medication

A detailed and complete list of a patient's current medication is required in the medical history. Often the patient cannot remember all the medication that they have been prescribed and it is useful if they can bring in a recent prescription, which can then be scanned into their notes.

There are too many drug interactions and side effects to mention here but the dentist should refer to the British National Formulary (BNF) if in doubt.

Respiratory disorders

These, obviously, are relevant to the dentist as certain respiratory disorders can make it more difficult for a patient when undergoing dental treatment. Conditions such as chronic obstructive pulmonary disease (COPD) can limit the patient's ability to tolerate long stints of dental treatment.

For patients with asthma, it is advisable to check that they have their inhaler with them in case of an asthmatic attack.

Pregnancy

It is important to check as to whether a patient is or could be pregnant. There is debate as to whether carrying out an amalgam filling during pregnancy can cause harm to the unborn child and, in view of this, it is wise to delay treatment if possible or to use an alternative material.

Other infectious diseases – HIV and hepatitis

Historically, patients with HIV or hepatitis were treated differently with added precautions; however, as identifying patients is difficult, current policies set out procedures that manage all patients in the dental surgery, and the UK Department of Health has produced a memorandum to advise the dental profession on local decontamination procedures: Health Technical Memorandum (HTM 01-05), 2009. *Decontamination in Primary Care Dental Practices*. Available at: www.gov.uk/government/publications/decontamination-in-primary-care-dental-practices

8 Equipment and operating positions

Figure 8.2 Dental chair with integral (under-patient) delivery unit
Source: Reproduced with permission of A-dec Inc.

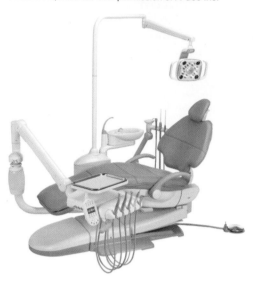

Figure 8.1 Free-standing delivery cart
Source: Reproduced with permission of A-dec Inc.

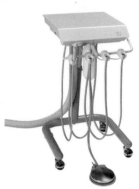

Figure 8.3 Over-patient delivery unit
Source: Reproduced with permission of A-dec Inc.

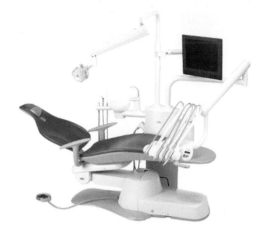

Figure 8.6 12 O'clock operating position

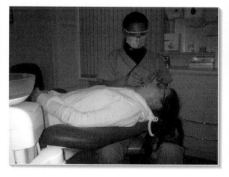

Figure 8.4 Operator standing to extract an upper tooth

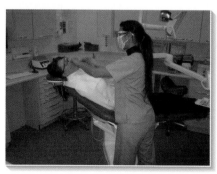

Figure 8.5 9 O'clock operating position

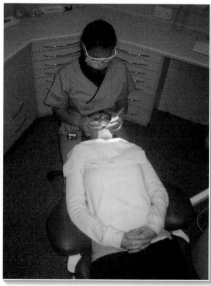

To deliver quality, appropriate dental care to patients, a dentist and support staff need to be able to have good access to the patient's oral cavity and to the equipment. This has, over the past 100 years, evolved from working standing in an upright position to today's approach, where the patient is reclined and the dentist and nurse are usually seated.

Surgery equipment

The key components of the surgery equipment associated with the delivery of patient care are:
- A dental chair
- An operating light to illuminate the area to be worked upon in the mouth

Dentistry at a Glance. First Edition. Edited by Elizabeth Kay. © 2016 John Wiley & Sons, Ltd. Published 2016 by John Wiley & Sons, Ltd.
Companion website: www.ataglanceseries.com/dentistryseries/dentistry

- A delivery unit to deliver handpieces and other powered instruments
- A spittoon to allow the patient to rinse out
- Suction – a selection of suction pipes of different volumes to allow water, saliva etc. to be removed from a patient's mouth to keep the patient comfortable and the operating area clear of fluids
- Operating stools for dentists and nurses to sit on.

These components may all come separately or can be combined in one unit. In Europe, it is now more common for these to be combined in one unit, designed to be used by both left- and right-handed dentists. This is made possible by the light, spittoon, suction and delivery units being on booms, which can be swung around under the chair.

Delivery units tend to be of two types:
- Separate – mobile carts (Figure 8.1)
- Combined – attached to the chair; these can either be side delivery or over the patient (Figures 8.2 and 8.3).

There are strengths and weaknesses of each system. It is a matter of personal preference and any issue relating to the surgery (e.g. size of room), which may determine what is used. In addition to these basic components, dentists may wish to have an X-ray machine close to the dental chair, a composite resin light-curing machine, a digital intraoral camera and liquid-crystal display (LCD) viewing screen (Figure 8.3). These items can be attached to the dental chair and delivery cart or can be kept elsewhere in the surgery.

Operating positions

The considerations relating to operating positions are as follows:
- Patient's needs, and their ability to lie back in a chair, this may be restricted due to medical conditions (such as heart conditions, arthritis or hiatus hernia) or nervousness, in which case they may need to be treated in a more upright position
- The procedure to be carried out
- Dentist's preference.

There are four operating positions that are commonly adopted:

1 Upright – patient is seated and their back is set in a vertical plane

2 Supine – the patient is lying back and their knees and feet are almost at the same level

3 Reclined – the chair is tilted back but the patient's knees are higher than their feet

4 Emergency position – the chair is tilted so that the patient's head is down and their feet higher than their head. This position is needed to manage a patient who has had a vasovagal (faint) incident.

Optimum access for individual areas of the mouth

For the dentist and dental nurse, the ideal operating position is determined by the procedure to be carried out and how to gain the best visual access to the operative site. Ideally, the dentist should have a straight line of visual access to the operative site, either directly or indirectly via a dental mirror. For example:
- To extract a tooth a dentist needs to be able to apply the maximum pressure possible in a straight line through the forceps onto the tooth. This may require the dentist to stand in front or above the patient (Figure 8.4).

- Placing a filling in an upper molar tooth is better carried out with the patient supine and the dentist seated and using a mirror to gain visual access. This provides greater comfort for the dentist and nurse during what might be a long procedure (Figure 8.5).

Asking the patient to rotate their head to left or right may be required to allow a straight line of sight to the area of the dental procedure.

Once the dentist has established a straight sight line to the operating site, either directly or via a mirror, they need to adopt a body posture that minimises strain on their neck, shoulders and back. The key to this is having the patient's mouth at the dentist's focal plane, usually 45 cm from the dentist's eyes, and the patient's head tilted slightly forward but in line with the trunk. The dentist's back should be straight and their feet flat on the floor (see Figure 10.5).

To understand the different seated operating positions, the analogy of a clock face is often used. The dentist and nurse may adopt different positions relative to the patient to gain access to the operative site and maintain their physical comfort.

If the patient's mouth is considered to be the centre of a clock, see Figure 10.6, with the top of their head being at 12 o'clock (Figure 8.6), then if the dentist is right handed they may be seated anywhere between the 12 o'clock position and nine o'clock positions, occasionally even 7 o'clock. A left-handed operator is likely to work from 12 o'clock to 4 o'clock.

Positions normally adopted for different area of the mouth

- Upper and lower anterior teeth: the dentist should sit in the 12 o'clock position. The patient's head should be tilted slightly back for operating on the upper incisors and slightly forwards for the lower incisors
- Upper and lower posteriors: the patient's head can be tilted backwards (towards 12 o'clock) or forwards as for the incisors, but in addition the patients head can be rotated slight to the left or right depending on whether it is the left molar or right molar region being operated on.
- Upper and lower incisors: the patient's head should be in a straight line with the operator and ideally the jaw where the work is being carried out should be at right angles to the patient's body.
- Upper and lower molar areas: the patient's head can be rotated slight to the left or right depending on whether it is the left molar or right molar region being operated on.

The likely outcome from not adopting an appropriate operating position

The outcome may be musculoskeletal problems, including headaches, painful neck, shoulders or back pain and sciatic nerve pain.

Over 90% of dentists report requiring treatment for neck and back pain during their careers. This is usually related to not adopting the optimum operating position on a regular basis. Keeping fit also helps to obviate occupationally related back pain.

Minimising back problems can be achieved by:
- Trying always to **adopt the optimum operating position**. This may not always be possible due to the patient being unable to position their head in a way that is comfortable for them.
- **Sit correctly with shoulders held up** so allowing the spine to curve inwards.
- **Get up and stretch and move around** between patients.
- **Keep fit**, especially the abdominal muscles which support the lower back.

9 Cross-infection control

Figure 9.1 Personal protective equipment

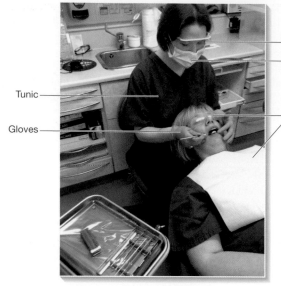

Eye shield
Facemask
Tunic
Gloves
Patient's eye mask and bib

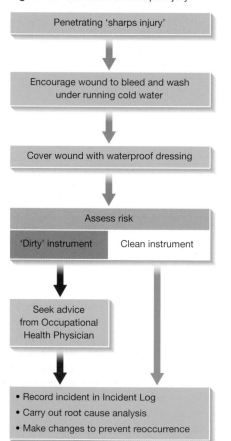

Figure 9.2 Protocol for 'sharps injury'

Penetrating 'sharps injury'
↓
Encourage wound to bleed and wash under running cold water
↓
Cover wound with waterproof dressing
↓
Assess risk
| 'Dirty' instrument | Clean instrument |
↓
Seek advice from Occupational Health Physician
↓
• Record incident in Incident Log
• Carry out root cause analysis
• Make changes to prevent reoccurrence

Figure 9.3 Decontamination of reuseable dental instruments

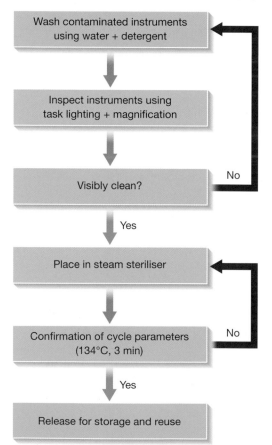

Wash contaminated instruments using water + detergent
↓
Inspect instruments using task lighting + magnification
↓
Visibly clean? — No
↓ Yes
Place in steam steriliser
↓
Confirmation of cycle parameters (134°C, 3 min) — No
↓ Yes
Release for storage and reuse

Dentistry at a Glance. First Edition. Edited by Elizabeth Kay. © 2016 John Wiley & Sons, Ltd. Published 2016 by John Wiley & Sons, Ltd.
Companion website: www.ataglanceseries.com/dentistryseries/dentistry

Infection control is crucial to the safe treatment of patients and for the safety of all members of the dental team. It is every member of the dental team's ethical responsibility to ensure that patients are protected from the risk of healthcare associated infections. Failure to adopt safe working practices can lead to a risk of prosecution by professional regulators. Protocols and procedures must be adopted in the dental surgery to minimise the risk of the transmission of infectious agents. Of particular risk are species of bacteria, viruses and prions. Infectious agents may spread by direct person to person contact, via intermediate inanimate objects known as fomites (such as contaminated instruments or surfaces) or via contaminated aerosols.

Personal protection

It is important to protect dental staff from becoming reservoirs of infection. This can be done by active or passive prevention.

Active prevention is usually by means of immunisation against a range of common or serious infections (Box 9.1). In particular, people working in a surgical discipline should be protected against hepatitis B, a blood-borne virus that is extremely infectious and has a very small infectious dose; as little as 1 picolitre (10^{-12} litre) of infected blood or body fluid can contain an infectious dose of this virus. Chronic infection with this virus can lead to terminal liver disease.

Passive prevention is by means of personal protective equipment (PPE), which acts as a barrier to prevent the penetration of microbes into the tissues of the operator. Essential PPE includes hand protection in the form of single-use surgical examination gloves, eye protection in the form of glasses or visors and face protection in the form of single-use surgical masks. All of these items are intended to protect the operator from contaminated splatter generated during dental procedures (Figure 9.1).

Good hand hygiene protocols are also an important part of personal protection, as well as reducing the risk of transmitting infection to patients. Hands should be decontaminated to remove transient microorganisms before and after touching patients, after touching the surgery environment and after any contact with body fluids. A combination of thorough washing using liquid soap and water and the use of alcohol gel is necessary, ensuring that all parts of the hands and wrists are treated. Disposable surgical examination gloves must be worn for each episode of patient treatment and disposed of after each use.

Sharps injuries must be dealt with promptly and appropriately (Figure 9.2).

Decontamination, sterilisation and disinfection

Disinfection is the killing or removal of all pathogenic micro-organisms with the exception of bacterial spores, which can only be inactivated by sterilisation.

Sterilisation is a process that provides an acceptably low probability ($<1:1\,000\,000$) that any microorganism, including spores, will survive the process.

Decontamination is a process that renders an item fit for reuse with an acceptably low risk of the transmission of infection.

Thorough cleaning of the dental surgery, including equipment and work surfaces, which may have become contaminated during dental procedures, both immediately before and immediately after treating each patient, is essential.

It is essential that all dental instruments used in the provision of dental treatment are safe from the risk of transmission of infection. For some instruments this will be accomplished by the selection of single-use items such as hypodermic needles, aspirator tips and triple-spray tips. This is particularly important where the item is difficult to clean thoroughly, such as lumened instruments.

Where instruments are relatively straightforward to clean and are made of materials that are able to withstand the effects of high temperature steam, these may be reprocessed. Reprocessing or decontamination of reusable dental instruments must be carried out in a designated and dedicated area of the surgery or preferably in a separate room. The process should be carried out in a methodical manner using a work-flow that is progressive, starting with cleaning of the contaminated used instruments and concluding with a sterilisation process. All staff engaged in the decontamination of instruments must be adequately protected from the risk of acquired infection and the use of appropriate PPE; this will include eye protection, heavy duty gloves, mask and disposable apron to protect the operator from splashes.

Cleaning instruments can be carried out in various ways. Manual cleaning of instruments must be done carefully using water and detergent in a sink dedicated for this purpose, and using a long-handled nylon brush to reduce the risk of injury. The instrument should then be rinsed in clean water in a separate sink to remove traces of detergent. The instruments should then be dried using a disposable cloth and visually inspected for cleanliness using an illuminated magnifier. It is vital that all traces of soiling, including biological matter and dental materials, are removed from the instruments if sterilisation is to be effective (Figure 9.3).

Other methods of cleaning instrument include the use of an ultrasonic bath or a fully automatic washer/disinfector. An automated washing process is to be preferred as it safer for the operator and is more reproducible and can therefore be validated.

Once the instruments have been thoroughly cleaned they must then be sterilised. In dental surgeries, the only practical method for sterilising instruments is high-temperature steam using a bench-top steam steriliser (autoclave). After each cycle the parameters (134°C held for 3 min) should be checked before the instruments can be released for storage and further use.

Following sterilisation, instruments should be stored in a way that minimises the risk of recontamination before further use.

Clinical waste

All waste that is potentially contaminated with biological soil must be stored and disposed of safely and in line with current legislation. The waste must be collected by licensed contractors and destroyed by incineration.

10 Examination of the mouth

Figure 10.1 Non-verbal and verbal communication

Non-verbal communication
- Dentist and patient meet in waiting room
- First impressions established

Appearance
- Uniforms/scrubs
- Reassuring or threatening?

Eye contact and facial expression

Interpersonal space
- Dentist often intrudes on this. Not normal in everyday encounters

Seating position
- Face to face, eye to eye, same level

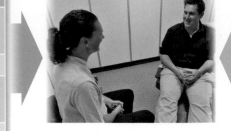

Verbal communication
- Medical and dental history, pain history, series of questions

Open questions
- What is the problem? Gives a broad answer

Specific question
- Can you describe the pain?
- Allows patient to reply in their words

Closed question
- Does the pain keep you awake at night?

Clarification
- Clarify patient's response

Active listening and empathise

Figure 10.2 Dentist and patient talking at the same level, with eye-to-eye contact and with no personal protective equipment being worn

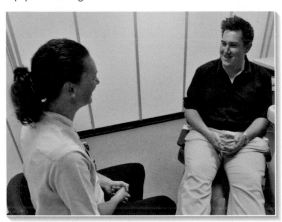

Figure 10.3 Personal protective equipment: gloves, eye protection and plastic apron worn by dentist and nurse

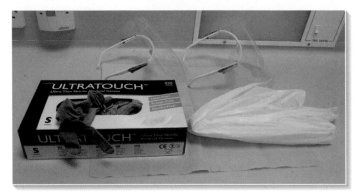

Figure 10.4 Personal protective equipment worn by all, that is dentist, patient and nurse. Positioning: note how the nurse is sitting higher than the dentist

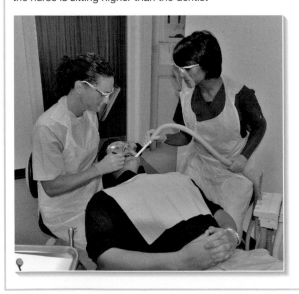

Figure 10.5 Saddle chair, which promotes your spine to adopt a natural S shape rather than slumped C shape

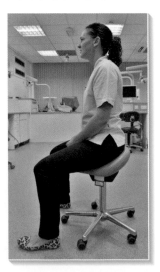

Figure 10.6 Patient's head as a clock-face. Dentist sits at 11 o'clock and is able to move between 1 o'clock and 8 o'clock

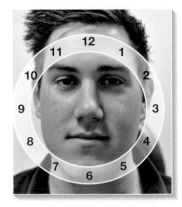

Dentistry at a Glance. First Edition. Edited by Elizabeth Kay. © 2016 John Wiley & Sons, Ltd. Published 2016 by John Wiley & Sons, Ltd.
Companion website: www.ataglanceseries.com/dentistryseries/dentistry

Collecting the patient

Your first encounter with the patient is normally in the waiting room when you collect them. As students you are encouraged to do this but in the practice setting it may change. You can learn a lot by observing the patient as they walk to the chair, in relation to medical and social aspects. Non-verbal communication is important in welcoming the patient and reassuring them. Verbal communication will take place and a history and questions will be asked whilst empathising with them and building rapport and trust (Figure 10.1).

Introductions

Introductions are key and the dental nurse should always be introduced as should any other staff who are present. Introduce yourself in a friendly manner, remembering that the majority of our patients don't like us. Once the patient is comfortable it is important to position yourself correctly, so that you can take a history and ask these important questions that will help you formulate a diagnosis. It is best to face the patient and ensure you are at the same level (Figure 10.2). If you stand above the patient or sit behind them, communication is difficult and the patient may feel at a disadvantage. During this initial conversation, do not wear gloves or personal protective equipment (PPE) (Figure 10.3). This stage is crucial in building rapport with the patient. One of the key aspects of being a good dentist is the ability to listen to your patient and utilise the information given.

Dentist and nurse positioning

Once the histories have been taken, it is time to examine the patient or carry out procedures. Whilst charting, the nurse will normally not wear PPE as they will input the information into a computer system.

Whilst carrying out procedures, PPE should be worn by the dentist, nurse and patient (Figure 10.4). It is important to ensure eye protection, in the form of a visor or glasses, is worn by all. Always advise the patient when the chair is going to be moved. The chair should be tilted back and raised so that the patient is horizontal. The patient's head should be on the headrest and approximately at the level of the dentist's waist. The dentist should not need to bend forward excessively to see into the patient's mouth.

The dentist sits behind the patient on either a chair or saddle seat with castor feet, which allow easy movement. Forearms and thighs are parallel to floor, with elbows close to the rib-cage, hip angle of 90°, and feet spread apart so that legs and chair base form a tripod. The operator's back should be straight (Figure 10.5).

The majority of chairs in use today are equipped for left or right-handed dentists.

If you are right handed, the nurse sits on the left-hand side, facing towards the patient, and vice versa for left-handed dentists. So that the nurse can see clearly into the patient's mouth, they normally sit approximately 10 cm higher than the dentist, as can be seen in Figure 10.4.

Whilst examining the patient, you will find that you will move around the patient to gain the best access. Over time, you will discover and identify the best position for you. As a guide, think of the patient's head as a clock face with the forehead being 12 o'clock and the chin at 6 o'clock (Figure 10.6). The dentist sits to the right of the patient at the 11 o'clock position, and is able to move around the patient between 1 o'clock and 8 o'clock. The dental nurse normally sits between 1 o'clock and 4 o'clock. Again for left-handed dentists, this is vice versa.

You can also ask the patient to move their head to facilitate access. The patient's head can be moved either to the left, right, up or down to make examination or treatment easier. When examining lower teeth, it may be easier to ask the patient to tip their chin down. With upper teeth, the patient should tip their head back.

Instrument positioning

Instruments are normally situated on the dentist's side or over the patient. The disadvantage in this is that the nurse is not able to pass instruments to you. This can be overcome by selecting the appropriate instruments before starting the procedure and passing them over to the nurse's side before commencing treatment.

Posture

Posture is key from your early days as a student and good habits should be encouraged from day 1 of treating patients. Following graduation, you will have 30–40 years working as a dentist and is important to adopt a work position and posture that looks after your back and neck. A high percentage of dentists are forced to retire early due to back problems. There are various pieces of equipment that can help you whilst working. A saddle chair can help you to sit in an ergonomic position and improve your posture (Figure 10.5). Magnification aids visibility and encourages the dentist to sit in an upright position. There are a variety of systems available and if possible you should trial these whilst at dental school so that you are able to make an informed choice when entering dental practice. It is important during the first few months of treating patients to experiment with positioning as there is no one rule and you will find that different dentists have different approaches. It is important to find what works for you and to maintain good habits.

Lighting

The clinic should be brightly lit and the patient's mouth lit adequately. The operating light is situated above the patient's head and its position and direction altered depending on the teeth being examined. The mirror is used to direct the light to difficult-to-see areas.

There is the option of using a headlight system, with loupes which deliver a focused beam for better visibility.

11 Special tests

Figure 11.1 Methodology for precussive testing. Gently tap or press each tooth and compare the patients reaction at each tooth

Figure 11.2 Methodology for cold testing. (a) Step 1: Hold the cotton pledget in the forceps spray the ethyl chloride onto the cotton pledget away from the patient and ideally over the sink at a distance of 2 cm from the distribution tube (b) Step 2: Place the chilled pledget against a neighbouring tooth to the 'suspect' one and ask the patient to raise their hand when they feel the cold. Record the patients response (c) Repeat step 1 and 2 on the suspect tooth and record the patient's response. NB: Take care not to touch the patient's soft tissue with the cold cotton pledget

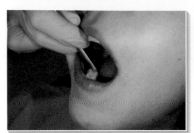
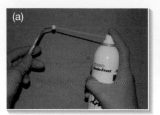
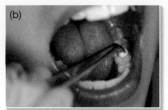
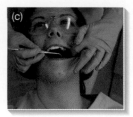

Figure 11.3 Electrical pulp testing. (a) Connect all cables and ensure that the EPT is fully charged as per manufacturer's instructions (b) Place the grounding lip clip over the patients mucosa Ensure that the EPT probe has a small amount of toothpaste on its tip to allow transmission of stimulus (c) Slowly increase the voltage to the threshold of the stimulus being felt and record the result.This should be repeated on several teeth in addition to the 'suspect' tooth

Figure 11.4 Tooth Sleuth. (a) Place the concave area of the pyramid on the suspected cusp (b) Ask the patient to bite down gently and observe the patient's reaction

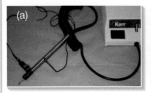
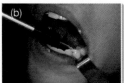
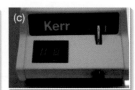
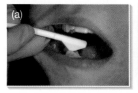
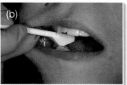

Box 11.1 An example of a full pain history

1 Where is the pain?
2 How frequent is the pain?
3 What makes the pain better?
4 What makes the pain worse?
5 What does the pain feel like?
6 Where is the pain located?
7 How long does the pain last?
8 Does the pain radiate?
9 Do analgesics relieve the pain?
10 Does the pain keep you awake at night?

Table 11.1 False readings following electrical pulp testing

False negative	False positive
Large restoration having an insulating effect on the pulp	Multirooted tooth with both vital and non-vital roots
Large amount of secondary dentine having an insulating effect on the pulp	Nervous or anxious patient responding in anticipation to stimulus
Nerve damage, however, blood supply intact	Pulp chamber full of pus

Table 11.2 Summary of vitality testing results

Response	Clinical implication
Normal: Response to stimulus is not exaggerated and does not linger	The pulp is 'normal' and is not yet showing any signs of pulpitis
Exaggerated: The stimulus evokes a response that is greater than neighbouring teeth and the sensation lingers	Reversible pulpitis: mild pain of short duration following removal of stimulus
	Irreversible pulpitis: severe pain that lingers in duration (often referred to as a throb) following removal of stimulus
Absence of response: No response from the patient following correct application of the stimulus	Indicative of pulpal necrosis; pulp absence; root canal therapy Further radiographic investigation is required

Dentistry at a Glance. First Edition. Edited by Elizabeth Kay. © 2016 John Wiley & Sons, Ltd. Published 2016 by John Wiley & Sons, Ltd.
Companion website: www.ataglanceseries.com/dentistryseries/dentistry

Patients presenting to the dentist with 'tooth pain' is the most common cause for attendance. Often the pain is poorly located and pain histories (Box 11.1) are limited in their degree of accuracy. Having a standard methodical approach to investigating pains aids the dentist in making a clear and accurate diagnosis. In this chapter special tests to aid in diagnosis are considered.

Vitality testing

The objective of vitality testing is to establish the vitality of a tooth's nerve and blood supply; however, it should be remembered that the blood supply is more important in the tooth's continued vitality. When performing any type of vitality test (as described in this chapter) it is essential that the full clinical picture is examined and the focus is not solely on the suspect tooth. In addition to performing tests on the tooth of interest, it is important that testing of neighbouring or adjacent teeth (similar in size and degree of restoration) are also tested to establish what is 'normal' for the patient you are examining.

Visual examination

Although not strictly a special test, visual examination can often be overlooked as a valuable clinical investigation. Prior to performing any form of special test or radiographic examination, it is essential that the clinician thoroughly examines the dentition under a bright light. Visual inspection will often reveal not only frank caries and cavitation but also periodontal, mucosal and other pathologies.

Percussive testing

Percussive testing (TTP) (Figure 11.1) requires no additional equipment beyond the dental instruments that are used in an inspection.
- **Equipment required**: dental mirror
- **Outcomes/implications**: if the patient displays a positive or increased response to gentle percussion this is suggestive of one of the following:
- tooth is extruded
- presence of periodontitis (apical or lateral)
- presence of a pulpitis.

Cold testing

Cold testing (Figure 11.2) is readily performed with very little additional equipment required. When placing a cold pledget on a patient's tooth it can occasionally evoke a definitive and painful response, which may make the patient jump. Ensure that the patient has been warned prior to beginning this test.
- **Equipment required**: ethyl chloride spray (EndoFrost ™); cotton pledget; college locking forceps
- **Outcomes/ implications**:
  - reaction to cold with no lasting effects and recognition equivalent to similar teeth = **normal**
  - mild pain displayed by patient to cold stimulus with short duration of pain following removal of stimulus = **reversible pulpitis**
  - severe pain displayed with increased duration following removal of stimulus = **irreversible pulpitis**.

Electrical pulp testing

Electrical pulp testing (EPT) (Figure 11.3) works on the principle that an electrical charge can stimulate the nerve fibres of the tooth and elicit a response in the patient. It is important that the correct technique is used (note this may vary between models) to ensure accurate responses. Ensure that the patient has been warned that they may feel a tingling sensation when the stimulus is applied.
- **Equipment required**: electrical pulp tester, toothpaste
- **Outcomes/ implications**: it is essential to remember that there is no empirical cut off or value associated with EPT. Each patient will vary in their response. It is essential that a clear 'normal' value is established with the patient to allow correct and accurate interpretation of the results. If trauma has occurred to the tooth, it can take between 4 and 6 weeks for the pulp to recover. There are several outcomes from EPT:
  - reaction to EPT with no lasting effects and recognition equivalent to similar teeth = **normal**
  - mild pain displayed by patient to EPT stimulus with the current being slightly increased= **reversible pulpitis**
  - exaggerated response that occurs with greatly increased current = **irreversible pulpitis**
  - no response to the EPT = indicative of **pulpal necrosis, pulp absence or root canal therapy.**

There are a number of instances in which an EPT can give either a false-negative or a false-positive reading; these are summarised in Table 11.1.

Tooth Sleuth™

The Tooth Sleuth™ (Figure 11.4) device is available commercially and is useful in the diagnosis of cracked tooth syndrome (CTS). It is of particular use when the patient reports sensitivity on biting that is both irregular and infrequent.
- **Equipment required**: Tooth Sleuth™
- **Outcomes/ implications**: pain on biting or release of biting indicates that a particular cusp or cusps are fractured. This is normally noted in teeth that contain large restorations. Other potential outcomes are:
  - presence of apical or lateral periodontitis
  - presence of a pulpitis.

Heat testing

Heat testing is mentioned for completeness; however, it is not commonly carried out. This method requires the dentist to melt a piece of gutta percha onto the patient's (Vaselined) tooth and record their response. This method is used to determine if the pulp is vital or non-vital. It is not sensitive enough to distinguish between reversible or irreversible pulpitis.

Other sensitivity tests

The following are mentioned as specialist tests that are available but are not covered here in detail.
- Transillumination: strong light used to detect changes in pulp colour
- Pulse oximetry: assesses blood gas concentrations in the pulp
- Laser Doppler flowmetry (LDF): assesses blood flow within the pulp
- Transmitted laser light: variant of LDF, thought to eliminate false positives.

Summary

It is important to remember that special tests alone will not give an empirical answer or definitive diagnosis, rather the information aids the dentist in reaching their diagnosis. Electrical and thermal testing of pulps are useful when attempting to determine if a tooth has pulpitis. The results of vitality testing can be categorised into one of three main responses. These are summarised in Table 11.2.

12 Reading and reporting radiographs

Figure 12.1 A traditional X-ray viewer

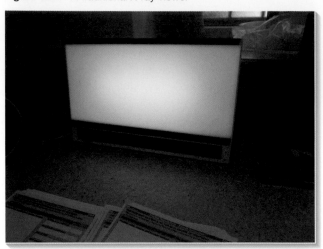

Figure 12.2 Example of a QA1 radiograph: no positioning, processing or film handling errors present

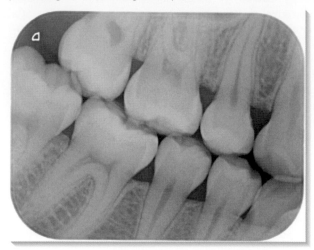

Figure 12.3 Example of a QA2 radiograph: a processing and film handling error has occurred but can still be used for diagnostic purposes

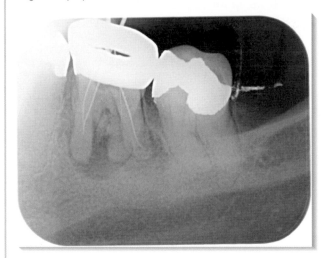

Figure 12.4 Example of a QA3 radiograph: a positioning error has occurred and has rendered this radiograph radiographically unacceptable

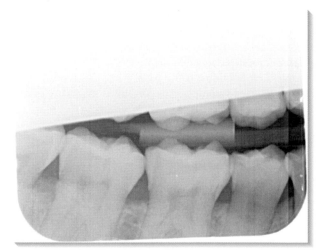

Dentistry at a Glance. First Edition. Edited by Elizabeth Kay. © 2016 John Wiley & Sons, Ltd. Published 2016 by John Wiley & Sons, Ltd.
Companion website: www.ataglanceseries.com/dentistryseries/dentistry

Reading radiographs

There are many necessary requirements for adequately reading and interpreting dental radiographs and some of these include:

• **Optimal viewing conditions**: for traditional radiographs, the requirements are a dry radiograph, an even, uniform, bright light viewing screen, a dark surround around the radiograph so that light only passes through the film and the use of a magnifying glass. For digital systems the requirements to view the radiograph are: optimal contrast, brightness and image enhancement, and use of a zoom facility. See Figure 12.1 for a traditional X-ray viewer.

• **Knowledge of the radiographic appearance of normal anatomical structures**: it is especially important to be able to differentiate between healthy teeth, normal periodontal tissues and other normal structures such as foramina, bone trabeculae, the inferior dental nerve canal etc., and pathological features.

• **Knowledge of the radiographic appearance of pathology that may affect the dental region**: it is important to recognise dental caries and periodontal disease on radiographs but also necessary to be able to recognise less common pathology such as cysts and tumours etc.

• **Knowledge and understanding of what dental radiographs should look like**: this is so that quality assurance and reporting can be carried out accurately.

• **Access to previous radiographs so that comparisons can be made**: this is important so that key features and the progression of lesions can be ascertained, e.g. caries, apical pathology, bone loss and the rate of development can be measured.

• **A systematic approach to viewing the entire radiograph and pathology-specific areas**: a systematic and logical approach is very important so that all relevant information is read and reported correctly. Suggestions for a systematic sequence for reporting radiographs should include:

- • **Teeth**
  - record missing teeth
  - record the findings relevant to the crowns of the teeth: caries/restorations etc.
  - record the findings relevant to the roots of the teeth: fillings, resorption, length, fractures, caries etc.
  - record the findings of the apices: nothing abnormal detected, radiolucencies, opacities, obturation material etc.
- • **Periodontal tissues**
  - record any calculus deposits
  - record bone loss, vertical and horizontal
  - note furcation involvement
  - record any widening of the periodontal ligament

  With dental panoramic tomographic (DPT) radiographs note the mandible shape, thickness, condyle anatomy, foramina, border, trabeculae, antra etc.
- • **Pathology**: a description of a pathological lesion should include:
  - location of the lesion, e.g. apex, crown, interdental, mesial, distal, horizontal, vertical, anterior, posterior, within an antrum etc.
  - size of the lesion, give a measurement in mm, e.g. 5 mm in diameter
  - shape and nature of the lesion, e.g. oval, round, regular, irregular, radiopaque, radiolucent etc.
  - proximity to other structures
  - when comparing to previous radiographs, try to ascertain the time that lesion has been present.

Reporting radiographs

Justification for the radiograph should always be recorded in the patient's notes, for example caries screen, bone levels, apical pathology etc. Radiographs should be labelled correctly (traditional films) with the name of the patient, date radiograph was taken, dentist who prescribed the radiograph and identification of the tooth that was X-rayed (e.g. Joe Bloggs, PA of LR7, 23rd October 2012 and initials of dentist).

The findings from the systematic and logical examination of the radiograph, including teeth, periodontal structures and pathology, should be documented in the patient's notes.

Quality assurance

The World Health Organisation (WHO) has defined radiographic quality assurance (QA) programmes as 'an organised effort by the staff operating a facility to ensure that the diagnostic images produced by the facility are of sufficiently high quality so that they consistently provide adequate diagnostic information at the lowest possible cost and with the least possible exposure of the patient to radiation'.

Rating a radiograph falls into one of three categories (Box 12.1). QA1 (Excellent) being the optimal score and when auditing radiographs should be no less than 70% of all radiographs. QA2 (Diagnostically acceptable) should be no more than 20% and QA3 (Diagnostically unacceptable) no more than 10%. Examples are given in Figures 12.2, 12.3 and 12.4.

Box 12.1 Quality assurance

Being able to report on radiographs is imperative to maintaining good quality and high standards of dental care.

• Quality assurance 1 (QA1) Excellent – no errors. Patient positioning is correct as well as the film being positioned correctly. Exposure time should be correct for size of patient and position of the tooth/ teeth with no processing or handling faults.

• Quality assurance 2 (QA2) Diagnostically acceptable. Some errors present. Patient positioning could be incorrect, exposure time, processing or film handling could be problematic. However, they do not detract from the application of the radiograph and a diagnosis can still be derived.

• Quality assurance 3 (QA3) Diagnostically unacceptable. Errors present such as patient positioning or tolerance of intraoral film by patient. Exposure time and setting could make film too pale or dark. Processing errors, such as inadequate chemicals in the processing machine or a fault with the digital equipment, can lead to the radiograph being deemed diagnostically undesirable.

13 Diagnostic 'surgical sieve'

Figure 13.1 White patch in floor of mouth

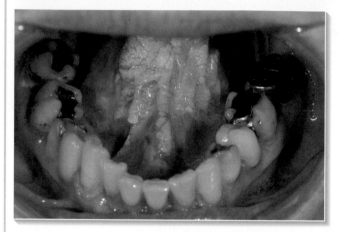

Figure 13.2 Ulceration on lateral border of the tongue

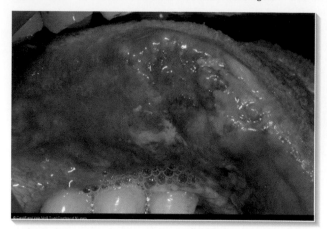

Figure 13.3 Tooth electrical vitality test

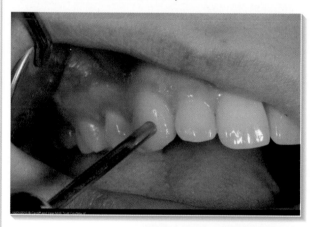

Figure 13.4 Venepuncture

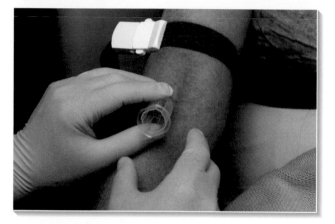

Figure 13.5 Incisional biopsy

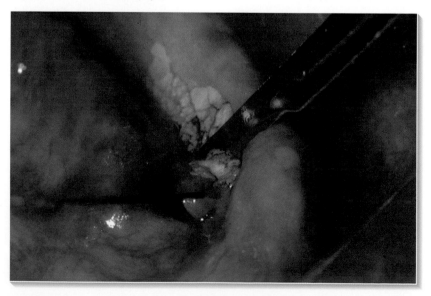

Dentistry at a Glance. First Edition. Edited by Elizabeth Kay. © 2016 John Wiley & Sons, Ltd. Published 2016 by John Wiley & Sons, Ltd.
Companion website: www.ataglanceseries.com/dentistryseries/dentistry

To ensure a thorough and organised examination of a patient, a process known as 'surgical sieve' is often applied. As in many aspects of medicine, a mnemonic is helpful in remembering a sieve approach to differential diagnosis. One such, mnemonic is 'VITAMIN C' (author unknown).

Vascular, Infection, Trauma / Toxicity, Autoimmune, Metabolic, Idiopathic, Neoplastic and Congenital

Consideration of each of the possible aetiologies can help ensure that all possible diagnoses are addressed. As a generalisation, it is also important to remember that conditions that occur frequently in the population will be seen frequently. So, to put possible diagnoses in perspective, list common conditions first then add rarities. There is an old saying 'If you hear a noise of "trotting hooves", think horse not giraffe'.

Examples of the use of a surgical sieve approach to an oral mucosal white patch or ulceration are shown in Figures 13.1 and 13.2 and in Tables 13.1 and 13.2.

Special investigations

Once the surgical sieve approach has been applied to the findings of the extraoral and intraoral examination, a list of differential diagnoses can be compiled. It is essential to take into account aspects of the history of the signs and symptoms. In addition, a thorough dental and medical history can provide valuable information. On occasions, determining the patient's condition may be straight forward from this information alone. However, more often it is necessary to undertake a series of special investigations to confirm the exact diagnosis. With regard to dental and oral disease, the following types of special investigation are often used.

- Tooth vitality (heat, cold, electrical) (Figure 13.3)
- Imaging techniques
  - plain radiographs (intraoral periapical view, orthopantomograph)
  - sialography
  - ultrasound
  - computed tomography (CT) scanning
  - magnetic resonance imaging (MRI)
- Needle aspiration
- Haematological investigations (Figure 13.4)
  - full blood count
  - vitamin B_{12}, ferritin and folate
  - glucose
- Microbiological investigations
  - smear
  - culture of plain swab, concentrated oral rinse or imprint
- Histopathological examination
  - incisional biopsy (partial removal) (Figure 13.5)
  - excisional biopsy (total removal)
  - labial gland biopsy.

Table 13.1 Surgical sieve approach to a white patch

Aetiology	Relevant	Possible diagnosis
Vascular	No	The appearance does not suggest presence of blood vessels
Infection	Yes	Candidal infection: hyperplastic candidosis Viral infection: Epstein–Barr associated with hairy leukoplakia
Trauma/ toxicity	Yes	Physical: frictional keratosis caused by chronic irritation Chemical: topical aspirin burn caused by low pH of drug
Autoimmune	Yes	Lichen planus
Metabolic	No	
Idiopathic	Yes	Leukoplakia
Neoplastic	Yes	Squamous cell carcinoma
Congenital	Yes	White sponge naevus

Table 13.2 Surgical sieve approach to ulceration

Aetiology	Relevant	Possible diagnosis
Vascular	No	The appearance does not suggest presence of blood vessels
Infection	Yes	Bacterial infection: Mycobacterium tuberculosis, Treponema Pallidum Viral infection: herpes simplex
Trauma/ toxicity	Yes	Physical: physical injury Chemical: topical aspirin burn
Autoimmune	Yes	Pemphigus vulgaris or mucous membrane pemphigoid
Metabolic	Yes	Uraemic stomatitis
Idiopathic	Yes	Recurrent aphthous stomatitis
Neoplastic	Yes	Squamous cell carcinoma or lymphoma
Congenital	No	

14 Charting the oral cavity

Figure 14.1 Diagrammatic representation of the oral mucosa

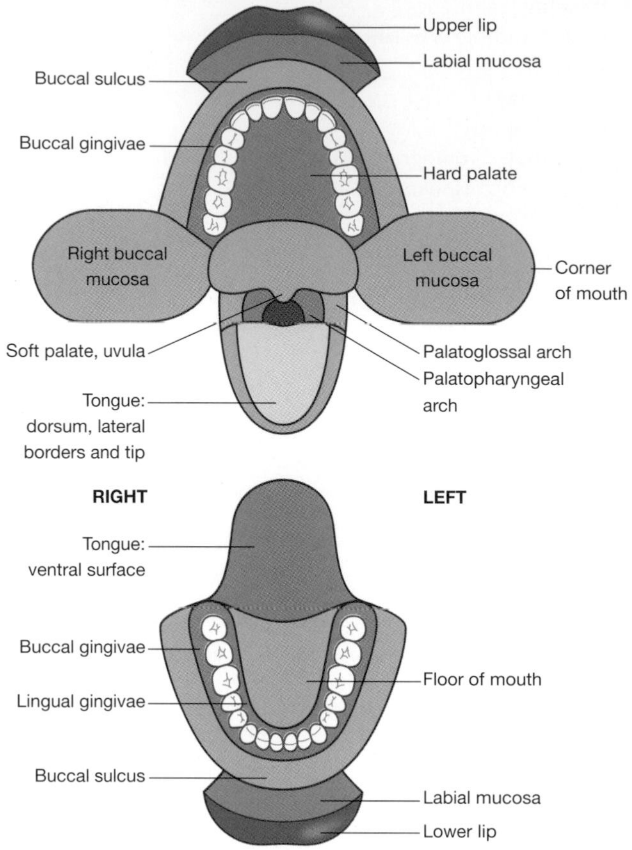

- Upper lip
- Labial mucosa
- Buccal sulcus
- Buccal gingivae
- Hard palate
- Right buccal mucosa
- Left buccal mucosa
- Corner of mouth
- Soft palate, uvula
- Palatoglossal arch
- Palatopharyngeal arch
- Tongue: dorsum, lateral borders and tip

RIGHT   **LEFT**

- Tongue: ventral surface
- Buccal gingivae
- Lingual gingivae
- Floor of mouth
- Buccal sulcus
- Labial mucosa
- Lower lip

Figure 14.2 The Palmar system for identification of the permanent and primary teeth

UR   UL
1 2 3 4 5 6 7 8
LR   LL

UR A B C D E UL
LR   LL

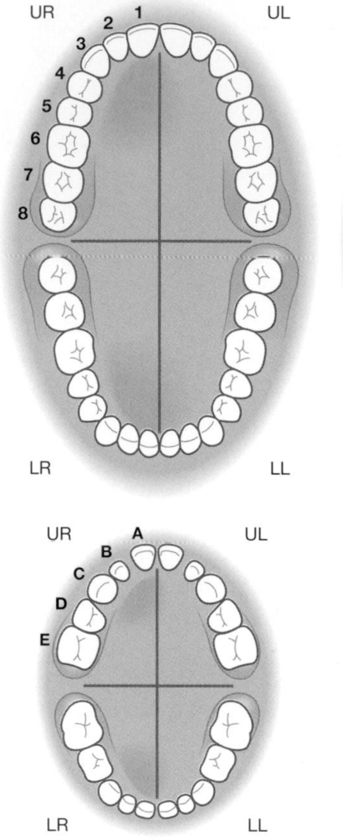

Figure 14.3 The FDI system for identification of the permanent and primary teeth

UL
12 11 21 22
13 23
14 24
15 25
16 Upper right 1 Upper left 2 26
17 27
18 28
48 Lower right 4 Lower left 3 38
47 37
46 36
45 35
44 34
43 33
42 41 31 32
LR   LL

UR 51 61 UL
52 62
53 63
54 64
55 Upper right 5 Upper left 6 65
85 Lower right 8 Lower left 7 75
84 74
83 73
82 81 71 72
LR   LL

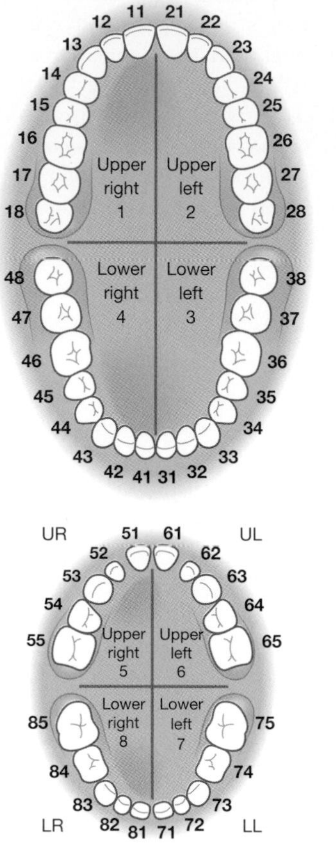

Figure 14.4 Tooth surfaces

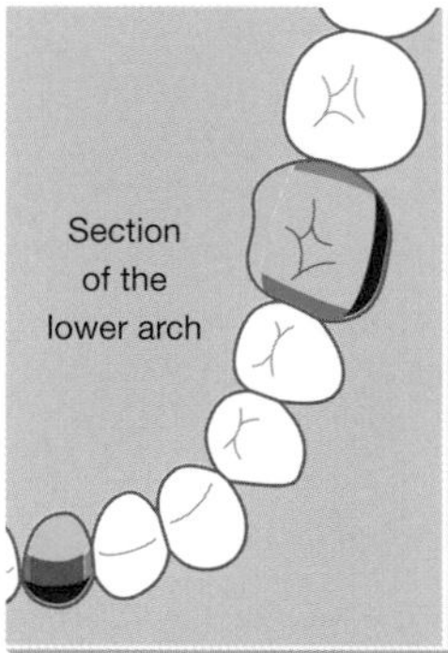

Section of the lower arch

Occlusal	Biting surface of premolars and molars
Incisal edge	Biting edge of incisors and canines
Buccal	Surface facing the cheeks/lips, may also be referred to as labial for incisors and canines
Lingual	Surface facing the tongue (lower arch)
Palatal	Upper arch, surface adjacent to the palate
Mesial	Surface closest to the centre line, around the arch
Distal	Surface furthest from the centre line, around the arch
Cervical	Area of the tooth nearest to the gingival margin

Figure 14.5 Example of baseline and treatment charts; see Table 14.2 for the key to symbols

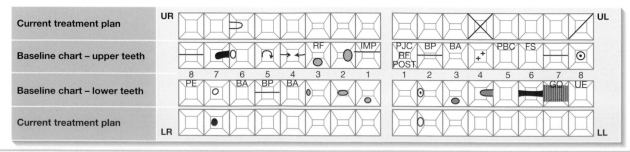

	UR															UL
Current treatment plan																
Baseline chart – upper teeth						RF	IMP	PJC RF POST	BP	BA		PBC	FS		
		8	7	6	5	4	3	2	1	1	2	3	4	5	6	7	8
Baseline chart – lower teeth		PE			BA	BP	BA								GO	UE
Current treatment plan	LR															LL

Dentistry at a Glance. First Edition. Edited by Elizabeth Kay. © 2016 John Wiley & Sons, Ltd. Published 2016 by John Wiley & Sons, Ltd.
Companion website: www.ataglanceseries.com/dentistryseries/dentistry

Accurate charting of the oral mucosa, teeth and periodontal tissues is essential to good clinical practice. Many different charting systems are available, both written and computerised. Clinicians must take time to become familiar with the systems available to them and adopt a systematic approach to clinical examination and relevant record keeping.

Oral mucosa

Visual inspection of the lips and all oral mucosa forms part of a thorough extraoral and intraoral soft tissue examination. Good lighting is required and any denture or other removable appliance taken out of the mouth. Labial, buccal, hard and soft palate, and dorsal, lateral and ventral surfaces of the tongue and the floor of the mouth are carefully visually examined and palpated when appropriate. The site, size, shape, colour, consistency, and the presence of ulceration, attachment or pain associated with any lesion recorded. It may be helpful, especially if the shapes of lesions are complex or extensive, to draw them on a diagram (Figure 14.1) and to take photographs. Some common terms for the description of lesions of the intraoral mucosa are listed in Table 14.1. If no abnormality is detected, this must be recorded.

Table 14.1 Common terms for the description of intraoral mucosal lesions

Bulla	Blister; visible fluid accumulation within or beneath epithelium, usually >5 mm in diameter
Desquamation	Loss of superficial epithelial thickness (commonly follows a blister)
Ecchymosis	Bruise; macular area of haemorrhage >2 cm in diameter
Erosion	Loss of superficial epithelial thickness (often follows a blister)
Erythema	Redness of mucosa (from atrophy, inflammation, vascular congestion or increased perfusion)
Fibrosis	Formation of excessive fibrous tissue
Fistula	Abnormal connection, lined by epithelium, between two epithelium-lined organs
Haematoma	Localised collection of blood
Leukoplakia	Predominantly white lesion that cannot be diagnosed clinically as any other oral mucosal disorder; will not rub off
Macule	Circumscribed alteration in colour or texture, not raised
Naevus	A coloured lesion present from birth
Nodule	Solid mass under or within the mucosa >5 mm in diameter
Papule	Circumscribed palpable elevation <5 mm in diameter
Petechia	Haemorrhagic spot 1–2 mm in diameter
Plaque	Elevated area >5 mm in diameter
Pustule	Visible accumulation of pus in epithelium
Scar	Fibrous tissue replacement of another tissue
Sclerosis	Induration of submucosal and/or subcutaneous tissues
Sinus	A pouch or cavity in any organ or tissue
Tumour	Swelling caused by normal or pathological material or cells
Ulcer	Loss of epithelium with loss of some underlying tissues
Vesicle	Small visible fluid accumulation in epithelium <5 mm in diameter

Charting the teeth

Several methods have been developed to facilitate the identification of individual teeth with numbers and/or letters. For permanent teeth the Palmar system (Figure 14.2) allocates the number 1 to the central incisor in each quadrant, rising in sequence for each tooth until the third molar is allocated number 8. Quadrants are separated by a vertical line between the central incisors and a horizontal line separating the upper and lower arches. Individual teeth are represented by their proximity to these lines; for example the permanent upper right first premolar is represented as 4⌋ or alternatively UR4 using letters to indicate the quadrant. Primary teeth are identified by quadrant in a similar way; the teeth are allocated letters from A, central incisor, to E, second molar. The primary upper left lateral incisor, for example, is represented by ⌊B or ULB.

The International Dental Federation (FDI) system allocates similar numbers to the permanent teeth (Figure 14.3) and identifies quadrants by number; the upper right quadrant is number 1 with the other quadrants rising in sequence clockwise. When representing an individual tooth the quadrant number is stated first, followed by the tooth number; the permanent lower left first molar, therefore, is tooth number 36. For the primary dentition (Figure 14.3), teeth are allocated numbers from 1 (central incisor) to 5 (second molar), the upper right quadrant is number 5 with the other quadrants rising in sequence clockwise. The primary lower right canine, for example, is 83.

Diagrams are used to record details regarding the history and condition of individual teeth and as an aid to treatment planning. These diagrams allow for all surfaces to be represented (Figure 14.4). A baseline chart is completed, on a grid, to record teeth present or missing, any rotations, restorations or cavities, where space has closed or tooth artificially replaced (Figure 14.5). Other details regarding the occlusion will be entered as text in the general notes. A separate outer grid is utilised to record details of treatment planned and procedures carried out as the treatment plan progresses. When radiographs have been exposed, it is essential to refer to them when completing the charts especially to record dental caries and also the presence of root fillings or posts. As items of treatment are completed the treatment plan grid is updated, providing, at a glance, most of the information needed to determine the progress of treatment. Table 14.2 provides details regarding the symbols in the example grids for the written charting in Figure 14.5. Computerised charting programs allow the use of colour to denote different restorative materials and separate shapes to distinguish types of bridge units.

Table 14.2 Symbols commonly used in baseline and treatment charts

Baseline chart

UR1	Tooth missing – replaced by implant	UL1	Root filling, post, porcelain crown
UR2	Mesial incisal tip composite restoration	UL2	Tooth missing – replaced by adhesive bridge pontic
UR3	Root filling and palatal restoration	UL3	Palatal adhesive bridge wing
UR4	Tooth missing – space closed	UL4	Tooth broken down – root present
UR5	Tooth rotated	UL5	Porcelain bonded crown
UR6	Distal carious lesion	UL6	Fissure sealant
UR7	Mesial occlusal (MO) amalgam restoration	UL7	Tooth missing – space not closed
UR8	Tooth missing	UL8	Secondary caries associated with an occlusal amalgam restoration
LR1	Labial glass ionomer cement restoration	LL1	Tooth present and sound
LR2	Incisal edge composite restoration	LL2	Secondary caries associated with a mesial composite restoration
LR3	Distal composite restoration	LL3	Buccal tooth coloured restoration
LR4	Porcelain fused to metal bridge abutment	LL4	Distal occlusal (DO) composite restoration
LR5	Tooth missing – replaced by bridge pontic	LL5	Tooth present and sound
LR6	Porcelain fused to metal bridge abutment	LL6	Mesio-occluso-distal (MOD) amalgam restoration
LR7	Occlusal carious lesion	LL7	Mesio-occluso-distal (MOD) gold onlay
LR8	Tooth partially erupted	LL8	Tooth unerupted

Treatment planned and carried out in this course of treatment

UR6	Distal occlusal (DO) restoration planned	UL4	Extraction carried out
		UL8	Extraction planned
LR7	Occlusal restoration carried out	LL2	Mesial restoration planned

15 Periodontal assessment

Table 15.1 BPE codes and criteria

BPE code	Criteria
0	• Healthy periodontal tissues • No bleeding after gentle probing
1	• Bleeding after gentle probing • Black band remains completely visible above gingival margin • No calculus or defective margins detected
2	• Supragingival and/or subgingival calculus and/or other plaque retention factor • Black band remains completely visible above gingival margin
3	• Shallow pocket (4 or 5 mm) • Black band partially visible in the deepest pocket in the sextant
4	• Deep pocket (6 mm or more) • Black band disappears in the pocket
*	• Furcation involvement

Figure 15.1 BPE probe

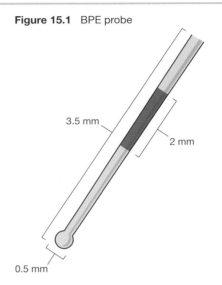

3.5 mm

2 mm

0.5 mm

Table 15.2 Example BPE grid

4*	0	3
1	2	3*

Figure 15.3 (a,b) BPE index teeth and sextants

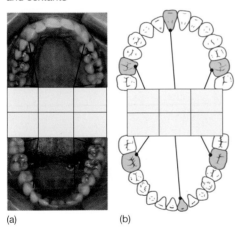

(a) (b)

Figure 15.5 *Left to right:* BPE probe; William's and UNC15 probes (both for measuring probing depth in millimetres); Naber's probe

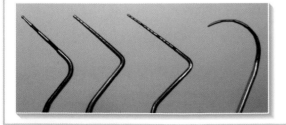

Figure 15.2 Use of probe and codes for BPE

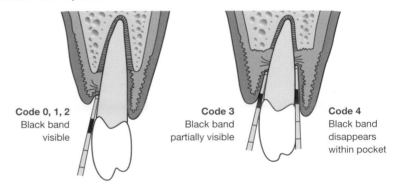

Code 0, 1, 2
Black band visible

Code 3
Black band partially visible

Code 4
Black band disappears within pocket

Figure 15.4 O'Leary plaque index chart; marks indicate presence of bacterial plaque on the tooth surface

8	7	6	5	4	3	2	1	1	2	3	4	5	6	7	8

Figure 15.6 Grading of furcation involvement

The probe is inserted between the roots of a multirooted tooth

F1 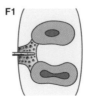 **F2**  **F3**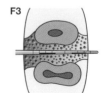

Class 1 involvement (F1) is where a probe can be inserted less than 3 mm between the roots

Class 2 involvement (F2) penetrates more than 3 mm but not fully through the furcation

Class 3 involvement (F3) extends completely between the roots

Sources for Table 15.1, Table 15.2, Figure 15.6, 15.8 and Box 15.1. Clerehugh V, Tugnait A, Genco RJ (2010). *Periodontology at a Glance.* Reproduced with permission of John Wiley and Sons, Ltd

Box 15.1 Grading of tooth mobility

Handles of two instruments placed on tooth and mobility graded according to movement in horizontal (buccolingual) and vertical direction:

- Grade I = 0.2–1 mm movement in horizontal direction
- Grade II = more than 1 mm movement in horizontal direction
- Grade III = more than 1 mm movement in horizontal direction + vertical movement

Figure 15.7 Probing a pocket depth, recession and clinical attachment loss

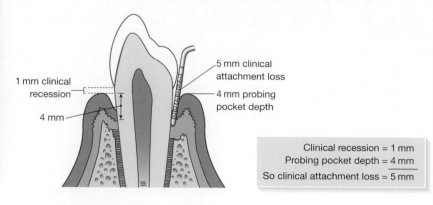

1 mm clinical recession

4 mm

5 mm clinical attachment loss

4 mm probing pocket depth

Clinical recession = 1 mm
Probing pocket depth = 4 mm
So clinical attachment loss = 5 mm

Figure 15.8 Example section of a 6-point periodontal chart for the upper and lower right second premolars to third molar

UPPER												
Buccal	UR8			UR7			UR6			UR5		
Probing point	D	B	M	D	B	M	D	B	M	D	B	M
Probing depth	1	1	2	2	2	4	6	2	4	3	1	2
FGM	0	0	0	0	0	1	3	1	1	1	0	0
Attachment	1	1	2	2	2	5	9	3	5	4	1	2
Bleeding					Y			Y				
Suppuration								Y				
Palatal	UR8			UR7			UR6			UR5		
Probing point	D	P	M	D	P	M	D	P	M	D	P	M
Probing depth	1	1	2	1	1	3	5	2	3	2	1	2
FGM	0	0	0	0	0	1	3	1	0	0	0	0
Attachment	1	1	2	1	1	4	8	3	3	2	1	2
Bleeding					Y			Y				
Suppuration								Y				
Furcation grade								1				
Mobility grade								1				
LOWER												
Lingual	LR8			LR7			LR6			LR5		
Probing point	D	L	M	D	L	M	D	L	M	D	L	M
Probing depth	1	1	2	2	2	3	2	2	4	3	2	2
FGM	0	0	0	0	0	0	0	0	2	1	1	0
Attachment	1	1	2	2	2	3	2	2	6	4	3	2
Bleeding								Y				
Suppuration												
Buccal	LR8			LR7			LR6			LR5		
Probing point	D	B	M	D	B	M	D	B	M	D	B	M
Probing depth	1	1	1	2	1	2	2	1	3	2	1	2
FGM	0	0	0	0	0	0	0	2	1	0	0	0
Attachment	1	1	1	2	1	2	2	3	4	2	1	2
Bleeding								Y				
Suppuration												
Furcation grade												

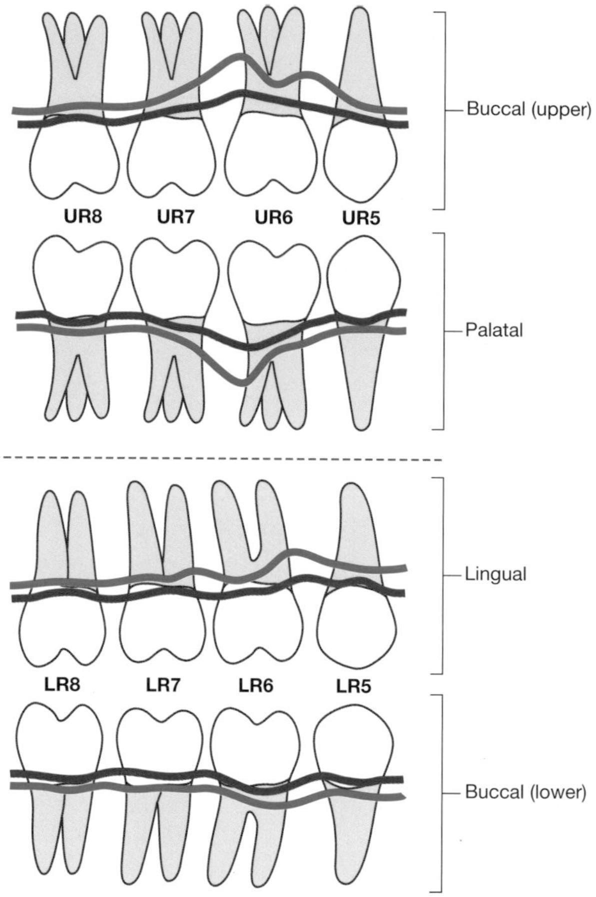

Buccal (upper)

UR8 UR7 UR6 UR5

Palatal

Lingual

LR8 LR7 LR6 LR5

Buccal (lower)

Periodontal screening

The periodontium is comprised from the gingivae, alveolar mucosa, alveolar bone and periodontal ligament. Periodontal diseases may cause irreversible damage to these tissues.

Screening the condition of the periodontal tissues is advised for all patients who are aged 7 years or over. More extensive clinical examination must be carried out for patients who are identified as susceptible to periodontal diseases, providing more detailed assessment and facilitating diagnosis, treatment planning, treatment provision and monitoring.

Following the recording of a general visual examination of the periodontal condition a Basic Periodontal Examination (BPE) should be completed. The BPE probe is shown in Figure 15.1, BPE codes in Figure 15.2 and Table 15.1, and an example grid in Table 15.2. The screening examination is carried out by gently walking the probe around the gingival crevice using a pressure equivalent to a weight of 20–25 g. The highest of codes 0, 1, 2, 3 or 4 are recorded for each sextant, together with * if furcation involvement is found.

For patients aged 7–11 years, six index teeth (Figure 15.3) are examined. Because false pockets (deepened gingival crevices due to excess gingival tissue coronal to the cement–enamel junction) may be associated with newly erupted teeth only codes 0, 1 and 2 are recorded unless an unusually deep pocket is identified. For patients aged 11–17 years the same index teeth are examined, adopting the full range of codes. For adults all teeth in each sextant (Figure 15.3), except third molars, are examined unless the highest possible score (4*) is found, in which case the examination can progress immediately to the next sextant.

With the exception of code 0, all BPE codes have implications for recording indices, for diagnosis and for treatment planning; however, codes 3 or 4 indicate the need for more detailed periodontal assessment. When a single code 3 is recorded, six-point periodontal probing depths for all teeth in that sextant should also be recorded. However, when more than one code 3, or any code 4 or code * are recorded, a full periodontal assessment should be carried out. If there are no teeth in a sextant, an 'X' is recorded; if there is only one tooth in a sextant, it is added to the neighbouring sextant.

Plaque and bleeding indices

BPE code 1, bleeding on probing, indicates the presence of bacterial plaque on the tooth surfaces causing inflammation at the gingival margin. It is helpful to record the presence of bacterial plaque around all the teeth. An index that includes disclosing plaque is recommended as deposits can readily be demonstrated to the patient. The O'Leary plaque index (Figure 15.4) records the presence or absence of plaque around the four surfaces adjacent to the gingival margin of every tooth. A percentage score is calculated by dividing the number of surfaces with plaque present by the total number of surfaces, then multiplied by 100 to give a percentage.

In the example, 32 teeth are present, with total number of surfaces 128, and plaque is present on 31 surfaces. Thus the index is:

$$\frac{31}{128} \times 100 = 24\%$$

A bleeding index may be calculated using a similar type of calculation from a chart of bleeding points, possibly following a full periodontal assessment; that is, number of sites with bleeding following probing, divided by the total number of sites, multiplied by 100.

Full periodontal assessment

In the absence of false pocketing, codes 3, 4 and * indicate true pocket formation due to deepening of the gingival crevice following destruction of the periodontal ligament and loss of alveolar bone. Full periodontal assessment includes the recording of:
- six-point pocket chart for all teeth, measured in millimetres, with a William's or similar, probe (Figure 15.5). Probing depth is measured at six points around every tooth, for a lower molar for example, at the centre of the buccal and lingual surfaces and as close to the contact points as possible keeping the probe parallel to the long axis of the tooth, mesio-buccal, disto-buccal, mesio-lingual and disto-lingual.
- plaque scores
- bleeding points (bleeding may appear to be delayed when a pocket is deep, indicating inflammation at the base of the pocket)
- gingival recession measured from the cement–enamel junction to the free gingival margin (FGM)
- suppuration; grading of furcation involvement (Figure 15.6)
- tooth mobility (Box 15.1).

Naber's probe, a curved probe, can be used to facilitate examination of furcation areas, especially the mesial and distal aspects of the palatal root of upper molars.

Computerised charting systems may automatically calculate clinical attachment loss (CAL; Figure 15.7) by adding pocket depth and gingival recession measurements at each site. Six point pocket charts usually display the upper teeth, buccal and palatal view and the lower teeth, buccal and lingual view. The example of a section of upper and lower posterior teeth in Figure 15.8 records significant CAL distally at UR6 and mesially at LR6; the blue line represents the free gingival margin demonstrating recession; the green line represents the position of the soft tissue base of the periodontal pockets; areas on the grid are provided to enter bleeding points, the grades for furcation involvement and tooth mobility. Some grids enable the position of the mucogingival junction to be recorded, allowing the width of keratinised gingiva to be assessed.

Radiographs to assess alveolar bone loss should be considered following a full clinical periodontal assessment once it is determined which teeth have significant clinical attachment loss.

16 Treatment planning

Figure 16.1 Key step in the treatment planning process

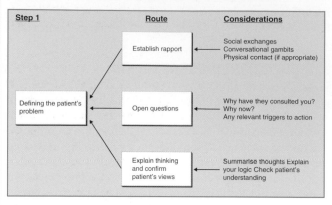

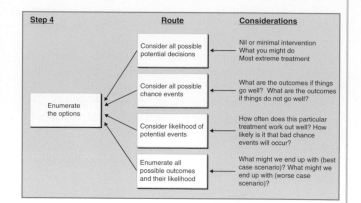

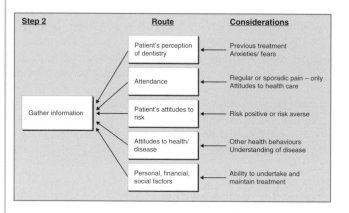

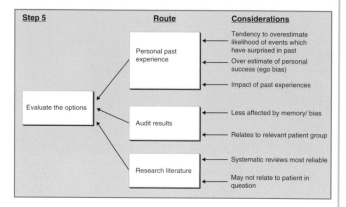

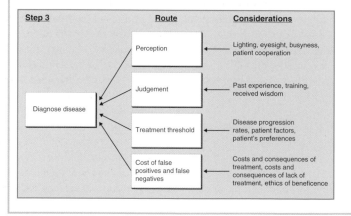

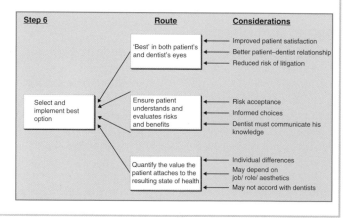

Figure 16.1 shows the key steps in the treatment planning process. Each of these steps involve clear logical thought, and each step's outcome is dependant upon the outcomes of the previous one.

The key to good treatment planning is to remember that there are not 'right' or 'wrong' treatment plans, just good and not so good ones. A **good** plan is one that raises the probability of an outcome which the patient regards as good whilst concomitantly reducing the probability of outcomes the patient would regard as bad.

Defining the patient's problem

It is important not to confuse problem identification with diagnosis. They are separate processes as will be described below. After introductions and social niceties (e.g. a handshake) have been made and rapport built, identifying the patient's problem involves asking open questions, listening carefully to the responses and following the clues given by what the patient says, and also by what they half-say or leave unsaid.

Phrases that are likely to elicit the maximum useful information include "How can I help you?" and "What brings you here today?". Identifying the patient's reason for attending, the duration of any symptoms and when the problem arose will give you an indication of its importance. If it is of long duration, you will need to understand why the patient has decided to consult you about it at this particular time. It is also very important for the dentist to understand what the patient's understanding of his problem, and its potential treatment, is. It is important to dispel mistaken beliefs about miracle cures and quick fixes at this stage.

Gather information

Patients' problems cannot be viewed in isolation from the context of the patient's life. Therefore the dentist needs to understand something about the patient's social history, the amount of time and money the patient is likely to wish to spend on maintaining their dentition and the patient's degree of commitment to oral homecare after the treatment is completed. This is necessary because embarking on courses of treatment that require effort beyond the patient's will or capabilities will lead to poor outcomes.

Diagnose disease

This is a crucial part of treatment planning, but contrary to popular belief is not as exact a science as we might wish to think. This is due to two factors: perception and judgement. If two people look at the same thing (for example a carious lesion or inflamed gingivae) what they 'see' varies from individual to individual. This can depend on light sources, eyesight or other factors. In addition, even when two dentists 'see' the same thing, they may still disagree about whether the disease has reached the point where intervention is necessary. That is, they make different judgements about the appropriate treatment for disease at a particular stage. All dentists set 'thresholds' at which they instigate treatment (treatment criterion), but good treatment planning involves adjusting this treatment threshold according to the patient's needs, behaviours and values.

Enumerate the options

Once the first three steps in Figure 16.1 have been completed, the dentist must then consider what courses of action are open to him or her. This consideration must include **all** possible courses of action (including doing nothing) and should not be limited to the first feasible option that is acceptable to the patient. Each potential option identified will have both good and bad potential outcomes. It is essential that the possible negative consequences of each option, as well as the positive ones, are considered.

Evaluate the options

Of the possible ways of solving the patient's problem, the dentist, in discussion with the patient, needs to evaluate each of the potential outcomes in terms of its potential value/disvalue to the patient. Here the dentist will need to use his or her knowledge of research evidence in order to tell the patient the likelihood of good and poor outcomes from treatment, and will also need to utilise his or her knowledge of physiology, pathology and the natural history of oral diseases in order to be able to explain to the patient the consequences of no or limited treatment, or indeed of treatment failure.

Select and implement the best option

The final stage of treatment planning is to select the best treatment plan for that particular patient, taking into account all the prevailing external and personal factors.

The 'best' option should be selected by weighing the risks against the expected gain. The dentist needs to determine the patient's commitment to the effort required to achieve the desired outcomes. Consideration of whether the patient can, and is willing to, afford the cost, time and, in some cases, discomfort, for each possible option is also essential. Finally, the dentist's limitations must be taken into account. It is essential that the dentist does not overestimate his or her ability to deliver treatments, which may be difficult. It is also necessary that the patient recognises that the stability of all dental interventions is dependent on the subsequent oral environment (oral hygiene/diet) in which they are placed.

Rational decision making

In order to make a treatment plan, values and costs need to be assigned to different possible outcomes. Using this rational approach focuses the dentist's thinking on the things that influence which outcome is achieved, thereby helping to structure organised thought. A rational approach uncovers hidden assumptions and ensures that all possible outcomes are considered. Planning treatment in this rational way also helps to provide an effective vehicle for communicating the options to patients. This, in turn, identifies where additional information might be needed by either dentist or patient before a rational decision can be made.

Most decisions dentists make are fairly routine and are encountered many times. However, some call for the dentist to choose between different risky strategies in order to solve difficult or undefined patient problems. The framework suggested here will help to ensure that you make decisions that are successful not only from a clinical point of view but will also satisfy the patient.

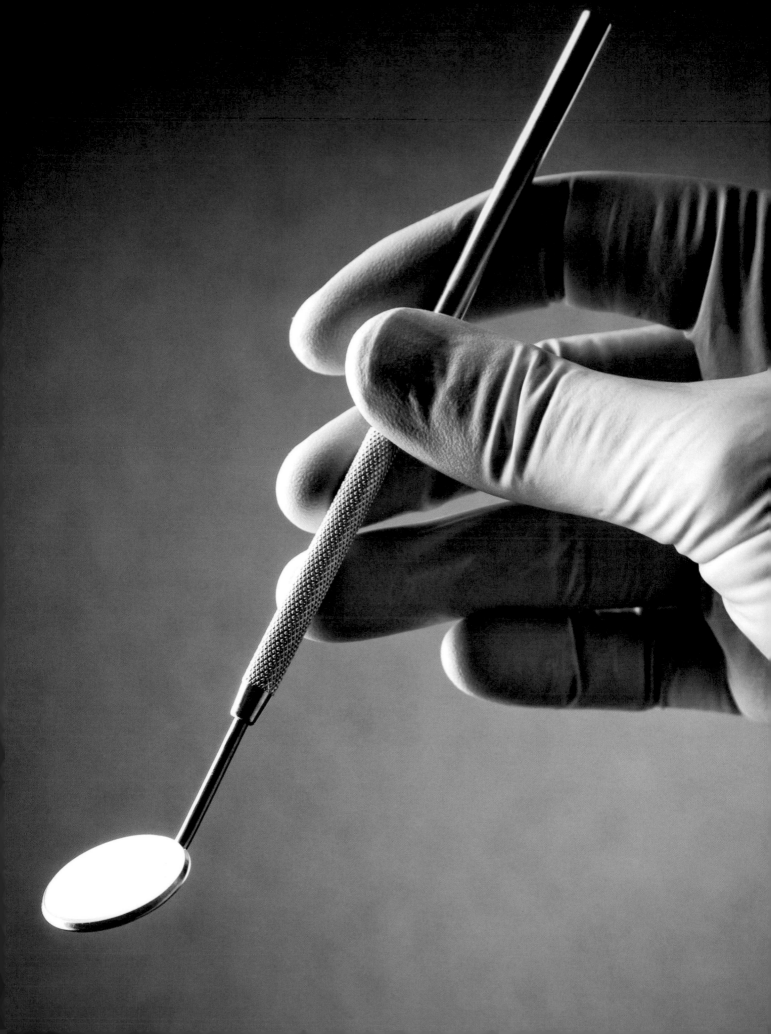

Clinical presentations

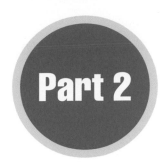

Part 2

Chapters

17 Sudden loss of consciousness

Figure 17.1   Head tilt and chin lift

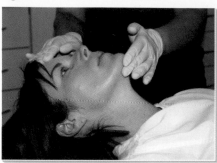

Figure 17.2   An oropharyngeal airway sized by placing against the angle of mandible and lip profile as shown

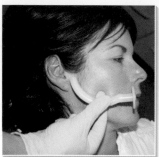

Figure 17.3   Non-rebreathing self-inflating oxygen mask to deliver 15 L/min oxygen

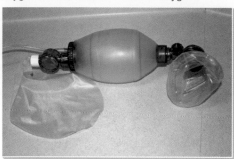

Figure 17.4   Taking the carotid pulse

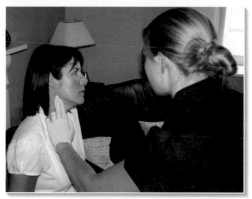

Figure 17.5   Capillary refill test

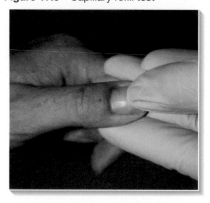

Box 17.1 The approach can be summarised as DR ABCDE R

D Check that all **D**anger to you and the patient is removed

R Elicit a **R**esponse if possible by tapping the patient's shoulders and speaking firmly, calling the patient's name if possible. If there is no response then you do need to call for assistance.

A Establish that the patient has a clear **A**irway.

B Assess that the patient is **B**reathing.

C Assess the **C**irculatory status.

D Look for signs of neurological **D**isability.

E Exposure to look for **E**verything else that may challenge the patient's health and survival.

R **R**epeat again as each cycle is a snap shot of the existing status and does not tell you what they will be like in another 5 minutes, that is commence steps A–E again.

Dentistry at a Glance. First Edition. Edited by Elizabeth Kay. © 2016 John Wiley & Sons, Ltd. Published 2016 by John Wiley & Sons, Ltd.
Companion website: www.ataglanceseries.com/dentistryseries/dentistry

It can be very frightening for a dental team when a patient loses consciousness. Fortunately, it is a rare event but this means that it is something that few dental teams encounter often enough to be confident about managing. A standard approach to the patient, which the whole team understands, must be adopted. The first response if you are sure that consciousness has been lost is to **call an ambulance**. Ensuring help is summoned as soon as possible is crucial. Once help is on its way, the guidelines provided by the UK resuscitation council should be followed.

A Airway

Assessing whether our patient has an airway is important. If they are still conscious and can talk normally, the airway is patent. If unconscious it is prudent to check in the mouth to ensure there is nothing obvious causing an airway obstruction, for example vomit, blood or dentures. If these are present, efforts should be made to remove them. If there is loss of consciousness and the patient cannot maintain their own airway, you will need to re-establish it by either: (1) performing the head tilt and chin lift procedure (Figure 17.1), which, by extending the neck (if there is no evidence of spine injury) and supporting the mandible, keeps the tongue away from the posterior pharyngeal wall; or by (2) inserting an oropharyngeal airway (Figure 17.2). This should be inserted after checking the size (as shown in the Figure 17.2) and, for an adult, inserting it upside down until the palate is felt and then turning 180° to rest behind the posterior border of the tongue. For children, the airway is inserted the normal way up and used as a tongue depressor to engage the correct space, thus avoiding soft palate and pharyngeal wall injury.

Once the airway is open, it is then vital to place a non rebreathing oxygen mask with a self-inflating bag, to deliver 15 L/min oxygen (Figure 17.3).

B Breathing

It is important to establish for certain whether the patient is breathing. Talking and interacting appropriately is clearly a sign of an open airway and normal breathing. But some checks are needed. Counting the respiratory rate, which should be less than 20 breaths per minute, and looking for other signs of distress can be informative, for example use of accessory muscles and tiredness. It is imperative to 'look, listen and feel'. Placing your ear over the patient's mouth, listening and feeling for air movement from the mouth (for up to 10 seconds), and placing your hand on their chest will give a good indication if breathing is taking place. If there is an oxygen saturation monitor available, that will provide evidence of levels of oxygen saturation but if cyanosis is present (there is more than 5 g/dL deoxygenated haemoglobin), there is no breathing detected and no response, this should be treated as a cardiac arrest (see Chapter 18).

C Circulation

The next stage is to assess how well the blood is being circulated. For the dental team this is challenging as we do not make these kinds of assessments regularly. If you are trained and confident at taking blood pressure readings. These should be performed. If blood pressure cannot be taken, look at the patient. Talking and appropriately responding implies enough blood with sufficient oxygen is being circulated to the brain. Skin colour can be misleading as sympathetic nervous activity can initiate selective vasoconstriction leading to a pale skin, whilst septic shock can lead to a red perfused skin. Other confirmation is therefore usually needed. Taking the carotid pulse in both adults and children is recommended, and gives a lot of information about the heart rate and rhythm and the volume of blood. The carotid pulse is taken by feeling the anterior border of the sternocleidomastoid muscle with at least two fingers and pressing backwards to engage the carotid artery against the lateral spinous processes (Figure 17.4). A rate of over 100 beats per minute signifies tachycardia (heart rate too fast) whilst less than 50 beats per minute indicates bradycardia (heart rate too slow). Another test the dental team can apply is the capillary refill test. To do this press the nail bed for 5 seconds to blanch the tissue then release. The tissues should reperfuse within 2 seconds, indicating sufficient blood flow (Figure 17.5). Hold the finger at the heart level when applying this test.

Reasons for circulatory collapse are failure of the heart (acute heart failure or severe myocardial infarction) or, more rarely, a loss of the blood volume from the intravascular compartment, for example from a bleed or because of anaphylaxis.

D Neurological disability

The next stage in your assessment is to judge neurological function, and whether it is working well. An alert and talking patient indicates good cerebral function. However, any deterioration in this will require assessment. The reliable method for the dental team is to use the AVPU system:

A patient is **A**lert and responding normally
V patient only responds to **V**ocal commands
P patient only responds to **P**ainful stimulation (knuckles pressed hard into the sternum or the glabella region)
U patient is **U**nresponsive.

If cerebral function appears to have deteriorated, the team will be expected to check the blood glucose level using the blood glucose monitoring machine (found in in the emergency equipment). The brain only uses glucose as a metabolite and deteriorating function can arise due to hypoglycaemia.

The team should again remember that this assessment gives information for the current status, not what the condition will be in 5 minutes, so it should be repeated until help arrives. If the patient is unconscious, continue to support the airway and breathing until the ambulance arrives.

E Exposure (everything else)

In the accident and emergency department the patient will be unclothed completely to check for other events that may be threatening the patient's wellbeing. However, in the dental chair the patient's dignity must be preserved. If possible, inspection of other areas is useful. For example the abdomen can be checked for swelling and bruising, bleeding or perforation of an ulcer or aneurysm, or the rash of anaphylaxis. Inspection of the legs might reveal bilateral swelling, which could indicate heart failure. The patient should be kept warm and their dignity maintained at all times.

R Repeat

Whilst the ambulance is coming repeat the A to E cycle every 5 minutes to ensure no further deterioration and to look for clues to the underlying problem, and to ensure that you are able to convey an up to the minute picture to the paramedic crew.

18 Acute chest pain and cardiac arrest

Figure 18.1 (a) Glyceryl trinitrate spray. (b) Dispersible asprin 300 mg

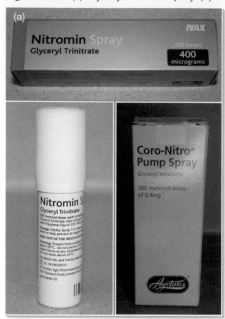

(a)

Nitromin Spray
Glyceryl Trinitrate
IVAX
200 Doses
400 micrograms

Coro-Nitro® Pump Spray
Glyceryl trinitrate
200 metered doses of 0.4mg

Nitromin S
Glyceryl Trinitrate

Ayrtons

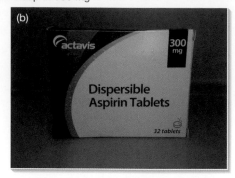

(b)

actavis
300 mg

Dispersible Aspirin Tablets

32 tablets

Figure 18.2 Chest compressions and rescue breaths via a ventilation mask; note the applied AED pads and machine

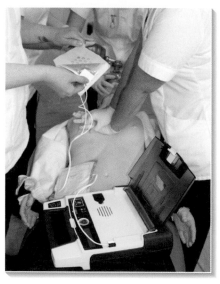

Figure 18.3 Chest compressions on a child, performed with the heel of one hand

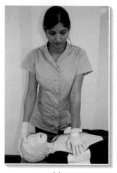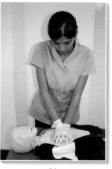

(a)   (b)

Figure 18.4 Chest compressions on a child performed with two fingers above the xiphisternum

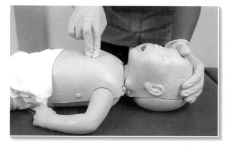

Source: Figures 18.2, 18.3, and 18.4. Jevon P (2013). *Basic Guide to Medical Emergencies in the Dental Practice*. 2nd Edition. Reproduced with permission of John Wiley and Sons, Ltd.

The advent of increased heart muscle demand for oxygen (increased exercise, effort and anxiety), which can be caused by a visit to the dentist for example, may lead to anaerobic metabolism in the heart muscle when there is narrowing of the coronary arteries by atherosclerosis. The subsequent build-up of tissue acid will lead to pain in the chest.

The pain is described as crushing in nature (vice like) spreading down the left arm and occasionally into the left side of the jaw. The dentist should (already knowing the medical history) recognise the cardiac symptoms, stop all treatment and quickly ask for oxygen (15 L/min) and arrange to deliver 800 micrograms of glyceryl trinitrate (GTN) sublingually (Figure 18.1). If the issue is a reversible ischemia of the muscle tissue the GTN will help the symptoms, although further doses during the next 5 minutes may be needed. If the patient recovers, you can be certain that this was a reversible ischemic event called

Dentistry at a Glance. First Edition. Edited by Elizabeth Kay. © 2016 John Wiley & Sons, Ltd. Published 2016 by John Wiley & Sons, Ltd.
Companion website: www.ataglanceseries.com/dentistryseries/dentistry

angina. The dental appointment should be abandoned, another appointment made and the patient asked to take GTN prior to any further dental appointments.

If the pain does not respond to the GTN, you must be suspicious that this is a non-reversible (infarctive) event called a myocardial infarction (MI). The heart muscle is not receiving blood or oxygen, and the tissue is becoming necrotic. The patient will feel nauseous and may even vomit. They will also be very frightened.

The dental team **must call an ambulance**, and whilst it is on the way the patient has to placed in a comfortable position (sitting up is recommended if possible), oxygen mask applied (15 L/min), a 300-mg aspirin (Figure 18.1) given to the patient to chew in the mouth (the dental team must inform the ambulance crew of this when they arrive) and the patient must be monitored. Aspirin should be given even if patient is already taking aspirin, warfarin or clopidogrel. The only reason not to give it is if they are allergic to aspirin. If the patient loses consciousness and stops breathing, management should be as for cardiac arrest.

The ultimate negative result of a medical emergency is the inability of the heart to ensure there is a sufficient supply of oxygenated blood to the brain and thereby preserve vital functions such as breathing. In adults this is usually due to cardiac events and in children to respiratory problems. The collapse of a patient as a result can be a frightening event but the dental team **must** recognise the condition and instigate a suitable treatment regime aimed at restoring the supply of oxygenated blood to the brain within 3 minutes.

Procedure for adults in cardiac arrest

The regimen currently recommended for **adults** is:
• Approach the patient after ensuring all danger has been removed and dental equipment turned off and moved away. Next ascertain a response by shaking the patient at the shoulders and shouting into both ears, calling their name. If there is no response, ensure help is called to provide you with some assistance. Next, establish an airway using the 'head tilt chin lift' method and listen for breathing for at least 10 seconds. This is performed by placing your head over the mouth (listening and feeling) and looking at the chest for any breathing movements. **If there is no response and no evidence of breathing by 10 seconds, call for an ambulance.**
• Cardiopulmonary resuscitation should then be commenced. Current recommendations suggest that 30 chest compressions are applied in the mid-chest region, compressing to a depth of at least 5 cm, from directly over the chest to avoid lateral pressure application. The rate of compression is between 100 and 120 per minute. After 30 compressions have been provided, two rescue breaths are administered via a pocket (ventilation) mask, each breath given with the neck extended, chin supported and each breath lasting 1 second. Chest compressions should not be interrupted for greater than 10 seconds. This cycle should continue until signs of recovery and normal breathing have been established, which may involve asking others to take over if they are available – including the ambulance crew when they arrive. (NB this guidance changes from time to time – you should attend emergency care training on a regular basis to ensure you are up to date on current practice.)
• The chances of a successful outcome are dramatically improved if you have access to and can apply an automated electronic defibrillator (AED). This portable rechargeable source of electric current needs to be applied whilst CPR is being performed **not** instead. Whilst the CPR is being performed as described above, the chest has to be completely exposed, dried (as there is likely to be excessive sweating due to sympathetic stimulation) and chest hair in the pad application sites removed (razors are provided within most AED machines). The machine and the pads should be removed from the bag and the AED turned on. It will then issue instructions that the clinician needs to follow. One pad is applied in the right subclavicular region whilst the second is applied in the mid-axillary line in the sixth intercostal space. The pads are then connected to the machine (Figure 18.2). CPR **must** continue uninterrupted whilst the pads are applied. The machine will then assess for any electrical activity in the heart and will ask at this point for the rescuers not to touch the patient. CPR should then be temporarily ceased. The AED will then decide if a shock needs to be delivered. If one is required (usually for a rhythm such as ventricular fibrillation or pulseless ventricular tachycardia) there will be a short period of charging during which CPR must restart and continue until the shock is ready to be delivered. When about to shock a patient, the operator must order everyone to stand clear. Once the shock is delivered, the AED will assess the outcome and will advise to continue CPR if required. This will continue for 2 minutes until the assessment cycle is repeated. If the rhythms detected are asystole or pulseless electrical activity (PEA), the machine will advise that no shock is required and to begin CPR.
• Resuscitation should continue until signs of recovery and normal breathing are detected, or the ambulance team take over. If recovery is achieved, the patient should then be placed into the recovery position.

Procedure for children and infants in cardiac arrest

The procedures for **children (1 year–puberty)** and **infants (0–1 year)** have some differences. The main issue is that most cardiac arrests in this age group are likely to be due to respiratory problems rather than cardiac events. Thus the procedure is as follows:
• Assess and clear any danger. Determine whether a response can be achieved. If there is no response, help should be summoned. An airway must be established but in children this means extending to the mid-extended position, whilst in infants neck extension is NOT recommended. The breathing is assessed for 10 seconds by placing your ear over the patient's mouth and looking for chest movements.
• If cardiac arrest is confirmed (no response and no breathing) then five rescue breaths must be given.
• If the patient does not respond to the five rescue breaths, a cardiac origin may be behind the collapse. You must therefore check for a pulse. In a child, find the carotid pulse whilst in an infant find the brachial pulse. If the pulse is not felt or is difficult to establish or is definitely less than 60 beats per minute, then CPR should be commenced.
• In younger patients, the regime is to apply 15 chest compressions at a rate of 100–120 per minute followed by two rescue breaths (Figures 18.3 and 18.4). CPR should be continued until recovery signs are noted and normal breathing achieved, or the ambulance crew take over.
• AED machines are also available for younger patients although the adult machines and pads can be used safely down to the age of 8 years and with caution to the age of 1 year but no younger.

19 Difficulty breathing

Figure 19.1 Salbutamol inhaler

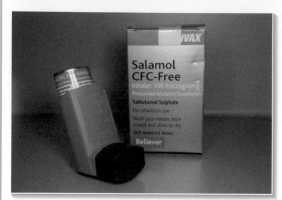

Figure 19.2 Spacer device

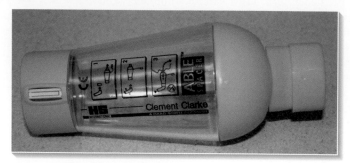

Figure 19.3 Volumatic spacer

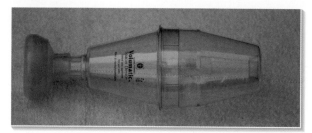

Figure 19.4 (a,b) Adrenaline ampoules

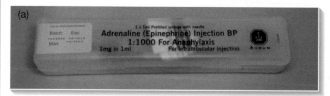

Figure 19.5 Where to administer an Epipen injection

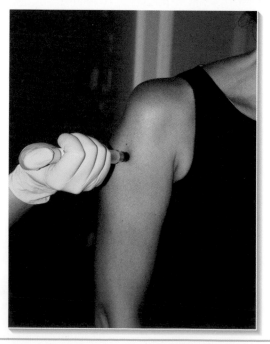

Dentistry at a Glance. First Edition. Edited by Elizabeth Kay. © 2016 John Wiley & Sons, Ltd. Published 2016 by John Wiley & Sons, Ltd.
Companion website: www.ataglanceseries.com/dentistryseries/dentistry

Shortness of breath can be due to a variety of causes:

- Wheeze
  - asthma, chronic obstructive airway disease (COAD), anaphylaxis, heart failure
- Stridor
  - acute epiglottitis, angio-oedema, trauma
- Clear chest
  - hyperventilation, pleural effusion, pulmonary embolism
  - pneumothorax (reduced or absent air sounds and hyper-resonant on percussion).

Asthma

The dental team needs to be alert to the challenges of treating a patient with asthma and be able to respond to the development of an acute event. Hopefully, the asthmatic patient will have been identified and risks anticipated. The key to successful management is to recognise **early** when the condition is starting to become serious. If the patient becomes **breathless and cannot finish sentences in one breath** then all work should be stopped and the patient give a couple of puffs of salbutamol inhaler (200 micrograms), which should help. Another couple of puffs will be required in 5–10 minutes (Figure 19.1). Most will recover at this point and the decision to halt the treatment can be made. It may be sensible to ask the patient to have a couple of puffs of salbutamol prior to the next appointment.

If the condition does not improve and the following symptoms develop, this is a serious emergency. The patient may be pale, fearful and sweating.

- Severe asthma
  - inability to complete sentences in one breath
  - pulse rate >110/min
  - respiratory rate >25/min
- Life-threatening asthma
  - silent chest, poor respiratory effort
  - cyanosis
  - heart rate <50/min
  - exhaustion
  - confusion.

When any of these signs or symptoms develops **call an ambulance immediately** (the earlier the better). The patient urgently needs support. Place an oxygen mask on them (15 L/min) and if they are struggling to use their own inhaler, quickly call for and assemble the (volumatic) spacer device (Figures 19.2 and 19.3). Administer up to 10 activations (1000 micrograms) and ask the patient to inhale over the next 5 minutes. This can be repeated every 10 minutes if the patient can tolerate it.

The patient must be monitored (ABCDE) until the ambulance crew arrive, when they may try a nebuliser to administer additional medication.

Anaphylaxis

Anaphylaxis is a significant risk in the modern day dental practice. The dental team must be aware of the risk and a good medical history may identify the patient with a history of sensitivities. If this is the case, care must be taken to avoid exposure to known allergens. Latex is probably the most common dental surgery allergen but others, such as preservatives in local anaesthetics and nickel, could potentially pose a problem. Unknown allergies are always a possibility and recent allergic reactions to chlorhexidine and Corsodyl mouth washes have highlighted the need to be vigilant.

The onset of anaphylaxis is immediate with the development of a range of signs and symptoms:

- Urticaria (due to histamine release)
- Angioedema (dilatation and increased permeability of small vessels)
- Pruritis (histamine related)
- Abdominal pain (swelling and constriction of the gastrointestinal tract)
- Conjunctivitis (dilated conjunctival blood vessels)
- Erythema (dilated blood vessels)
- Hypotension (loss of intravascular blood volume due to fluid loss and reduced peripheral resistance, may lead to cardiac arrest)
- Vomiting (swelling of the intestinal walls)
- Rhinitis (dilatation of nasal mucosal vessels)
- Wheezing and stridor (bronchospasm and laryngeal swelling, may lead to cardiac arrest).

As soon as you suspect a patient is having an anaphylaxis reaction **call an ambulance immediately**. Then monitor the patient and place them in the head down position, place an oxygen mask on them (15 L/min) and deal with any airway issues appropriately. If the symptoms are clearly advancing, epinephrine (adrenaline) should be administered intramuscularly (IM). The dose for an adult is to give 0.5 mL of 1 : 1000 solution (ampoules are provided in the emergency drug box; Figure 19.4). This is equivalent to 0.5 mg, and can be repeated every 5 minutes. The site of injection is the anterolateral thigh, through the clothes in an emergency. There are autoinjector preparations available (e.g. Epipen; Figure 19.5), which administer 300 micrograms automatically. The Epipen is a suitable alternative to an epinephrine ampoule but as less epinephrine is administered the dental team should only wait 3–4 minutes before considering a repeat injection. If wheezing develops and the patient can manage, then salbutamol can be administered either via a inhaler or volumatic spacer.

The doses of epinephrine for children are:
- Child older than 12 years: 500 micrograms IM (0.5 mL)
- Child 6–12 years: 300 micrograms IM (0.3 mL)
- Child younger than 6 years: 150 micrograms IM (0.15 mL).

The ambulance team are responsible for the remainder of the care, which may involve:
- Chlorphenamine 10 mg IM (an antihistamine)
- Hydrocortisone 200 mg IM (an anti-inflammatory)
- Salbutamol 400 microgram by inhaler every 5 minutes (a beta 2 agonist to relax the bronchioles and bronchi)
- Head down and elevate legs (watch airway) (to maintain blood flow to brain)
- IV fluids (against the severe hypotension)
- Recurrence within 24 hours – need to be admitted to hospital.

Hyperventilation

The anxiety and stress felt by patients attending the dental surgery can precipitate hyperventilation. Driven centrally, the patient will begin breathing very quickly and is unable to stop themselves. Exhaling will reduce the levels of carbon dioxide in the blood, leading to a rise in the pH with a metabolic compensatory exchange of hydrogen ions (into the blood from bone to reduce the pH) and calcium (into the tissues, e.g. bone), resulting in a reduction in the levels of calcium in the blood. This leads to the development of a tetany-like state and the developments of tingling, light headedness and feeling very faint.

Reassurance will usually suffice but using a rebreathing device, such as breathing into a paper bag, will increase the level of inhaled carbon dioxide and reverse the biochemical events. Reassurance is crucial to calm the patient down and reduce the driver of the anxiety.

20 Convulsions and choking

Figure 20.1 Buccal administration of midazolam

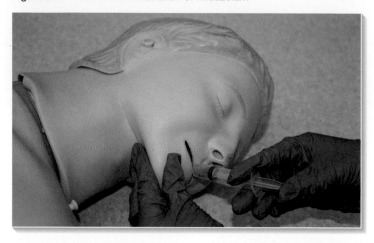

Figure 20.2 (a) Abdominal thrusts and (b) back slaps in adult choking

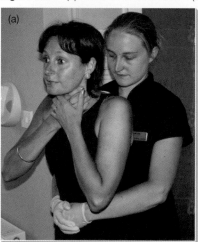

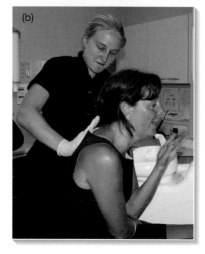

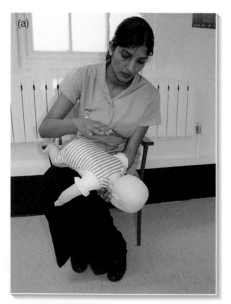

Figure 20.3 (a) Back slaps and (b) chest compressions in an infant

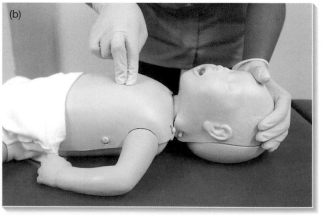

Source: Figures 20.1 and 20.3, Jevon P (2013). *Basic Guide to Medical Emergencies in the Dental Practice.* Reproduced with permission of John Wiley and Sons, Ltd.

Dentistry at a Glance. First Edition. Edited by Elizabeth Kay. © 2016 John Wiley & Sons, Ltd. Published 2016 by John Wiley & Sons, Ltd.
Companion website: www.ataglanceseries.com/dentistryseries/dentistry

Epilepsy

Epilepsy has a spectrum of events that can lead to altered consciousness of which the most demanding in the dental surgery is the grand mal (tonic–clonic) seizure. Representing a global brain electrical activity, it usually presents with a rigid phase (tonic) followed by, and alternating in some cases with, a convulsive stage (clonic)

The dentist must stop all treatment and make the environment safe. Lower the chair closer to the ground and, without restraining the patient, prevent them from hurting themselves. Try and apply an oxygen mask (15 L/min oxygen) or at least hold the mask close to the patient's face. Most seizures will be over in a few minutes, at which point the patient should be placed in the recovery position. They will be tired and drowsy (postictal) and may have been incontinent or possibly bitten their tongue. Obviously, they need to be handled with care and their dignity preserved.

If the fit continues beyond 3 minutes then it is worth the dentist checking the blood glucose (blood glucose monitoring machine) to ensure the seizure is not caused by hypoglycaemia. The pulse should not be below 40 bpm (hypoxic seizure).

If the seizure finishes before 5 minutes, after consideration the patient could go home. If they are a known epileptic patient, they must not drive home but should be taken by someone who is going to be with them overnight (i.e. not a taxi driver). However, not everyone should go home. Those patients include:
* Those for who this is the first seizure
* Those for who there is a risk of recurrent fits
* Those for who monitoring is difficult and responses do not seem to suggest full recovery
* Those who may have injured themselves by falling at the start of the seizure
* Those for whom the seizure goes on for more than 5 minutes (status epilepticus).

All these patient should be taken to hospital in an ambulance.

If the seizure continues for more than 5 minutes then the dental team must ring for an ambulance. Whilst the ambulance is on route, administer 10 mg of buccal midazolam, with a syringe (with no needle) 5 mg onto each buccal mucosa slowly (Figure 20.1). The dose for children is 5 mg (1–5 years), 7.5 mg (5–10 years) and 10 mg (>10 years). Then monitor the patient until the ambulance crew arrive, when they may administer IV diazepam.

Choking

Choking can be a challenge in dentistry with so much activity taking place in the mouth. The use of rubber dams has reduced this risk but challenges to the air way still exist (e.g. in oral surgery).

If an object does disappear from view you must consider whether it has been inhaled. Two scenarios can be considered:
Scenario 1: The object is inhaled but the patient is not compromised and can still breathe and talk. Remove any foreign bodies visible from the mouth and pharynx. The patient is asked to cough vigorously to see if the object can be encouraged to come out and a salbutamol inhaler will help if there is underlying asthma. If not, then the patient must be sent for a chest X-ray straight away. You must ensure that they attend and have the X-ray taken. A phone call to the department would be advisable to inform them of what has happened. If the object is in the lungs (probably in the right main bronchus), then it must be removed.
Scenario 2: The patient has aspirated and is severely compromised and is choking. Encourage them to cough if possible but if this is not possible then the patient should be bent over with arms crossed and up to five sharp back blows between the shoulder blades delivered to dislodge the object. If that fails, then stand behind the patient and deliver up to five abdominal thrusts (Figure 20.2), and alternate with the back slaps until the object is delivered or the patient loses consciousness and stops breathing, when the case is managed as a cardiac arrest.

Children (age 1 year to puberty) are treated the same except that they can be treated whilst sitting in a chair with a firm back support. Infants (<1 year) are held in the head down position on the dentists legs and alternating back slaps and chest compressions delivered, checking each time to ensure the object emerges (Figure 20.3). No abdominal thrusts should be attempted on infants or very small children.

21 Other emergencies

Figure 21.1 Trendelenburg position

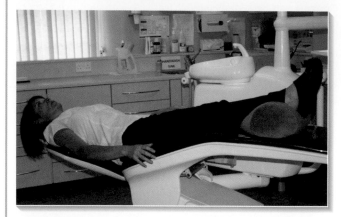

Figure 21.2 Blood glucose monitor

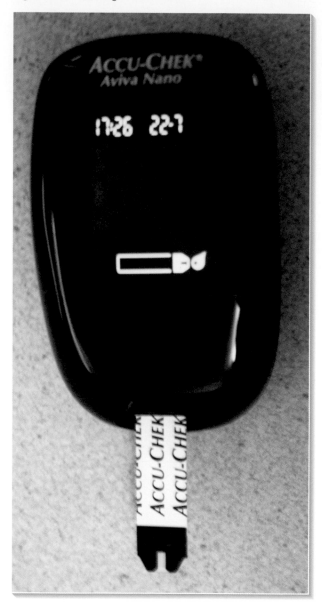

Figure 21.3 Glucogel

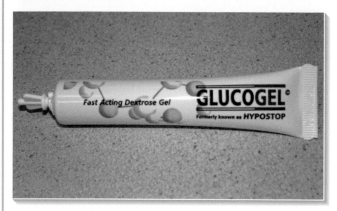

Figure 21.4 IM glucagon, which has to be reconstituted with the powder and fluid provided

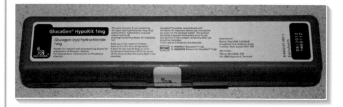

Figure 21.5 Prednisolone: an example of a commonly taken steroid prescription

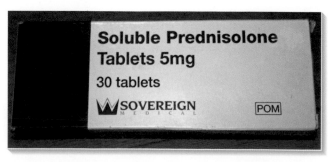

Dentistry at a Glance. First Edition. Edited by Elizabeth Kay. © 2016 John Wiley & Sons, Ltd. Published 2016 by John Wiley & Sons, Ltd.
Companion website: www.ataglanceseries.com/dentistryseries/dentistry

There are further medical emergencies the dental team is expected to manage in the dental surgery. These are:

- Faint
- Hypoglycaemia
- Angina
- Myocardial infarction
- Addisonian crisis
- Hyperventilation.

Fainting

The precipitant for these vasovagal episodes can be multiple and the dental surgery may be one of them! The patient will develop the signs associated with activation of the sympathetic nervous system in response to the perceived threat, including pale skin, sweating, increased heart rate dry mouth and nausea. Then, for some unknown reason, the sympathetic stimulation is turned off, the blood pressure plummets and the patient loses consciousness.

The dental team will apply the ABCDE approach but if they recognise it is a faint, the patient should be placed in the head down (Trendelenburg) position and an oxygen mask (15 L/min oxygen) applied, whilst ensuring circulation is sufficient (Figure 21.1). Any tight clothes are loosened and the patient should improve within 60 seconds or less. They can then slowly sit up. The appointment should be brought a close and the patient given a sweet drink over the next 15–30 minutes before going home.

Hypoglycaemia

Diabetic patients present significant challenges for all forms of care, especially surgical procedures. The brain is dependent on glucose for all its metabolic needs, and therefore changes will be noticed if the glucose levels decrease below 3 mmol/L. This may arise as a result of not having breakfast whilst taking normal insulin/ hypoglycaemia medication. This can be compounded by making the patient wait for their treatment once they arrive. Faced with a reduction in glucose, the patient goes through a number of changes including:

- Shaking and trembling
- Pale skin
- Nausea
- Increased heart rate and respiratory rate
- Sweating
- Headache
- Difficulty in concentration / vagueness
- Slurring of speech
- Aggression and confusion
- Fitting/ seizures
- Unconsciousness.

At the first sign of changes the patient can usually recognise the onset and will probably have a supply of sugar on their person, which they should take. However, if they do not have any sugar, the dentist should ask the nurse to prepare a glucose drink with at least 10 g of glucose in the fluid. The blood sugar level should also be confirmed as soon as possible (Figure 21.2), to ensure that the correct diagnosis has been made. The drink should be repeated every 15 minutes for 30 minutes before letting the patient go home.

If, on the other hand, the patient becomes drowsy and refuses to swallow the drink, a tube of Glucogel (Figure 21.3) should be administered (10 g glucose) into the buccal mucosa. Each tube has 25 mL of gel so it is better to divide the amount and administer to both sides in equal volumes.

If the patient loses consciousness and blood sugar has confirmed the diagnosis, the dental team must administer 1 mg of IM glucagon (Figure 21.4), which activates glycogenolysis, mobilising the glucose stores. For children >8 years or >25 kg, 1.0 mg is administered; for children <8 years or <25 kg, 0.5 mg is given. Beware of patients with no glucose stores, for example anorexic and alcoholic patients.

Check the blood glucose levels at 10 minutes to ensure the levels have risen above 5 mmol/dL and continue to give glucose drinks until it rises to this level. **If a patient remains unconscious 2–3 minutes after the injection, call an ambulance** and continue to monitor the patient (ABCDE R) until help arrives.

Adrenal insufficiency

The range of medical conditions requiring medium or long-term steroid management is increasing. The dental team thus need to be able to recognise the issue of possible steroid-related adrenal suppression. The suppression lasts for an unpredictable amount of time following cessation, making prediction of responses difficult.

External steroids potentially suppress the adrenal gland's release of cortisol. Cortisol is responsible for increasing blood pressure (via mineralocorticoid effects) and blood sugar (glucocorticoid effects) to help the body deal with any stress. Thus, if the natural release of adrenal gland steroid is suppressed, there is only the external steroids to help respond to stress events. If this is not sufficient, there will be a collapse with hypotension and hypoglycaemia at the heart of the event (Figure 21.5).

General dentistry is not felt to be likely to cause a problem but it is currently thought that surgical events, such as extractions or implant placements, may be sufficient to precipitate a collapse. Also, patients with systemic infection should also be recognised to be at risk. These patients need to be managed according to the Addison's Clinical Advisory Panel (http://addisons.org.uk). In essence, if the risk exists, patients are told to double their preoperative dose of steroid and continue this for 24 hours after the event.

If the patient does collapse due to adrenal insufficiency, a range of symptoms will be evident.

- Shock
- Tachycardia
- Pallor
- Sweating
- Hypotension
- Weakness
- Confusion
- Hypoglycaemia
- Loss of consciousness.

The dental team should manage such a collapse in a manner similar to other emergencies, that is DR ABCDE R, but **if it is likely that it is an adrenal insufficiency, an ambulance must be called immediately**. An oxygen mask must be applied (15 L/min) and the patient placed in the head down position. The ambulance crew will administer the required IM hydrocortisone (200 mg) and IV dextrose fluids (titrated against the blood pressure and blood sugar).

22 Caries prevention

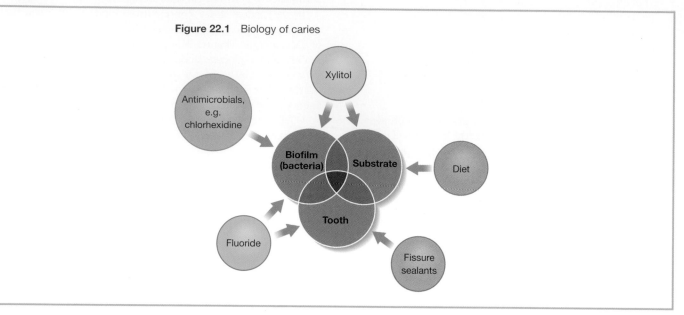

Figure 22.1 Biology of caries

Xylitol

Antimicrobials, e.g. chlorhexidine

Biofilm (bacteria)

Substrate

Diet

Fluoride

Tooth

Fissure sealants

Caries is the localised destruction of susceptible dental hard tissues by acidic by-products from the bacterial fermentation of dietary carbohydrates. It is one of the most common diseases worldwide and people remain susceptible throughout life.

Despite significant improvements in oral health in the UK over the past 30 years, the burden of caries remains unacceptably high in many communities and has wide **social and economic consequences**. Dental professionals have an important role in delivering prevention in the clinical setting for individual patients. However, effectively preventing caries in the population requires policies that address all **risk factors** at all levels of society.

The caries process is multifactorial and dynamic and it is possible to arrest or reverse early lesions before cavitation occurs. The contemporary view of the caries process is that it is **controllable,** and as such all patients should receive preventive advice and treatment. Caries **risk assessment**, where a patient is assigned to a risk category (usually high or low) is an essential element of caries control.

Caries control

Figure 22.1 shows the biology of caries. There are two broad approaches to caries control: (1) strengthening or protecting the tooth and (2) behaviour modification to reduce the availability of substrate and to promote the regular removal of plaque. In practice, caries control is achieved through the following actions.

Plaque control

Regular disturbance of the biofilm by tooth brushing prevents plaque accumulation and is the principle vehicle for introducing fluoride to teeth. Brushing twice per day is a social norm for the majority of people. For some patients, physical plaque removal is problematic and it may be supplemented by the use of the antimicrobial chlorhexidine. While regular professional prophylaxis has been shown to be effective, it is neither a practical or cost-effective caries control measure.

Diet

The aim of dietary advice is to reduce the amount of sugar consumed and the frequency of its intake. Free sugars found in food and drinks are the most important dietary factors. Standard advice is to restrict their intake to mealtimes only (three to four times a day) and not within 1 hour of going to bed. For dietary advice to be effective it must be personal, concise and positive and a 3-day diet diary is a method of working with patients to modify their diet. Dietary advice should also include information on healthy nutrition and should always be given in the wider context of general health.

Fluoride

Fluoride has proven effectiveness in caries prevention (Table 22.1). It has a systemic and topical anticaries effect, providing greatest protection to the smooth surfaces of teeth when present topically in the mouth at frequent low doses. It has several anticaries properties but the principal action when present in plaque fluid is to promote remineralisation over demineralisation in the caries process. The effectiveness of fluoride is dose (concentration) dependent, with higher concentrations offering greater caries reductions. However, this must be balanced against its associated risks. Swallowing and eating toothpaste during dental development can lead to mottling (fluorosis), which in severe cases can be unaesthetic. Acute overdose can also occur if fluoride ingestion is excessive, leading to systemic toxicity at

Table 22.1 Fluoride vehicles for caries prevention

Vehicle	Fluoride concentration	Application	Caries prevention	Advantages	Disadvantages
Toothpaste	Standard formulation is 1350–1500 ppm Low and high strength formulations available	Twice daily tooth brushing at home for 2 min	On average a 24% reduction in caries	Widespread availability Socially acceptable	Compliance – frequency of use, duration of brushing, and rinsing behaviour limit effectiveness
Water	1 ppm	Public water drinking supplies	On average a 15% reduction in caries	Population coverage No compliance required Safe Sustainable	Politically sensitive Freedom of choice removed Capital outlay for plant equipment
Salt	250 ppm	Addition to table salt or salt used in food manufacture	Similar effectiveness to water fluoridation	Population coverage Safe Freedom of choice	Promotes salt intake
Milk	2–5 ppm	School based milk schemes	Some effectiveness but limited availability of evidence	Community coverage Nutritional benefit Safe	Multiagency approach Distribution network Sustainability
Tablets/drops	Varies depending on fluoride exposure. Range from 0.25–1.0 mg per day	Allowed to slowly dissolve in mouth	On average a 40–50% reduction in caries	May be effective in high-risk children	Increased risk of fluorosis Poor compliance
Varnish	22 600 ppm	In surgery, applied to smooth surfaces of susceptible teeth	On average a 33% reduction in the primary dentition and 46% in the permanent	Simple to apply Well tolerated High fluoride dose	Regular application required (2–4 times per year) Professional use only
Mouth rinse	230 ppm (0.05%) or (0.2%) 920 ppm	1 min rinse daily (0.05%) or weekly (0.2%)	On average a 30% reduction in caries	Ease of use	Compliance Not suitable for children <8 years

doses of 1 mg/kg or even death if doses exceed 5 mg/kg. For this reason, prescribing fluoride should be according to caries risk and with knowledge of existing exposure. National guidelines are available to assist in this process.

Sealants

Fissure sealants can be applied to the non-cleansing pit and fissure surfaces of susceptible teeth. For maximum benefit they should be applied as soon as possible after eruption. There is good evidence that sealing permanent molar teeth in children and adolescents at high risk of caries is an effective preventive measure. However, placement of fissure sealants is technique sensitive, and even when successfully applied they require careful monitoring and repair to ensure the all-important seal is maintained.

Xylitol

Xylitol is an artificial sweetener commonly used as a replacement for sugar. Xylitol is non-acidogenic and has anticaries properties due to antimicrobial actions. When contained in gum, the action of chewing also stimulates saliva flow for additional caries protection. Chewing sugar-free gum after meals is therefore recommended for at-risk patients. Its use, however, should be avoided in young children and can produce side effects if used to excess in other age groups.

The dental team

The adoption of a preventive philosophy is fundamental to caries control. Important factors include the use of skill mix (the wider dental team) to support patients in adopting new behaviours and habits, early diagnosis of caries using radiographs as appropriate and conservative management of early lesions in an attempt to prevent their progression to cavitation. It is important to implement relevant prevention strategies based on the best available evidence. Clinical guidelines aid treatment planning based on an individual's caries risk assessment. The interval for dental recall should also be linked to a patient's risk status so those at high risk of caries are recalled more frequently for examination and preventive care.

The public health approach

Clinical practise is only partially successful in caries prevention because individual behaviours are shaped by social and environmental factors – the **social determinants of health**. Professional actions are also only relevant to those people regularly accessing dental care. For this reason, partnership working and the use of multidisciplinary teams is vital to engaging communities to reduce risk factors for caries. This involves working with other health professionals, such as health visitors and school nurses, and alongside other programmes to ensure activities to reduce caries is integral to general health improvement activities. Outreach working has grown in recent years whereby dental professionals support or deliver interventions in the community setting. Programmes may include fluoride in their design via supervised tooth brushing clubs or the professional application of fluoride varnish to the teeth of children in nurseries and schools.

23 Plaque reduction

Figure 23.1 Manual toothbrushing

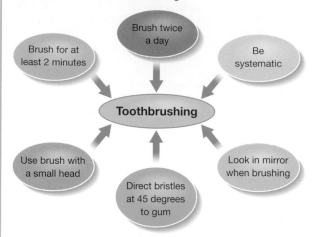

- Brush twice a day
- Brush for at least 2 minutes
- Be systematic
- **Toothbrushing**
- Use brush with a small head
- Direct bristles at 45 degrees to gum
- Look in mirror when brushing

Figure 23.2 Once recession has occurred interdental brushes are much more effective than floss in removing interdental plaque

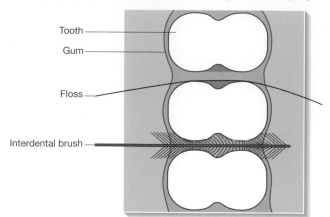

- Tooth
- Gum
- Floss
- Interdental brush

Figure 23.3 Interdental brushes come in a variety of sizes

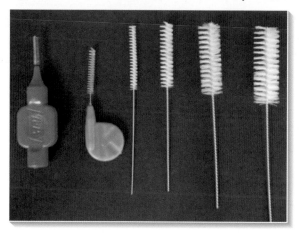

Box 23.1 Features of an ideal manual toothbrush

- Handle size appropriate to user age and dexterity
- Head size appropriate to the size of the patients mouth
- Use of round-ended nylon or polyester filaments not larger than 0.23 mm in diameter
- Use of soft or medium bristles
- Use of bristle pattern that enhances plaque removal in the approximal spaces and along the gum line.

Box 23.2 Patient factors in oral hygiene advice

- Age of subject
- Susceptibility of subject to gingivitis and periodontitis
- Past periodontal disease experience
- Manual dexterity
- Knowledge and motivation in oral hygiene practices

Figure 23.4 The use of plaque charts is an excellent method of patient motivation

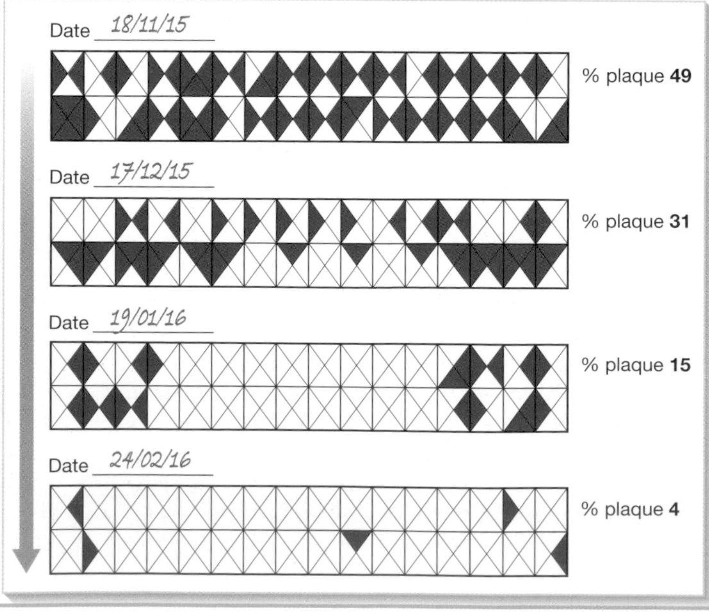

Date _18/11/15_   % plaque **49**

Date _17/12/15_   % plaque **31**

Date _19/01/16_   % plaque **15**

Date _24/02/16_   % plaque **4**

Table 23.1 Adjunctive benefit of chemical plaque control

Dentifrice	Effect on plaque	Effect on gingivitis
Chlorhexidine gluconate	45–61%	27–67%
Triclosan with co-polymer	20–58%	20–32%
Essential oils	19–56%	20–36%
Cetylpyridinium chloride	20–23%	17–19%
Stannous fluoride	–	20–30%

Mechanical
Tooth brushing

Manual toothbrushing is currently the most commonly used oral hygiene measure (see Figure 23.1 for relevant factors). Twice daily toothbrushing for 2 minutes should be performed to ensure removal of plaque. A medium-filament small flat-headed brush is recommended and some authorities recommend changing the toothbrush every 3 months, although there is no evidence that this is critical to plaque removal (Box 23.1 lists the features of an ideal manual toothbrush). Modifications to the shape of the head, including concave heads and double and triple-headed brushes, have also been proposed. Double and triple-headed toothbrushes have been shown to be more effective in the removal of plaque on lingual surfaces but these are not widely used.

A number of toothbrushing techniques have been described but there is no good evidence for one technique over another. Where a patient's toothbrushing technique requires modification, the modified bass technique has been found to be effective. This involves brushing with the bristles angled at a 45° to the tooth with a small circular or vibrating motion. A systematic approach should ensure that all areas of the mouth are covered. In clinical studies, toothbrushing alone has been shown to remove between 39% and 50% of plaque and to result in a 35% reduction in gingival bleeding.

Powered toothbrushes that work in an oscillating, rotating fashion have been recently shown to have improved efficacy when compared with manual toothbrushes. Brushes using sonic technology are also available and are also effective at removing plaque. These brushes utilise acoustic vibrations and dynamic fluid activity to remove plaque. Patients with limited manual dexterity, those caring for mentally handicapped patients or orthodontic patients could consider a powered brush. Powered brushes have also been shown to enhance long-term compliance and so might be suitable for patients who are unable to achieve good plaque control using a manual brush. The cost of high-end powered toothbrushes needs to be balanced against the perceived clinical benefit.

Box 23.2 indicates the factors that need to be taken into account when offering advice about oral hygiene to a patient.

Interdental cleaning

Effective toothbrushing can only clean around 65% of the tooth surface as it only removes plaque from the buccal, lingual and occlusal surfaces. Periodontitis occurs primarily between teeth; therefore, interdental cleaning is always necessary. Interdental cleaning can be performed using dental floss, dental tape, interdental brushes, toothpicks or powered irrigation devices. Studies have shown that the addition of intercleaning reduces bleeding on probing by 67% compared with 35% using toothbrushing alone. Interdental plaque should be removed at 12 to 48-hour intervals so daily interdental cleaning is therefore recommended.

Flossing can be carried out using either waxed floss or tape and there is no evidence to suggest either is more efficient at plaque removal. Floss is best used in sites where there has been little or no interdental recession and where the papilla fills the interdental space. Triangular toothpicks or wood sticks with a low surface hardness and high strength have been shown to be most effective where there is some recession.

Where there is space for interdental brushes these are to be preferred as they are better suited to cleaning grooves on exposed root surfaces. Interdental brushes can remove plaque up to 2.5 mm below the gingival margin and can clean areas that would be inaccessible to floss once recession has occurred (Figure 23.2). In addition, patients are more likely to comply with interdental brush use than floss. Interdental brushes come in a variety of sizes and advice from a dental professional will help the patient choose the correct brush size (Figure 23.3). Interdental cleaning aids should be reviewed as treatment progresses because resolution of inflammation will lead to recession and an increase in the size of interdental embrasure spaces.

Irrigation devices provide a pressurised pulsing or steady stream of water through a nozzle. These have been shown to have only modest adjunctive effects on plaque removal and gingival condition but can be used in areas that are not easily cleansed by conventional mechanical methods.

Chemical plaque reduction

Levels of dental plaque can also be reduced by chemical anti-plaque agents. While these can be administered through a variety of vehicles, toothpaste and mouthrinses are the most commonly used. The efficacy of antiplaque agents is not directly related to antimicrobial action but rather seems to be related to persistence of action or substantivity. Table 23.1 and Figure 23.4 shows the effects of various chemicals on plaque control.

Chlorhexidine gluconate

Chlorhexidine was the earliest and one of the most effective anti-plaque agent available. It is a dicationic bisbiguanide and is available in 0.12% and 0.2% preparations for twice daily use. Adverse effects reported include staining of teeth, mucositis, reversible epithelial desquamation, alteration of taste, salivary gland swelling and increased supragingival calculus.

Quaternary ammonium compounds

Cetylpiridinium chloride (0.05%) is the most studied of the quaternary ammonium compounds. The duration of action is only 3–5 hours and, although some plaque inhibitory effect has been shown, most studies have concluded that it has a minimal effect on gingivitis when used in conjunction with toothbrushing. Cetylpyridinium chloride is also associated with staining of the teeth with regular use.

Phenolic compounds and essential oils

Triclosan: This is a non-ionic antimicrobial. It is found mainly in toothpastes and mouthrinses at 0.2–0.3% and has a substantivity of 5 hours. The activity of triclosan is increased by the addition of zinc citrate or polyvinylmethyl ethyl maleic acid ((PVM/MA). Long-term reduction in plaque averaged between 20 and 40% and in gingivitis 20–40%. Some studies have shown that triclosan and co-polymer has an anti-inflammatory effect that is independent of its antimicrobial effect. Studies have shown a modest beneficial effect on the progression of periodontitis.

Essential oils: Combinations of essential oils have been shown to be effective chemical adjuncts to plaque control. Strong taste, a low pH, burning sensation in the mucosa and a high alcohol concentration are reported.

Stannous fluoride

Stannous fluoride has been shown to reduce gingival inflammation and bleeding, although it has less of an effect on plaque levels. It is possible that it exerts its anti-inflammatory effect through modifying the plaque rather than removing it.

Other antiplaque and gingivitis agents that have been evaluated include metal salts, oxygenating agents, detergents, amine alcohols (delmopinol), salifluor, acidified sodium chlorite and hexetidine.

Prevention of periodontal disease

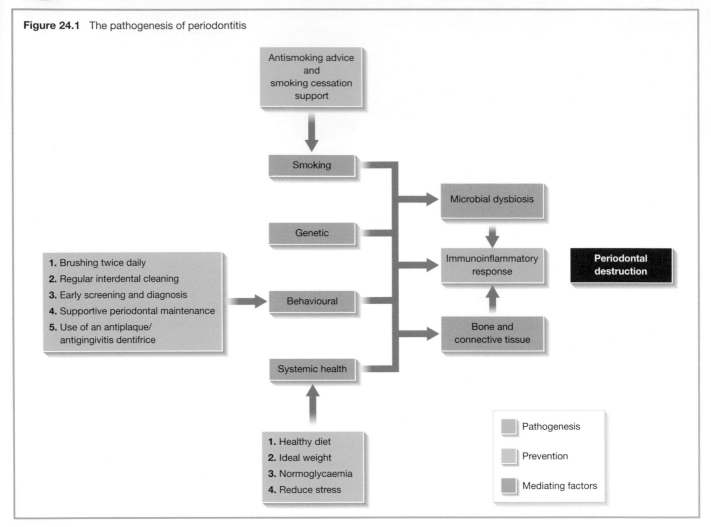

Figure 24.1 The pathogenesis of periodontitis

The pathogenesis of periodontitis is multifactorial and is shown in Figure 24.1. Theoretically, if we could intervene at any level of the causal pathway then we could reduce the burden of periodontitis to individuals and society. Despite much investigation, only a few of these risk factors are currently modifiable in order to prevent the occurrence of disease.

Microbial complexes

Bacteria are present on teeth in microcolonies within an amorphous mass of biofilm known as dental plaque. Dental plaque is the main aetiological factor in the development of gingivitis and periodontitis.

Gingivitis

There is good evidence that chronic gingivitis does not occur in the absence of plaque and that where plaque is allowed to accumulate gingivitis almost invariably occurs. Removal of plaque has been shown to lead to resolution of experimentally induced gingivitis in all cases. Chronic gingivitis can be prevented by meticulous self-performed plaque removal and chemical plaque control.

Periodontitis

Periodontitis is a chronic inflammatory disease caused by inflammation of the supporting tissues around the teeth. The infection begins with a microbial shift within the dental plaque from Gram-positive bacteria, which are compatible with periodontal health, to a dysbiotic biofilm characterised predominately by Gram-negative anaerobes and spirochaetes. This pathogenic biofilm induces an inflammatory response that, if ineffective, leads to formation of periodontal pockets and destruction of the alveolar bone and periodontal ligament.

Primary prevention

Animal studies have established that clinical attachment loss occurs at sites of plaque accumulation over time, although some animals were resistant to periodontitis despite the presence of plaque. In humans, periodontitis occurs interproximally in sites of plaque accumulation and on teeth where plaque removal is more difficult. In one deprived population without access to dental treatment and who did not practice regular tooth brushing, periodontitis occurred in all of subjects although there was wide variation in the extent and severity of attachment loss. In patients who have low levels of plaque and gingival inflammation, the development and progression of periodontitis is rare. Periodontitis is a complex multifactorial disease associated with multiple risk factors but dental plaque is necessary, although not on its own sufficient, to cause severe periodontitis. The daily removal and inhibition of the biofilm is key to the primary prevention of periodontitis.

Secondary prevention

Although plaque formation happens relatively quickly after toothbrushing or polishing, the re-infection of periodontal pockets takes longer to occur. Once periodontal health has been established it has been shown that in the absence of optimal oral hygiene measures it can still take months for a periodontopathic biofilm to be re-established on the root surface. It is the prevention of the formation of this mature subgingival plaque that is essential for periodontal health.

Once periodontal treatment is complete periodontal health can be maintained for many years if patients continue to practice excellent oral hygiene and comply with a supportive periodontal care regime. Recurrence is common in those who do not.

Needs-based professionally performed supportive care and prophylaxis, including monitoring of plaque levels, plaque removal and targeted oral hygiene advice, has been shown to reduce periodontal bone loss to negligible levels. Three-monthly visits seem to be an optimal time interval for professional care.

Smoking

Smoking has been shown to be associated with an increased risk of periodontal disease, which increases depending on the frequency and duration of the habit (risk ratio 3.25–7.28). It is estimated that smoking accounts for 50–80% of all periodontal disease. Patients who smoke have also been shown to be more resistant to treatment and are more likely to see recurrence and progression of their periodontal disease after it has been treated. Smoking is also an independent risk factor for tooth loss in patients with treated periodontitis and smoking cessation has been shown to be associated with better periodontal outcomes.

Strategies to prevent periodontal disease should include avoidance of smoking and smoking cessation advice for those who do. Dental professionals should ask all patients about their smoking habits and should advise them of the effects on the periodontium. Patients with periodontitis should either be given a brief intervention from the dentist or referred on to the appropriate service.

Local factors

Gingivitis and periodontitis can be caused by subgingival restoration margins and poorly contoured restorations that are plaque retentive. Care and attention in the contouring of interproximal restoration and ensuring an excellent marginal fit of all indirect restoration will minimise their periodontal effects. Partial dentures also contribute to periodontitis and care should be taken in the design of dentures to enable cleaning, minimise gingival coverage and maximise tooth support to mitigate against this effect.

Other measures

Periodontitis is associated with obesity, diabetes, stress and nutritional deficiency and deprivation, as well as other systemic factors. Taking a holistic approach to general health measures to ensure good systemic health, including a healthy balanced diet, maintaining a healthy weight, maintaining normoglycaemia and measures to address social inequalities, should have an overall effect of reducing periodontal diseases.

Challenges

One of the challenges in the reduction of plaque is the compliance of patients with suggested oral hygiene regimes. There are patient groups for whom compliance is difficult or impossible, including those with a mental or physical disability. In the general population, oral hygiene is poor and use of interdental aids, including floss, is low. In the UK, 62% of patients who opted to brush their teeth immediately prior to examination still had visible plaque. Just under a quarter of all teeth in the study had visible plaque.

Public health funding must be in place to ensure training and remuneration of the dental team is adequate and that appropriate educational and motivational strategies are applied at both a population and individual level.

25 Prevention of dental trauma

Figure 25.1 Increased overjet

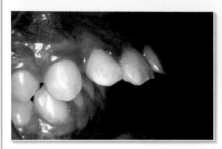

Figure 25.2 Gumshield

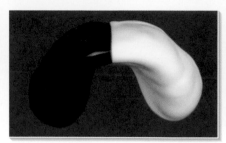

Figure 25.3 Clear mouthguard material

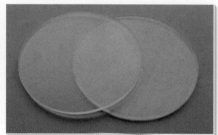

Figure 25.4 Mouthguard construction

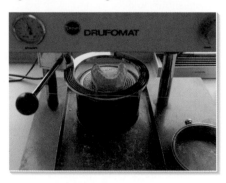

Figure 25.5 Colour mouthguard material

Table 25.1 Aetiology of dental trauma

Age	Aetiology			
	Fall	Sports	Bicycle/road traffic accident	Assault
Preschool	**62%**	6%	4%	9%
Mid-childhood	19%	14%	**39%**	6%
Adolescence and adult	7%	20%	20%	**46%**

Table 25.2 Categorising preventive strategies

Category	Primary	Secondary	Tertiary
Method	Alter the circumstances leading to the injury to prevent it occurring	Provide protection to diminish the severity of the injury when it does occur	Provide treatment for the injury to prevent or reduce complications from occurring
Examples	Playground design Reducing overjet Highlight suspicions of non-accidental injury	Mouthguards Headwear Avulsion kits	Adhere to trauma guidelines at www .dentaltraumaguide .org

Table 25.3 Features of a sports mouthguard

Feature	Benefit
Double thickness of mouthguard material in the anterior region only, extending into the full functional depth of the labial sulcus Inner layer using clear material and outer layer in colour (Figure 25.3)	To protect the upper anterior teeth and associated soft tissues Bulk in the posterior region comparatively reduced to ensure comfort of wear
Mouthguard created on model (Figure 25.4) then articulated against opposing model to obtain balanced occlusion	Even distribution of forces between the lower and the upper teeth to reduce risk of supporting bone/base of skull injuries
Various colours and designs (Figure 25.5)	Team branding and affiliation encourages wear and use

Dentistry at a Glance. First Edition. Edited by Elizabeth Kay. © 2016 John Wiley & Sons, Ltd. Published 2016 by John Wiley & Sons, Ltd.
Companion website: www.ataglanceseries.com/dentistryseries/dentistry

Dental trauma is a common occurrence, with both children and adults succumbing. Reported rates show the incidence of a person suffering a traumatic dental event is greater in childhood (around 80% of injuries occurring under 20 years of age) with a particular preponderance in the age bands of 1–3 years and 7–10 years.

In order to prevent dental trauma, it is necessary to be aware of the causative mechanisms for such trauma occurring in the first instance in order that preventive strategies can be suitably aligned.

Aetiology of dental trauma

There are myriad aetiologies for dental trauma, many of which account for a very small number of injuries; however, the main causes and their corresponding percentage incidence figures can be seen in Table 25.1 in relation to age of occurrence.

Categorising preventive strategies

It is possible to categorise the means of preventing trauma, and this may be done based on the medical model of prevention as shown in Table 25.2.

There is overlap between primary and secondary prevention whereby some preventive measures designed to prevent injuries occurring in the first instance can also reduce the severity of an injury where it occurs. Similarly, interventions aimed at reducing the severity of injuries may go so far as to prevent the injuries occurring in the first place.

The role of the dental team in the prevention of dental trauma

Preventive measures which can be undertaken by the dental team include:
- Reduction of increased overjets
- Raising concerns about suspicion of neglect and non-accidental injury
- Provision of mouthguards
- Provision of advice to patients, schools and clubs regarding prevention and emergency treatment
- Adhering to trauma treatment guidelines such as those available at www.dentaltraumaguide.org

Reducing increased overjet

Typically, just under 10% of children in the UK have an increased overjet greater than 7 mm. Whilst this is a relatively small percentage of the population, an overjet of just 3 mm or greater increases the likelihood of suffering dental trauma. For those with an overjet of 9 mm or greater (Figure 25.1), the risk for trauma doubles. With up to a quarter of children traumatising their adult teeth, doubling a child's risk is a significant additional burden of jeopardy.

The reduction of an overjet in the mixed dentition for a non-crowded arch requires the use of a functional appliance during the accelerated growth phase of early puberty, at which time the greatest incidence of trauma is over. In a crowded arch, to achieve overjet reduction in the mixed dentition requires a more prolonged period of orthodontic treatment involving removal of the primary canines, reduction of overjet, followed by further appliance therapy and extractions of posterior teeth when entering the complete secondary dentition. The need for such prolonged treatment must be carefully weighed against the potential preventive benefits. Large skeletal-based overjets cannot be fully corrected until growth ceases in early adulthood.

Raising concerns of suspicion of neglect and non-accidental injury

The importance of procedure in raising concerns of child welfare are discussed in Chapter 76.

Mouthguards

Mouthguards, or gumshields as they are otherwise known, (Figure 25.2) are recommended for the prevention of dental trauma by the World Dental Federation (FDI) who report the overall risk of oral injury during athletic activity to be between 1.6 and 1.9 times greater for those not wearing a mouthguard in comparison with those wearing one. The FDI also promotes the use of custom-made mouthguards over off-the-shelf or 'boil-in-the-bag' guards that the lay person moulds to fit their teeth. Custom-made guards have been shown to result in fewer injuries being sustained.

Features of a sports mouthguard: It is important to note the difference in construction between a bite-raising splint made for the treatment of bruxism and a sports mouth guard (Table 25.3).

Provide advice to patients, schools and clubs regarding prevention and emergency treatment

Advice regarding the need to access treatment expediently and what can be done immediately by those present at the site of injury can be highlighted to patients, parents, carers and service providers via information displayed in the surgery, at schools and in clubs and sports grounds where athletic activities take place.

General dental practice reception staff are ideally placed to give immediate advice to those contacting the practice regarding dental avulsion. The need to either replant an avulsed tooth or have it placed in milk or other suitable medium as soon as possible cannot be overstated. Having a written practice protocol and script available for such staff is a key method of providing tertiary prevention of the sequelae of dental trauma.

The 'normal' dentitions

Figure 26.1 The ugly duckling stage of dental development: (a) the maxillary lateral incisors are distally splayed and there is a midline diastema; (b) the radiograph shows that the distal splaying is due to pressure on the lateral incisor roots by the developing canines

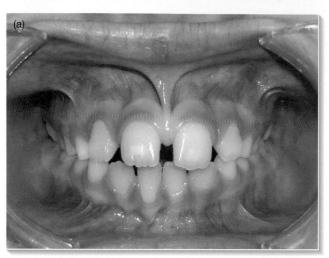

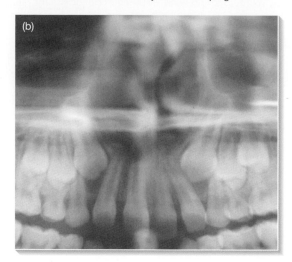

Source: Gill D (2008). *Orthodontics at a Glance*. Reproduced with permission of John Wiley and Sons, Ltd.

Table 26.1 Development of the primary dentition

Tooth (in order of eruption)	Start of calcification	Eruption	Root completion (12–18 months after) eruption)
Central incisors	14 weeks	6 months	2 years
Lateral incisors	14 weeks	7 months	2 years
First molars	15 weeks	12 months	2.5 years
Canines	16 weeks	18 months	3 years
Second molars	20 weeks	24 months (6–12 month's variation is normal)	4 years

Table 26.2 Development of the secondary dentition

Tooth (in order of eruption)	Start of calcification (5–6 years prior to eruption)	Eruption (+ 1)	Root completion (3+ years after eruption)
First molar	Birth	6 years	9 years
Mandibular central incisors	3 months	7 years	10 years
Maxillary central and mandibular lateral incisors	3 months	8 years	11 years
Maxillary lateral incisors	12 months	9 years	12 years
Mandibular canines	4 months	10 years	13 years
Maxillary first premolars	18 months	11 years	14 years
Mandibular first premolars	22 months	11 years	14 years
Maxillary canines	4 months	12 years	15 years
Maxillary second premolars	24 months	11 years	14 years
Mandibular second premolars	28 months	12 years	15 years
Second molars	32 months	12 years	15 years
Third molars	Variable	Variable	Variable

The first signs of tooth formation can be seen in the dental laminas when a foetus is 6–7 weeks old.

The deciduous dentition

At around 7 months of age the deciduous dentition begins to erupt, starting with the lower central and then the lateral incisors (Table 26.1). The teeth tend to be spaced and this spacing increase as the jaw grows. At 12–14 months of age the first deciduous molar (D) erupts, then the canines (C) at 18–20 months. The last tooth to erupt in the deciduous dentition is the second molar (E), which erupts between the ages of 2 and 3 years. The spacing is greatest in the maxilla distal to the lateral incisors. In the mandible the space is greatest distal to the canines. These widened gaps are known as the primate spaces. The deciduous dentition often occludes edge-to-edge or nearly so and as toothwear occurs this tendency to an edge-to-edge occlusion increases.

Eruption of permanent teeth

The lower central incisors erupt at around the age of 6 years and this coincides fairly closely with the eruption of all four first permanent molars (Table 26.2). This is followed by the eruption of the upper central and lower lateral incisors around the age of 7 years. The upper lateral incisors then appear at age 8 (or thereabouts). The exact timing may vary somewhat, but the sequence of eruption is relatively ubiquitous. If the central incisor does not erupt in sequence, radiographs should be taken to ascertain whether a supernumerary or altered morphology is causing the delay.

The lower canine erupts between 9 and 10 years, as do the first premolar teeth. The upper canine and second premolars erupt at 11 and the second molars at 12. Both the presence and the eruption of third molars is very variable.

The deciduous molars are larger mesiodistally than the permanent premolars which replace them. This is known as the 'leeway space' (width of C + D + E − width of 3 + 4 + 5) and is usually 1.5 mm in the upper and 2.5 mm in the lower.

Stages of eruption

There are four stages to the eruption of the permanent teeth.

Stage 1: As soon as root development begins, eruption starts. At the same time, resorption of the bone (and in the case of secondary teeth the primary tooth roots) needs to occur. If the two processes do not coincide, eruption will not progress.

Stage 2: When the root is about two-thirds complete, the tooth erupts into the mouth. The tooth moves approximately 0.4 mm/week and continues to erupt until aligned with the occlusal plane.

Stage 3: The maxilla and mandible continue to grow after the teeth have erupted into position and teeth continue to erupt to keep pace with this, with a speeding up of the eruption rate at the time of the adolescent growth spurt.

Stage 4: Teeth continue to erupt to compensate for occlusal wear and further growth. If there are no opposing teeth, over eruption will occur.

Early mixed dentition

The mixed dentition phase commences when the first permanent teeth, the mandibular lower incisors, erupt. The incisors often erupt slightly lingually to the deciduous tooth. As the upper centrals erupt, because of the position of the canine tooth close to the root of the lateral incisor, the lateral incisors are often distally inclined. This is a normal stage of development, commonly (and rather unfairly!) called the 'ugly duckling stage' (Figure 26.1).

The permanent incisors are considerably bigger that the deciduous ones. They are accommodated partly because of the spacing found between deciduous incisors and by being slightly more proclined than the very upright deciduous teeth. There is also an increase in intercanine width – in the mandible due to the permanent canine erupting to occupy the primate space. There is, therefore, often some incisor crowding until the canines erupt.

Late mixed dentition

This phase begins when the lower canine erupts, along with the premolar teeth, around the age of 11 years. The upper canines should be palpable buccally from the age of about 9 years. Because they erupt after the upper premolars, any shortage of space will cause them to be crowded out of the arch. If the canines erupt successfully, the incisors become less splayed and small diastemas will be likely to close.

27 Variations in the number of teeth

Figure 27.1 A 4-year-old boy with two missing mandibular incisors; there are double teeth of 72, 73 and 82, 83 in his primary dentition

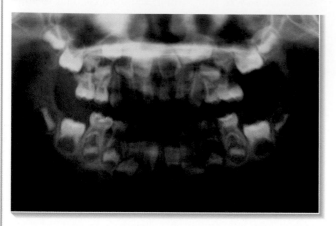

Figure 27.2 An erupted conical-shaped mesiodens

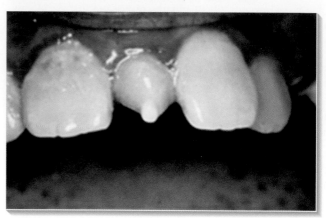

Figure 27.3 (a) A tuberculate supernumerary in relation to 11; (b) the surgically extracted tuberculate supernumerary

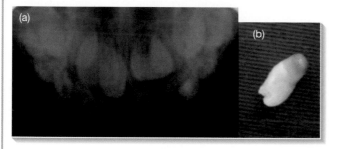

Figure 27.4 (a) The superrnumerary in relation to 16 looks like an odontome in the radiograph; (b) the supernumerary was surgically extracted and found to be a paramolar

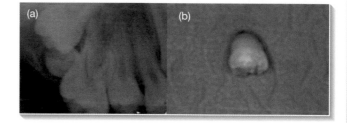

Figure 27.5 Two conical-shaped supernumerary teeth apical to 51 (inverted) and 61, respectively

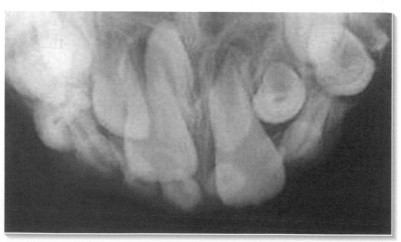

Decreased number of teeth – hypodontia

The following terms are used to refer to progressive degrees of tooth absence:

Oligodontia refers to six or more congenitally missing teeth.

Anodontia refers to the complete congenital absence of teeth.

The term **hypodontia** is generally preferred because it is inclusive of any number of missing teeth. A person is said to exhibit hypodontia when one or more teeth fail to develop, resulting in the congenital absence of one or several teeth (Figure 27.1).

Hypodontia is a condition that is rarely seen in other mammalian species, including other primates. The congenital absence of teeth may occur because of the adverse effects of local factors, an endocrine disorder, or bone fusion problems. However, more significantly, congenitally missing teeth are considered by some investigators to be the expression of an evolutionary trend. A reduction in the number of teeth in the dentition would thus signify an attempt by nature to fit the teeth into a smaller dental arch. In support of this theory is cited the high frequencies with which the third molars, in the posterior region of the arches, and the maxillary lateral and mandibular central incisors, in the anterior region, are missing. Also, it is now well established that the congenital absence of teeth may result from genetic factors; however, the modes of inheritance remain unclear. Many authors have suggested a Mendelian patterns of inheritance, whereas others have proposed that hypodontia may result from the interaction of multiple genetic factors.

Hypodontia is common in the permanent dentition where a prevalence of between 2.5% and 11.3%, excluding the third molars, has been reported. The prevalence of persons lacking one or more third molars varies from approximately 1% in some Black African and Australian aboriginal samples, to an estimated 30% in the Japanese population. The prevalence in Caucasian populations varies from 10% to 25%. Some scholars conclude that these population frequencies indicated a genetic basis for third molar agenesis in humans.

The gender difference consistently reported in the literature is that the prevalence of hypodontia is higher in women. With the exception of the third permanent molars, the second premolars have been found, by many investigators, to be the most commonly missing teeth in the permanent dentition. However, some reports have shown the maxillary lateral incisors to be the most frequently missing teeth, with frequency values within the range 0.8% to 2.5%. It is noteworthy that the mandibular incisor teeth have been observed to be missing in 6.4% of Chinese people.

Increased number of teeth – hyperdontia

Hyperdontia refers to any normal tooth or tooth-like structure formed from a tooth germ that is in excess of the usual number of teeth for a given region of the dental arch. These have been referred to as **supernumeraries**.

Supernumerary teeth can be classified by **shape**, **position** and **orientation**. The shapes include:

Conical (also called 'peg shaped'): this shape of supernumerary is most commonly found. It develops with root formation ahead of, or at an equivalent stage to, that of permanent incisors and usually presents as a mesiodens (Figure 27.2).

Tuberculate (also called '**barrel shaped**'): the tuberculate type of supernumerary possesses more than one cusp or tubercle (Figure 27.3). Root formation is usually delayed compared to that of the permanent incisors. Tuberculate supernumeraries are often paired and are commonly located on the palatal aspect of the central incisors. They rarely erupt and are frequently associated with delayed eruption of the incisors.

Supplemental (where the tooth has a normal shape for the teeth in that series): the supplemental supernumerary refers to a duplication of teeth and is found at the end of a tooth series. The most common supplemental tooth is the permanent maxillary lateral incisor, but supplemental premolars and molars also occur.

Compound odontomes (multiple small tooth-like forms of odontogenic tumour): the malformation bears some superficial anatomical similarity to a normal tooth.

Complex odontomes (a disorganised mass of dental tissue): a diffuse mass of dental tissue, which is totally disorganised.

When classified by position, a supernumerary tooth may be referred to as a **mesiodens**, a **paramolar** (Figure 27.4) or a **distomolar**. Among them, the most common type is a mesiodens, which occurs between the maxillary central incisors.

When classified by orientation, a supernumerary tooth may be referred to as **normal**, **inverted** (Figure 27.5) or **transverse**.

Hyperdontia often occurs as an associated symptom of a number of syndromes, all of which are rare. The best known of these is cleidocranial dysplasia. In the normal healthy individual, there are considered to be four possible aetiologies for hyperdontia. Firstly, the developing tooth germ may split into two separate units. Secondly, the dental lamina, as a result of early histodifferentiation, may undergo further budding, so initiating the development of an additional tooth. Thirdly, the existence of hyperdontia may represent a reversion to a primitive dentition, which contained a greater number of teeth than the 32 teeth of the permanent dentition or the 20 teeth of the primary dentition of modern man. Fourthly, some unknown inherited or environmental factor may have been responsible for causing hyperdontia. Nevertheless, whatever the true aetiology, it is interesting to note that men consistently exhibit this trait more frequently than women. Heredity has been put forward as an explanation for hyperdontia. Although no clear mode of inheritance has been established, polygenic factors probably need to be combined with environmental factors for hyperdontia to occur.

Hyperdontia in the permanent dentition for Caucasian people ranges from 0.4% to 2.1%; while they are lower than 3.4% for Japanese and 6% for African Americans.

28 Variations in tooth morphology

Figure 28.1 (a) Decayed double tooth 61 and 62; (b) extracted double tooth 61 and 62; (c) the permanent successor 21 and 22 is also a double tooth

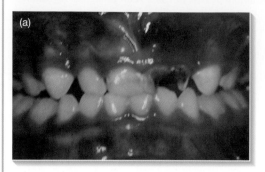

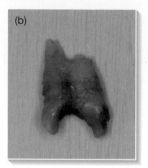

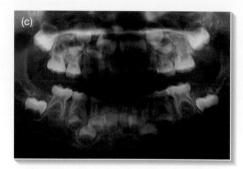

Figure 28.2 (a) Dilacerated 21 with a history of trauma to the primary upper central incisors when the child was 4 years old; (b) CT scan of the maxilla revealed the morphology of the dilacerated 21

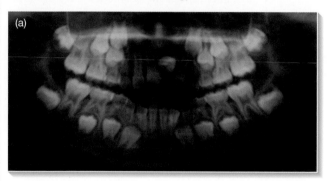

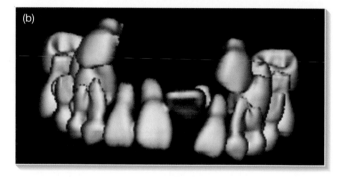

Figure 28.3 Dens evaginatus in a mandibular first premolar

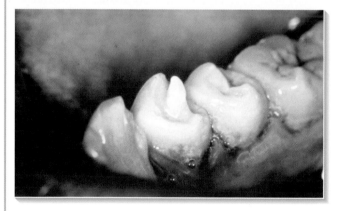

Figure 28.4 Talon cusp in maxillary central incisors

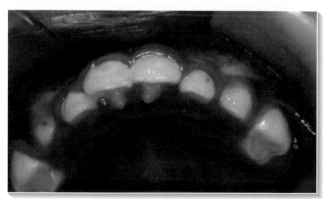

Morphological anomalies

Developmental variations in the dentition are frequently observed during a routine dental examination. If the word anomalous is taken to mean an irregularity of the norm, a **dental anomaly** is a feature of the dentition that can be expected to occur in the minority of a given population.

Double tooth

Double tooth is manifested as a structure resembling what appears to be two teeth that have been joined together. It can be diagnosed clinically by the presence of incisal notching and a groove on the labial surface. Radiographically, there is evidence of pulpal bifurcation. Reports on the inheritance of double teeth have been published, which suggest this characteristic has an aetiology of genetic origins.

Double teeth may occur, firstly, because of **fusion** of two normal teeth; hence, the dentition is reduced in number, unless a tooth is fused to a supernumerary tooth. Generally, this type of double tooth has two independent pulp chambers. The second possible cause is the apparent partial splitting of a single tooth, which is referred to as **gemination**, in which case the number of teeth is normal. It is possible that any one, or all, of these terms may be appropriate. However, because the aetiology and ontogeny are uncertain the term '**double tooth**' is probably the most appropriate.

The double tooth anomaly, unlike most other anomalies, is more common in the primary dentition than the permanent dentition. The prevalence of double teeth ranges from 0.1% to 0.8% in the permanent dentition, and 0.1% to 4.5% in the primary dentition. It has been proposed that there may be an inter-relationship between primary and permanent double teeth. A double tooth in the primary dentition has also been associated with disturbances in the permanent dentition, varying from a double tooth (Figure 28.1), to supernumerary teeth or even missing teeth.

Dilaceration

The term 'dilacerations' is used to describe a dental developmental anomaly characterised by a crease, an angulation or a sharp bend in the crown at the amelocemental junction, or by tortuous roots with abnormal curvatures. Although teeth are not all straight and most have multiple planes of curvature throughout the length of their root, dilacerated teeth present with an abrupt change in the axial inclination between the crown and the root in various degrees of severity. They were also called 'scorpion tooth' or described as 'the hand of a traffic policeman' because their roots often bent into a tight curve, with palatal surface of the crowns facing forward (Figure 28.2). Traumatic injury to the primary predecessors is the most often suggested cause of dilacerations; 3% of traumatic injuries to the primary teeth have been reported to result in dilaceration. This is due to the close anatomical relationship between the primary teeth and their developing permanent successors, which are positioned palatally to the roots of the primary teeth. Because of the trauma, the calcified portion of the developing tooth germ is displaced, resulting in a change in the axial inclination. It rotates, usually upwards, around the cellular and highly vascular dentine papilla. Death of the developing tooth germ does not usually occur and the root remains in position and tends to continue developing along its original axis, forming at an angulation to the rotated calcified portion.

The affected tooth, when fully formed, has a marked change in its longitudinal axis. Because the axis of the calcified portion is inclined in one direction and the axis of the later developing part in another, the tooth usually fails to erupt. A number of treatment options have been suggested in the literature, including surgical exposure and orthodontic traction, extraction followed by prosthesis, implant or space close-up, extraction followed by autotransplantation, and observation for spontaneous eruption followed by restorative treatment.

Dens evaginatus

Dens evaginatus, which is found in permanent teeth, is an enamel-covered tubercle which projects from the occlusal surface of a premolar and very occasionally from a canine or molar (Figure 28.3). Teeth with dens evaginatus usually occur bilaterally, and more frequently in the mandible than the maxilla. Dens evaginatus can be classified according to the location or form of the projection. Based on the location, the tubercle can arise from the lingual ridge of the buccal cusp or from the centre of the occlusal surface. On the basis of form, the evagination may be smooth, grooved, terraced or ridged. The grooved form has a definite groove or fissure surrounding the base, while the smooth form has no groove surrounding the base so it is continuous with the occlusal surface. The other types, which are less common, have a terraced like base or minute ridges on the sides.

Radiographic examination in one study showed that 42% of evaginations contain pulp tissue. The pulp tissue in the tubercle is normal unless the tubercle has been fractured, or worn down, thereby permitting bacterial invasion, with consequent pulpal necrosis. The necrosis of the pulp tissue can, subsequently, lead to an acute or chronic dentoalveolar abscess, or even osteomyelitis. The dens evaginatus trait is more frequently seen in people of Mongoloid origin, and here the reported prevalence ranges from 0.1% to 6.3%. (Compare dens invaginatus which is not described here.)

Talon cusp

Talon cusp is a palatal accessory cusp, which extends at least half the distance from the cementoenamel junction to the incisal edge. A large talon cusp may project with connection to the incisal edge of the tooth to give the crown a 'T' (Figure 28.4) or 'Y' shape. Questions have been asked about this anomaly and its association with dens evaginatus. Both are projections covered by enamel that contain pulp tissue and it is possible that a talon cusp could be the ultimate expression of a dens evaginatus. Therefore, the term 'dens evaginatus of the anterior teeth' has also been used instead of the well known 'talon cusp'.

It has been suggested that this anomalous accessory cusp has a multifactorial aetiology, combining both genetics and environmental factors. There is also an increased incidence of talon cusp associated with Mohr and Rubinstein–Taybi syndromes and with anomalies such as complex odontomes and impactions. Permanent maxillary incisors are reported to be the teeth that are most frequently affected by talon cusps. The prevalence of talon cusp ranges from 0.9% to 7.7% in the permanent dentition.

29 Enamel and dentine defects

Figure 29.1 Clinical appearance of dentinogenesis imperfecta in deciduous dentition

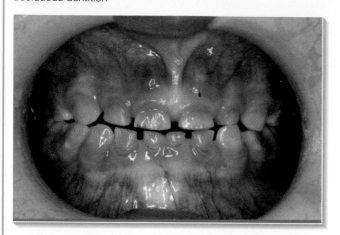

Figure 29.2 Radiographic appearance of dentinogenesis imperfecta in deciduous dentition

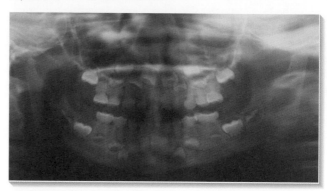

Figure 29.3 (a, b) Clinical appearance of dentinogenesis imperfecta in permanent dentition

(a)

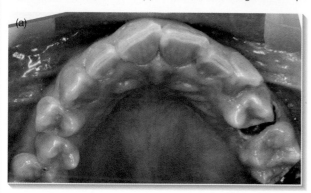

(b)

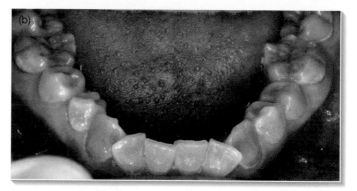

Figure 29.4 Radiographic appearance of dentinogenesis imperfecta in permanent dentition

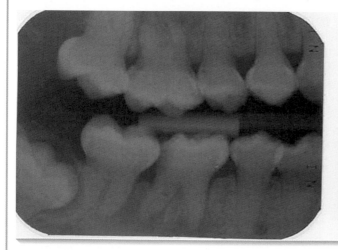

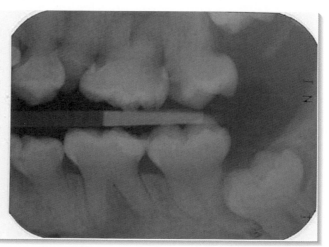

Dentine defects

There are three main causes of defects in the dentine of teeth. These are:

- Dentinogenesis imperfecta (linked to osteogenesis imperfection)
- Dentinal dysplasia
- Vitamin D resistant rickets

These diseases are not common. Other causes of defects in the dentine are excessively rare.

Dentinogenesis imperfecta

Dentinogenesis imperfecta is an autosomal dominant genetic defect. It can occur alone or linked to the condition of osteogenesis imperfect. Dentinogenesis imperfect is also known as 'hereditary opalescent dentine'.

The condition affects both the deciduous and the permanent dentition. The teeth are grey-brown and have an opalescent appearance. The enamel separates easily from the disturbed dentine thereby exposing it. The dentine is then prone to severe attrition and teeth may be worn to gingival level (most commonly in the deciduous dentition) (Figures 29.1–29.4).

Radiographically, the teeth are seen to have rather bulbous crowns and shortened, sometimes rather thin, roots. Often the pulps cannot be seen. It is thought that this is due to disorganised deposition of dentine.

Osteogenesis imperfecta

Children with this condition suffer from multiple fractures, which occur after very minor trauma. The sclera of the eyes appears bluish and they often develop hearing problems and deafness. The extent of dentine disturbance in osteogeneis imperfecta cases is very variable.

Dentinal dysplasia

Dentinal dysplasia is also an autosomal dominant genetically determined condition. The teeth on radiograph appear to have no, or very short, roots although the teeth in the mouth may look normal. The pulps tend to be very small or non-existent due to large amounts of abnormal dentine being deposited in the pulpal space. The shortness of the roots leads to mobility, and on occasions this is the first sign of the condition.

Vitamin resistant rickets

Vitamin D resistant rickets is a genetic condition. It is X-linkcd. Males have skeletal changes and tend to be of short height and have deformed lower limbs (bowed legs).

One of the presenting features of the condition to dentists may be the presence of periapical abscesses in the absence of any identifiable dental pathology (caries or periodontal disease). In vitamin resistant rickets, in the mouth, it is the dentine that is primarily affected, consisting largely of interglobular dentine. On radiographs the pulps of the teeth are very large and are abnormally shaped.

Other dentine defects

Local affects can disrupt the formation of the dentine. These may include chemotherapy, tetracycline use and severe nutritional deficiencies. These are all uncommon.

Developmental defects of enamel

Dental enamel is a unique calcified structure within the human body, which contains the largest crystals in a biological tissue. Recently, it has been suggested that the process of enamel formation by ameloblasts (**amelogenesis**) can be divided into three broad stages:

- **Matrix formation:** when the water and three major structural proteins, the amelogenin, ameloblastin, and enamelin, which are involved in amelogenesis, are produced
- **Calcification:** when the newly secreted matrix almost instantly becomes mineralised to approximately 30%, as the crystals of hydroxyapatite grow within the extracellular matrix, and calcium phosphate salts may accumulate on the crystals
- **Maturation:** the newly mineralised enamel undergoes final calcification, hydroxyapatite crystals increase in size, and the remaining water and proteins are removed.

Ameloblasts are particularly sensitive to changes in their environment. Dysfunction of ameloblasts may occur during the long process of amelogenesis, resulting in changes in the appearance of the enamel. These are now known as **developmental defects of enamel** (**DDE**). DDE may range from slight abnormalities of the colour, to a complete absence of the enamel (Figure 29.5a–g). The stage of amelogenesis at which the dysfunction occurs, the severity of the insult leading to temporary or permanent inactivity of the cells, the duration of the insult, the phase of ameloblast activity during the relevant period, and the specific agent involved may affect the final appearance of the defects.

There are three fundamental reasons to develop a general-purpose index for DDE based on descriptive rather than aetiological criteria. Firstly, the aetiology of many defects is unknown, and therefore documentation other than by appearance is impossible. Secondly, there is a scientific value in understanding the full range of DDE. Thirdly, unlike classifications based on aetiology, descriptive classifications do not presume cause, but they do have the potential for retrospective evaluation for identification of the aetiology. After reviewing previous studies and classifications of DDE, the working group of the FDI Commission on Oral Health, Research and Epidemiology, finalised a descriptive index in 1992, which was known as the Modified Index of Developmental Defects of Enamel (**Modified FDI DDE Index**). The definition of DDE is clarified as 'deviations from the normal appearance of tooth enamel resulting from enamel organ dysfunction'. This coding system included two formats, one for general screening surveys and one for epidemiological studies (Tables 29.1 and 29.2). Moreover, the recording system allows investigators to record the information on the extent of DDE (Table 29.3).

The Modified FDI DDE Index is based on a simple classification and uses simple terminology, which is effective for measuring almost the entire range of enamel defects on the basis of their macroscopic appearance. The Modified FDI DDE Index plays a role in establishing baseline data, and provides a common language and means of communicating about developmental defects of enamel. Thus, it is not surprising that this index was recommended by the World Health Organisation in 1997 for use in oral health surveys.

Figure 29.5 (a) White demarcated opacities on 11 and 21; (b) brown demarcated opacities on 31; (c) diffuse lines and patchy on maxillary incisors; (d) confluent diffuse opacities; (e) confluent/patchy plus loss of enamel on maxillary central incisors; (f) hypoplasia – pits and diffuse opacities; (g) hypoplasia – missing enamel on maxillary central incisors and mandibular incisors, and diffuse opacities on all teeth

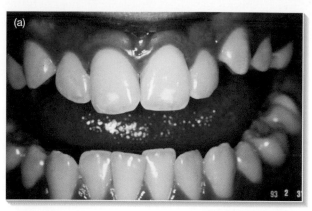

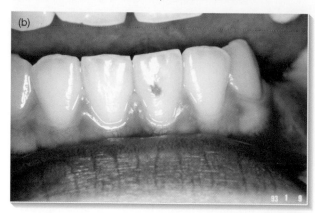

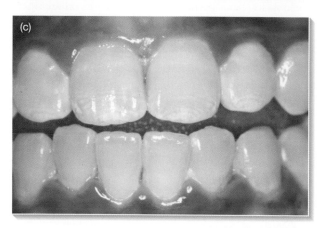

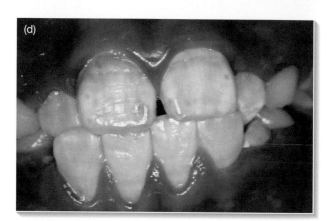

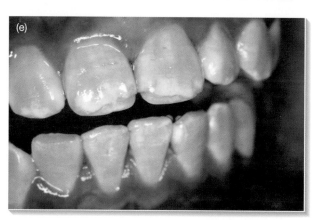

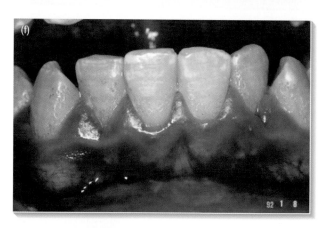

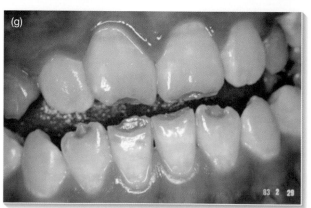

Table 29.1 Modified FDI DDE Index for screening surveys

Category	Description
Demarcated opacity	A defect which involves an alteration in the translucency. The defective enamel is of normal thickness with a smooth surface. It has a distinct and clear boundary with the adjacent normal enamel. Some maintain a surface translucency while others are dull in appearance.
Diffuse opacity	An abnormality which involves an alteration in the translucency of the enamel. The defective enamel is of normal thickness and at eruption has a relative smooth surface and is white in colour. It has no clear boundary with the adjacent normal enamel.
Hypoplasia	A defect which involves the surface of the enamel and is associated with a reduced localised thickness of enamel. The enamel of reduced thickness could be translucent or opaque.
Other defects	–

Table 29.2 Modified FDI DDE Index for epidemiological studies

Category	Description
Demarcated opacities (white/cream)	Demarcated opacities which are white or cream in colour.
Demarcated opacities (yellow/brown)	Demarcated opacities which are yellow or brown in colour.
Diffuse opacities – lines	Distinctive white lines of opacities which follow the lines of development of the teeth. Confluence of adjacent lines may occur.
Diffuse opacities – patchy	Irregular, cloudy areas of opacities which lack well defined margins.
Diffuse opacities – confluent	Diffuse patchiness which merges into a chalky white area extending from mesial to distal margins. It can cover the entire surface or be confined to a localised area.
Confluent/patchy plus both staining and or loss of enamel	Posteruptive change of colour and or loss of enamel related only to the hypomineralised zone of confluent opacities.
Hypoplasia – pits	Hypoplasia occurs in the form of pits, which can be single or multiple, shallow or deep, scattered or in rows arranged horizontally across the surface.
Hypoplasia – missing enamel	Single or multiple, narrow or wide grooves (maximum 2 mm), or partial or complete absence of enamel over a considerable area of dentine.
Any other defects	–

Table 29.3 Extent of defects for the modified FDI DDE Index

Category	Description
1	Less than one-third of the tooth surface
2	At least one-third to two-thirds of the tooth surface
3	At least two-thirds of the tooth surface

(30) Fluorosis

Figure 30.1 (a) Questionable fluorosis; (b) very mild fluorosis; (c) mild fluorosis; (d) moderate fluorosis; (e) severe fluorosis

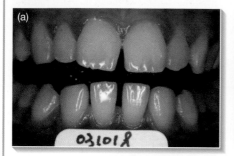

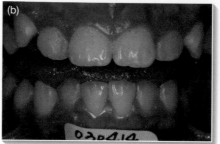

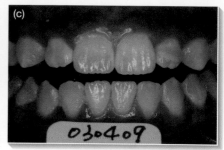

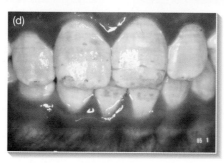

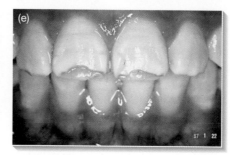

Dental fluorosis is a developmental disturbance of dental enamel caused by excessive exposure to high concentrations of fluoride during tooth development. Teeth are generally composed of hydroxyapatite and carbonated hydroxyapatite; as the intake of fluoride increases, so does the teeth's complement of fluorapatite. Excessive fluoride can cause white spots and, in severe cases, brown stains, pitting or mottling of the enamel (Figure 30.1a–e). The severity of dental fluorosis depends on the amount of fluoride exposure and the age of the child when exposed.

Many well-known sources of fluoride may contribute to overexposure. Public water fluoridation is directly or indirectly responsible for 40% of all fluorosis. Severe cases can be caused by exposure to water that is naturally fluoridated to levels well above the recommended levels, or by exposure to other fluoride sources such as brick tea or pollution from high-fluoride coal.

Dean, in 1934, was the first investigator to develop and publish an index for measuring the presence and severity of fluorosis (Table 30.1). It is a specific index, which presumes an aetiological factor of the defects and a unique cause-and-effect relationship. When using Dean's Index, the examiner must first decide whether the defects that are present are due to an excessive fluoride intake. Defects due to fluoride are considered to have a number of distinguishing characteristics, such as an opaque white colour and a generalised distribution within the dental arch (Table 30.2), plus a history of chronic ingestion of excessive amounts of fluoride during tooth development. When it is decided that a subject indeed has some fluorotic enamel, its

Table 30.1 Dean's Index

Score	Category	Description
0	Normal	Normal enamel represents the usual translucency
0.5	Questionable	Occasional white flecks or spots that are 1–2 mm in diameter
1	Very mild	Small, opaque, white areas cover up to 25% of tooth surface
2	Mild	More extensive white, opaque areas cover at least 50% of the tooth surface
3	Moderate	All of the tooth surfaces are involved, and minute pitting is often present; brown stain is common
4	Severe	All enamel surfaces are affected and hypoplasia is so marked that the general form of the tooth may be affected; the pits are dipper and confluent; stains are widespread and range from a chocolate brown to almost black

severity is recorded by the allocation of a score to the subject based on the two most severely affected teeth in the dentition.

Furthermore, Dean assigned a statistical weight (ranging from 0 to 4) to each category within the classification so that a Community Fluorosis Index (CFI) could be calculated for any given group or community. Below 0.4, it was said not to have any

Dentistry at a Glance. First Edition. Edited by Elizabeth Kay. © 2016 John Wiley & Sons, Ltd. Published 2016 by John Wiley & Sons, Ltd.
Companion website: www.ataglanceseries.com/dentistryseries/dentistry

Table 30.2 The differential diagnosis of the milder forms of dental fluorosis (questionable, very mild, and mild) and non-fluoride opacities of enamel as proposed by Russel in 1961

Characteristic	Milder forms of fluorosis	Non-fluoride enamel opacities
Area affected	Usually seen on or near tips of cusps or incisal edges	Usually centred in smooth surface; may affect entire crown
Shape of lesions	Resembles line shading in pencil sketch; lines follow in enamel, form irregular caps on cusps	Often round or oval
Demarcation	Shades off imperceptibly into surrounding normal enamel	Clearly differentiated from adjacent normal enamel
Colour	Slightly more opaque than normal enamel; 'paper-white'; incisal edges, tips of cusps may have frosted appearance; does not show stain at time of eruption (in these milder degrees, rarely at any time)	Usually pigmented at time of eruption; often creamy-yellow to dark reddish-orange
Teeth affected	Most frequent on teeth that calcify slowly (cuspids, bicuspids, second and third molars); rare on lower incisors; usually seen on 6 or 8 homologous teeth; extremely rare in deciduous teeth	Any tooth may be affected; frequent on labial surface of lower incisors; may occur singly; usually 1 to 3 teeth affected; common in deciduous teeth
Gross hypoplasia	None; pitting of enamel does not occur in the milder forms; enamel surface has glazed appearance, which is smooth to point of explorer	Absent to severe; enamel surface may seem etched, rough to explorer
Detection	Often invisible under strong light; most easily detected by sighting tangentially to tooth crown	Seen most easily under strong light on line of sight perpendicular to tooth surface

public health significance; while between 0.4 and 0.6, fluorosis is of some concern. The value of CFI can be calculated using the following equation:

$$\text{CFI} \quad \frac{\text{number of individuals} \times \text{statistical weight}}{\text{total number of individuals examined}}$$

Dean's Index has been widely used in epidemiological studies worldwide, probably because of its value when making comparisons with previously published studies. However, due to the concern that Dean's system was inefficient at recording dental fluorosis at both extremities of the fluoride intake range, an alternative index was proposed by Thylstrup and Fejerskov in 1978 (Table 30.3).

The authors were interested in the exact relationship between fluoride exposure and the whole range of clinical as well as histological changes. Therefore, this index requires that the teeth are dried before examination to improve sensitivity at low diagnostic thresholds. Owing to the drying, almost all teeth tend to show a very mild degree of fluorosis, so it is arguable to evaluate aesthetics with the Thylstrup–Fejerskov Index.

In order to record fluorosis from a public health and aesthetic viewpoint, research workers at the National Institute of Dental Research in the United States developed the Tooth Surface Index of Fluorosis (TSIF) in 1984 (Table 30.4). The TSIF records the prevalence of fluorosis on a tooth and tooth-surface basis, and so it appears to be more sensitive than Dean's Index.

Table 30.3 Thylstrup–Fejerskov Index

Score	Description
0	Enamel is normally translucent and glossy after drying
1	Thin white opaque lines run across the enamel surface, corresponding to the position of the perikymata; 'snow-capping' of cusps/incisal edges may also been seen
2	The opaque lines are pronounced, and may merge to form cloudy areas over the whole surface; 'snow-capping' is common
3	Merging of the lines occurs and cloudy opacities spread
4	The entire surface exhibits a marked opacity; parts of the surface exposed to attrition may appear to be less affected
5	The entire surface is opaque; there are round pits (focal loss of the outermost enamel) less than 2 mm in diameter
6	Pits may be seen merging in the opaque enamel to form bands less than 2 mm in vertical height
7	Irregular loss of outermost enamel; less than half of the surface is involved; the remaining intact enamel is opaque
8	The loss of outermost enamel involves more than half the surface; the remaining intact enamel is opaque
9	The loss of the main part of the enamel results in a change of the anatomical shape of the tooth/surface; a cervical rim of opaque enamel is often noted

Table 30.4 The Tooth Surface Index of Fluorosis (TSIF)

Score	Description
0	Enamel shows no evidence of fluorosis
1	Enamel shows areas with parchment-white colour covering less than one third of the visible surface
2	Parchment-white fluorosis covers one-third to two-thirds of surface
3	Parchment-white fluorosis covers more than two-thirds of surface
4	Enamel staining is in connection with any of the above condition
5	Discrete pitting of enamel exists; no staining of the intact enamel
6	Pitting and staining of the intact enamel exist
7	Confluent pitting exists; large areas of enamel may be missing; dark-brown stain is usually present

Tooth eruption and exfoliation

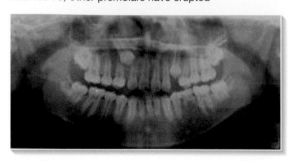

Figure 31.1 A 12-year-old boy with missing 35 and retained 75; other premolars have erupted

Table 31.1 The chronological course of deciduous tooth development

Tooth type	Calcification begins		Crown completed		Eruption		Root completed	
	Maxillary (months in utero)	Mandibular (months in utero)	Maxillary (age in months)	Mandibular (age in months)	Maxillary (age in months)	Mandibular (age in months)	Maxillary (age in years)	Mandibular (age in years)
Central	3.5	3.5	1.5	2.5	10	7	1.5	1.5
Lateral	4	4	2.5	3	11	13	2	1.5
Canine	4.25	4.25	9	9	19	20	3.25	3.25
1st Molar	3.75	3.75	6	5.5	16	16	2.5	2.25
2nd Molar	4.75	4.5	12	10	29	27	3	3

Table 31.2 The chronological course of permanent tooth development

Tooth type	Calcification begins		Crown completed		Eruption		Root completed	
	Maxillary	Mandibular	Maxillary (years)	Mandibular (years)	Maxillary (years)	Mandibular (years)	Maxillary (years)	Mandibular (years)
Central	3–4 months	3–4 months	4–5	3.5–4.5	6.5–8	5.5–7	10–11	9–10
Lateral	10–12 months	3–4 months	4.5–5.5	4–5	7.5–9	7–8	11	10
Canine	4–5 months	4–5 months	6–7	5.5–6.5	11–12	9–10	13–15	12–14
1st Premolar	18–22 months	18–22 months	5.5–7	5–6.75	9.5–11	10–12	12–14	12–14
2nd Premolar	24–27 months	24–27 months	6–7	6–7	10–12	10.5–12	12–14.5	13–15
1st Molar	at birth	at birth	2.5–4	2.5–3.75	5.5–7	5–7	9–11	9–11
2nd Molar	29 months	29 months	7–8	7–8	12–13	11–13	14–16	14–16
3rd Molar	7–9 years	8–10 years	12–16	12–16	17–22	17–22	18–25	18–25

Tooth eruption

The process of eruption involves the movement or change of position of the tooth from the deeper portion of the jaws into the oral cavity until it achieves occlusal contact with adjacent and opposing teeth. Tooth eruption has three broad stages. The first, known as **primary dentition** stage, occurs when only primary teeth are visible. Once the first permanent tooth erupts into the mouth, the teeth are in the **mixed** (or transitional) **dentition**. After the last primary tooth falls out of the mouth, the teeth are in the **permanent dentition**. The chronological course of development for primary and permanent teeth is shown in Tables 31.1 and 31.2.

Dentistry at a Glance. First Edition. Edited by Elizabeth Kay. © 2016 John Wiley & Sons, Ltd. Published 2016 by John Wiley & Sons, Ltd.
Companion website: www.ataglanceseries.com/dentistryseries/dentistry

Rate of tooth eruption

The rate of eruption represents a balance between forces tending to move the tooth into the mouth (**eruptive force**) and forces tending to prevent this movement (**resistive force**). Resistance may be produced by overlying soft tissues and alveolar bone, the viscosity of the surrounding periodontal ligament and occlusal forces. However, little is known about the nature, source and magnitude of either the eruptive or resistive forces.

The rate of tooth eruption also depends on the phase of movement. In the **intraosseous phase**, the rate of tooth eruption is 1–10 μm/day; in the **extraosseous phase** it is 75 μm/day. It takes approximately 2–3 years after eruption for permanent teeth to finish calcification. In radiographic studies it was found that the interval between crown completion and beginning of eruption until the tooth is in full occlusion is approximately 5–6 years for permanent teeth.

Mechanism of tooth movements

Tooth eruption is traditionally considered to be a developmental process. However, eruption can be regarded as a lifelong process because a tooth will often move axially in response to changing functional situations. This is shown in overeruption, resulting from the removal of an opposite tooth, or compensatory eruption related to attrition.

The theories advanced to explain the mechanism of tooth eruption can be divided into two main groups: (1) the tooth is pushed out as a result of forces generated beneath and around it, either by alveolar bone growth, root growth, blood-pressure/tissue fluid pressure, or cell proliferation; and (2) the tooth may be pulled out as a result of tension within the connective tissue of the periodontal ligament. Although the exact mechanism of eruption is still debatable, there are four important factors that are considered to be responsible for the eruption of teeth:

- Bone remodelling (deposition vs. resorption)
- Root growth
- Vascular (hydrostatic) pressure
- Periodontal ligament traction.

Sequence of eruption

The eruption or appearance of the teeth follows a general pattern or schedule. In general, the mandibular teeth precede the maxillary teeth. Homologous teeth in the same arch erupt at roughly the same time. A time period of more than 6 months between the eruption of homologous teeth should not be considered normal.

- The most common eruption sequence of the primary dentition is:

$$\frac{\text{AB} \quad \text{D} \quad \text{C} \quad \text{E}}{\text{A} \quad \text{B} \quad \text{D} \quad \text{CE}}$$

- The most common eruption sequence of the permanent dentition is:

$$\frac{6 \quad 1 \quad 2 \quad 4 \quad 5 \quad 3 \quad 7 \quad 8}{6 \quad 1 \quad 2 \quad 3 \quad 4 \quad 5 \quad 7 \quad 8}$$

Exfoliation of primary teeth

The physiological process responsible for the loss of deciduous or primary teeth is known as exfoliation or shedding. The roots of primary teeth begin to resorb approximately 3 years after completion. Resorption of a primary tooth root is the gradual dissolving away of the root due to the underlying eruption of the successors that will replace it. Root resorption continues as the successors move closer to the surface until the primary teeth eventually become loose and finally fall out. When a primary tooth is shed, the crown of the successors is close to the surface and ready to emerge. The interval between shedding of the primary teeth and emergence of the permanent teeth is usually 3–6 months.

Pattern of resorption and shedding

For a primary incisor or canine, root resorption initially occurs on the lingual surface adjacent to the developing permanent tooth. With subsequent movement and relocation of the teeth in the growing jaws, the developing permanent tooth comes to lie directly beneath the primary tooth and further resorption occurs from the apex. For a primary molar, root resorption often commences on the inner surfaces where the permanent premolars initially develop. The premolars later come to lie beneath the roots of the primary molar and further resorption occurs from the root apices. The shift in position of the primary tooth relative to the permanent successor may account for the intermittent nature of root resorption.

Mechanism of resorption and shedding

The initiation of root resorption may be an inherent developmental process, or it may be related to pressure from the permanent successor against the overlying bone or tooth. To examine which of these theories is correct, researchers have surgically removed permanent tooth germs and found that resorption of the predecessors still occurred, though the resorption process was delayed. This finding is also consistent with the clinical observation that shedding of a primary tooth still occurs but is retarded where the successor is congenitally missing (Figure 31.1), impacted or ectopically positioned. In this case, a primary tooth may exfoliate when the patient is older than 30 years.

It has also been suggested that increased masticatory loads may affect the pattern and rate of primary tooth resorption. It has been shown in experiment that, if primary teeth were splinted following the removal of the developing permanent teeth, there was less root resorption compared with removal of the permanent teeth alone.

32 Caries

Figure 32.1 Stages in the formation of an oral biofilm community
Source: Lamont RJ (2010). *Oral Microbiology at a Glance*. Reproduced with permission of John Wiley and Sons, Ltd.

Naked surface
Host salivary glycoproteins
Conditioning film
e.g. *Streptococcus*
Linking film
e.g. *Actinomyces*
Coaggregation, Re-conditioning film
e.g. *Fusobacterium*
Accumulation, Shedding

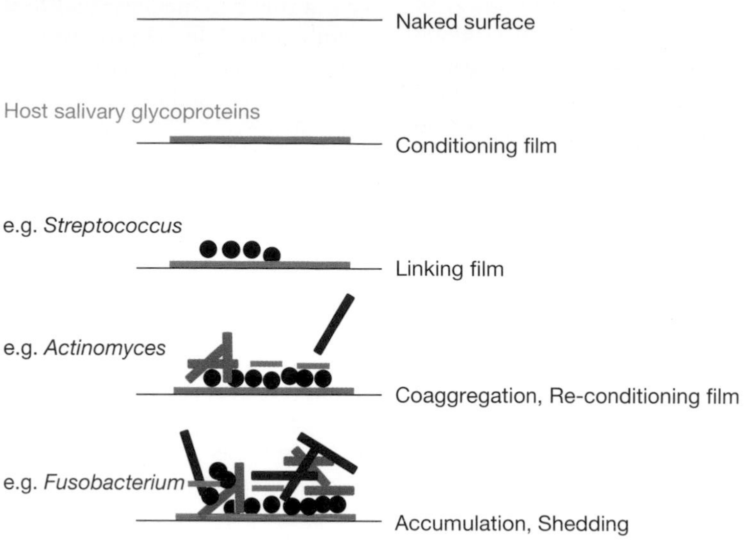

Figure 32.2 Schematic illustration of progressive stages of lesion formation: (1) reactive dentin; (2) sclerotic reaction or translucent (transparent) zone; (3) zone of demineralisation; (4) zone of bacterial invasion and destruction; (5) peripheral rod direction
Source: Fejerskov O et al. (2008). In: Fejerskov O, Kidd E (eds). *Dental Caries: The Disease and Its Clinical Management*, 2nd edn. Reproduced with permission of John Wiley and Sons, Ltd.

5
2
5 3 2
5 3 2 1
5 3 2 1
5 3 2 1
5 4 3 2 1

Dentistry at a Glance. First Edition. Edited by Elizabeth Kay. © 2016 John Wiley & Sons, Ltd. Published 2016 by John Wiley & Sons, Ltd.
Companion website: www.ataglanceseries.com/dentistryseries/dentistry

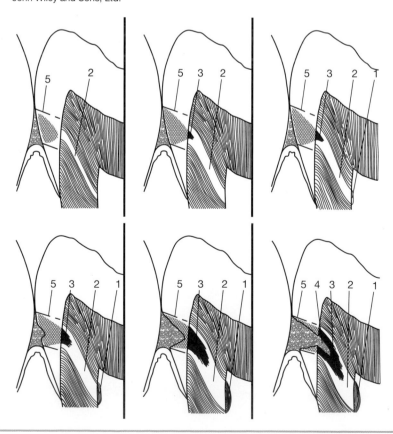

ental caries develops where biofilms form from deposits of microbes (Figure 32.1). This occurs at sites in the dentition where mechanical action fails to remove bacteria.

What happens?

After a week of enamel being in juxtaposition with an undisturbed biofilm, although no changes would be seen macroscopically (or clinically), microscopically the outer enamel surface can be seen to have signs of dissolution, making the enamel slightly more porous (Figure 32.2).

After 14 days, with completely undisturbed plaque, the enamel will appear whitish and opaque to the naked eye after air drying. This is because the enamel porosity has increased some more, but this time the porosity has increased because mineral underneath the outer surface has been preferentially removed, creating a subsurface lesion.

After 4 weeks, an active enamel lesion, or white-spot lesion, will have a chalky surface because the demineralisation and increased porosity cause loss of translucency. It is also partly due to surface erosion. At this stage, careful brushing to remove plaque can reverse the process and surface hardness can be re-achieved.

Dentine reactions to enamel lesions

The dentine underneath the deepest part of an enamel lesion will be the first to show signs of tubular sclerosis. When the enamel lesion reaches the enamel–dentine junction, demineralisation of the dentine along the junction occurs.

Lesion progression

Whilst subsurface mineral loss occurs, the enamel is still a highly mineralised tissue. Surface breakdown appears to occur due to the demineralised enamel being traumatised. This is why **it is particularly important not to disturb enamel surfaces with a probe** as this will introduce bacteria into the microcavity created by the probe tip, thereby transforming a demineralised area into a cavity. Once the microcavity is formed, bacterial will lodge within it and will be unlikely to be dislodged by mechanical cleaning.

Thus, the enamel cavity is enlarged by the combined effect of acid production by undisturbed bacteria and mechanical breakdown.

Following exposure of the dentine to the bacteria in the cavity (which is still confined to enamel), the most superficial dentine is relatively easily damaged by the acids being produced. After this, the bacteria invade the dentinal tubules (Figure 32.3).

Pulp reaction

The pulp can stimulate reactionary or reparative dentine to form even before the bacterial invasion reaches the dentine. When the demineralisation of the dentine reaches 0.5–1 mm from the pulp, an inflammatory reaction in the pulp will occur. The pulp is not yet infected but the pulp reacts to bacterial products.

Microbiology of caries

More than 700 different types of bacteria have been detected in the mouth. Different areas of the mouth are populated by different types of bacteria. The mouth is largely an aerobic environment but anaerobic bacteria can exist in biofilms on oral surfaces. The bacteria have to bond to a surface in order not to be washed away with saliva and ultimately ingested.

Figure 32.3 (a) Vertical sections showing major components of the tooth; (b) caries begins as reversible demineralisation (white spot); (c) if demineralisation continues the enamel decays and destruction eventually spreads through the dentin to the pulp chamber, which can lead to a periapical abscess

Source: Lamont RJ (2010). *Oral Microbiology at a Glance*. Reproduced with permission of John Wiley and Sons, Ltd.

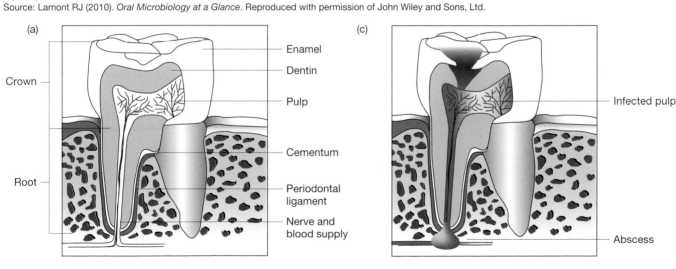

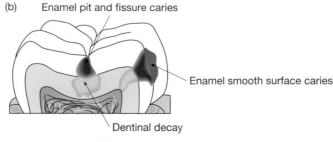

Carbohydrates increase the growth of many oral bacteria and increase acid production. This in turn makes the environment conducive to the more acidophilic bacteria.

Biofilm formation in the mouth

Teeth are covered by a film known as the pellicle. This film is comprised of glycoproteins, phosphoproteins, lipids and other materials and may be 1 μm thick after a period of 24 hours. It appears that bacteria are initially attracted to the tooth's pellicle by weak physicochemical forces but then adhesins on the cell wall interact with the pellicle.

The first colonisers of the tooth surface are usually *Streptococcus. sanguinis*, *S. oralis*, and *S. mitis* alongside *Actinomyces* and Gram-negative bacteria such as *Haemophilus*.

As the biofilm ages, the biomass ceases to be largely streptococci and becomes dominated by *Actinomyces* – a process known as microbial succession. As the bacterial deposits increase, the oxygen concentration lessens – thus plaque on teeth starts life composed of aerobic species but increasingly shifts to being made up of greater numbers of facultative anaerobes.

Bacteria and non-milk extrinsic sugars

Some acid-producing bacteria are found in dental biofilms, but if the pH is neutral they form only a small proportion of the total biomass. Whilst this is the case, any acid produced as a result of bacterial activity is minimal and its demineralisation effect can be counteracted. Thus demineralisation and remineralisation are in equilibrium. However, when non-milk extrinsic sugars (NMES) are eaten, or if salivary flow reduces, pH may fall below pH 5.5 (the critical point for demineralisation) for a sufficient amount of time for enamel demineralisation to occur. This has two effects. The low pH encourages the growth of acid-loving and producing bacteria (mutans streptococci and lactobacilli) and continues to favour demineralisation. Mutans streptococci and lactobacilli, in turn, cause more acid to be produced at a greater rate and thus demineralisation is further favoured. Thus, caries is a result of a change in the balance of the bacterial ecology, which comes about because the oral environment has changed (that is, become more acid because excess NMES is available) (Figure 32.4).

Summary

Understanding that caries occurs because of alterations in the ecology of the oral biofilm is important as it provides a clear theoretical basis for the preventive activities described in other parts of this book.

The importance of tooth brushing and the importance of sugar control are evidence based and biologically based.

Figure 32.4 The ecological plaque hypothesis and the aetiology of dental caries; MS, mutans streptococci
Source: Marsh PD, Nyvad B (2008). In: Fejerskov O, Kidd E (eds). *Dental Caries: The Disease and its Clinical Management*, 2nd edn. Reproduced with permission of John Wiley and Sons, Ltd.

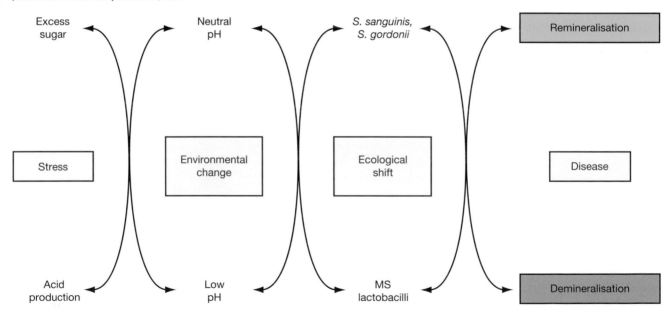

33 Tooth wear

Figure 33.1 Clinical features of severe multifactorial tooth wear in a young adult

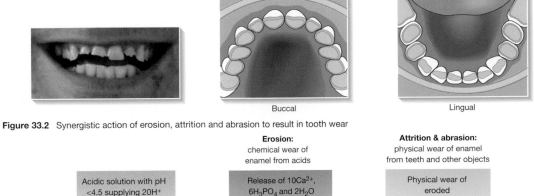

Buccal   Lingual

Figure 33.2 Synergistic action of erosion, attrition and abrasion to result in tooth wear

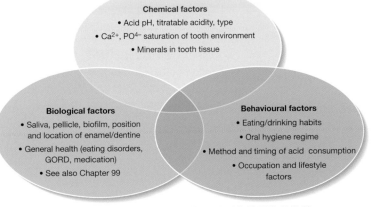

Erosion:
chemical wear of
enamel from acids

Attrition & abrasion:
physical wear of enamel
from teeth and other objects

Acidic solution with pH
<4.5 supplying $20H^+$

Release of $10Ca^{2+}$,
$6H_3PO_4$ and $2H_2O$
soften and roughens
enamel surface

Physical wear of
eroded
enamel surface

Enamel
hydroxyapatite
$Ca_{10}(PO_4)_6(OH)_2$

Erosion

Enamel
hydroxyapatite
$Ca_{10}(PO_4)_6(OH)_2$

Abrasion &
attrition

Enamel
hydroxyapatite
$Ca_{10}(PO_4)_6(OH)_2$

Figure 33.3 Interplay between chemical, biological and behaviour factors in the development and progression of tooth wear

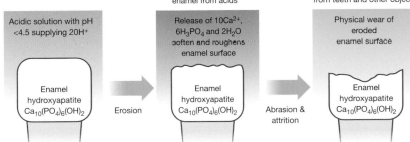

Chemical factors
• Acid pH, titratable acidity, type
• Ca^{2+}, PO^{4-} saturation of tooth environment
• Minerals in tooth tissue

Biological factors
• Saliva, pellicle, biofilm, position and location of enamel/dentine
• General health (eating disorders, GORD, medication)
• See also Chapter 99

Behavioural factors
• Eating/drinking habits
• Oral hygiene regime
• Method and timing of acid consumption
• Occupation and lifestyle factors

Source: Figure 33.3, Adapted from Magalhães AC et al. *J Appli Oral Sci* 2009; 17: 75–86

Table 33.1 Aims and recommendations for prevention of wear

Aim	Recommendations
Reduction of extrinsic acid exposure (i.e. dietary erosion)	Reduce the frequency of intake of acidic drinks and snacks. Acidic beverages should be drunk quickly
Reduction of intrinsic acid exposure (stomach acid)	Evaluation of the aetiology of acid exposure, therapy of physiological (e.g. reflux, xerostomia) or psychological (e.g. bulimia nervosa) disorders
Reduction of demineralisation, enhancement of remineralisation	Increase salivary flow (Chewing of sugar-free gum. Patients with xerostomia: systemic medication (cholinergic drugs), use of saliva substitutes Behaviour after acid contact (Rinsing of the oral cavity with water, milk or fluoride solutions); Consumptions of neutralising food (cheese, milk). Frequent fluoridation (Use of fluoridated toothpaste including higher fluoride concentrations of 2800/5000 ppm NaF, mouthrinse and gel)
Reduction of abrasion and attrition	No toothbrushing immediately after acid consumtion Use of manual toothbrushes or electric toothbrushes applied with gentle pressure Reduction of griding and parafunctional activity

Source: Adapted from Magalhães AC et al. J Appli Oral Sci 2009; 17: 75–86.

Dentistry at a Glance. First Edition. Edited by Elizabeth Kay. © 2016 John Wiley & Sons, Ltd. Published 2016 by John Wiley & Sons, Ltd.
Companion website: www.ataglanceseries.com/dentistryseries/dentistry

Definition: The irreversible, non-traumatic loss of dental hard tissues due to erosion, attrition and abrasion.

Prevention is paramount

Effective prevention of tooth surface loss protect enamel and dentine before aesthetic or functional concerns negatively impact oral health-related quality of life (Figure 33.1). Complex and costly restorative dentistry can improve aesthetics if prevention fails; however, the restoration of missing tooth tissue with restorative dental materials will not address the causes of the disease.

Epidemiology

The prevalence of tooth wear is increasing (especially in young adults) with 76% of adults having some degree of tooth wear and 15% of having moderate tooth wear. Severe tooth wear (Fig 33.1) is rare.

Aetiology

There are three main causes of tooth wear, which act synergistically (Figure 33.2):
• Erosion is chemical loss of tooth minerals as a result of extrinsic (e.g. dietary) acids or intrinsic (i.e. regurgitated from stomach) acids acting on the surface of enamel and dentine.
• Attrition is physical wear as a result of the action of antagonistic teeth removing the demineralised and softened tooth tissue.
• Abrasion is physical wear as a result of mechanical processes involving foreign bodies, such as tooth brushing, oral soft tissues and food during mastication wearing eroded tooth tissue.

Pathophysiology

Initially, acid erosion causes enamel mineral loss, which results in the surface softening and roughening without bulk tissue loss. The fragile surface is then prone to mechanical wear from oral soft tissues, tooth contact or tooth brushing. In dentine, acids demineralise the inorganic component of the dentine, which initiates metallomatrix proteases, degrading the exposed collagenous component of the dentine and resulting in bulk tissue loss.

Chemical, biological and behavioural factors all interact to modify these processes (Figure 33.3). For example, factors such as saliva quality and quantity, pellicle composition, calcium and phosphate content of food and drinks, and fluoride content of oral care products interact to either promote protection or loss of the enamel and dentine.

Clinical features

Clinically, erosive tooth wear appears as smooth silky-shining glazed surfaces with distinct cupping occlusally so restorations rise above the level of the adjacent tooth surface (Figure 33.1). In cases of severe tooth wear, the whole surface is affected and dentine is exposed.

The **basic erosive wear examination (BEWE)** assessment is a screening tool which outlines 4 risk levels according to the clinical presentation of the tooth wear. The clinical appearance of each grade is as follows:
0 = No tooth wear
1 = Initial loss of surface features

2* = Hard tissue loss <50% of the surface area
3* = Hard tissue loss >50% of the surface area
*In grades 2 and 3 dentine is often involved.
Sensibility testing, study models and intraoral photographs aid diagnosis.

Investigations

• Dietary analysis using a diet diary may reveal frequency of consumption of acid drinks (soft drinks, fruit juices, sport drinks) and foods (citrus fruits, salad dressing).
• Medical history questioning may reveal gastrointestinal diseases (especially gastro-oesophageal reflux disease, GORD), eating disorders (especially anorexia nervosa and bulimia nervosa) or alcohol abuse. Many systemic diseases affect salivary flow rate including:
  • diseases of salivary glands, radiation of the head and neck region, Sjögren syndrome, diabetes mellitus, chronic renal failure.
• Medications may be erosive (acetylsalicylic acid, vitamin C) or affect saliva flow rate such as:
  • antidepressants, anticholinergics, antihistamines, antiemetics, Parkinson medications, recreational drug abuse.
• Other risk factors include:
  • tooth brushing of excessive frequency, method, or duration
  • oral care products such as highly abrasive toothpastes, low fluoride content of mouthrinses and toothpastes.
• Oral habits exacerbate the effects of erosion, including brushing soon after acid intake; brushing soon after vomiting; acid intakes last thing at night and retaining acid drinks in mouth before swallowing (i.e. frothing, sluicing, sipping, ruminating).

Prevention

Risk assessment helps patients to understand their oral health status and encourages them to take ownership and responsibility for their own oral health. Effective communication requires taking time to establish rapport, which enables patients to feel they can trust their practitioner and that they are in control of their care. Patients should be empowered to take responsibility to change those factors within their control that are increasing their risk of tooth wear.

Counselling and behaviour change

There is likely to be wide individual variation in response to preventative advice. The variation may be due varying factors such as quantity and quality of saliva, features of the pellicle, individual habits with regard to frequency of eating and drinking, timing, oral swishing, frothing and retention, and toothbrushing after acid intake. Therefore, tailored specific advice is required for each individual patient based upon the information gained (Table 33.1).

Reduction of extrinsic acid exposure: Patients should be advised to avoid frequent intake of acidic foods and drinks and keep them to mealtimes. The following have erosive potential:
• Drinks containing citric acid (e.g. orange, grapefruit, lemon, blackcurrant); carbonated drinks; alcopops and designer drinks; cider; white wine; fruit teas (but not camomile); some sports drinks containing acid; acidic fresh fruit (lemons, oranges, grapefruit, which are consumed with high frequency); pickles; chewable vitamin C tablets; aspirin; some iron preparations.

Reduction of intrinsic acid exposure:

• A sensitive investigation of the patient's diet should be carried out to exclude extrinsic sources of acid.

• Liaison with the patient's general medical practitioner for management of regurgitation may be necessary (this may also involve a gastroenterology unit or an eating disorders unit).

Reduction of demineralisation and enhancement of remineralisation: Patients should be advised to:

• Use toothpaste containing 1450 ppm stannous/sodium fluoride twice daily

• Enhance salivary flow with sugar-free chewing gum and management of xerostomia

• Modify habits occurring concurrently with acid contact (e.g. no brushing immediately after eating or drinking acidic food or drinks, no brushing immediately after vomiting).

Reduction of abrasion and attrition: The following should be discussed with patients:

• Use of manual toothbrushes or electric toothbrushes applied with gentle pressure

• Use of fluoridated toothpastes with low relative enamel abrasion/ relative dentine abrasion (REA/RDA) value

• Use of custom-made soft bite guards, possibly in conjunction with placing a fluoride toothpaste into the mouthguard to protect the teeth during regurgitation/ vomiting and at night from parafunction.

Restorative treatment

In cases where the patient has continuing aesthetic or functional concerns regarding the remaining tooth structure or if the regurgitation erosion is rapidly progressing, possible restorative treatment includes:

• Minimally invasive restorative procedures, including direct composite bonding to seal and protect tooth surfaces from acids

• Complex fixed prosthodontics, including porcelain/metal crowns and onlays with or without surgical crown lengthening

• Occlusal splints to protect restorations from further attrition.

34 The normal gingivae

Figure 34.1 Normal gingivia: a, the mucogingival junction identifies the border between the gingiva and the mucosa, which has a redder appearance and visible blood vessels; b, gingival margin; c, interdental papilla

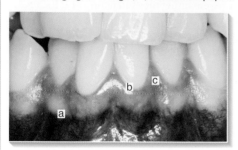

Figure 34.2 Gingival that has pigmentation related to a long-term smoking habit

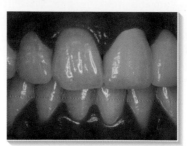

Figure 34.3 Gingival tissue with intrusive gingival frenum reducing the width of the gum.

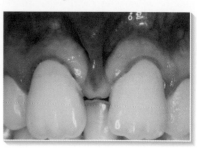

Figure 34.4 Thin gingival tissues in a teenager; note the blood vessels visible through the thin labial gingival tissue of the lower right central incisor

Figure 34.5 Gingival recession in the same patient 18 months later

Figure 34.6 Probing a normal gingival sulcus; the sulcus is 1 mm deep measured with a conventional periodontal probe with Williams markings (1, 2, 3, 5, 7, 8, 9 mm); note no bleeding in response to gentle probing

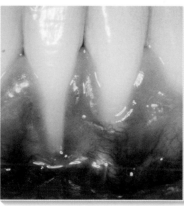

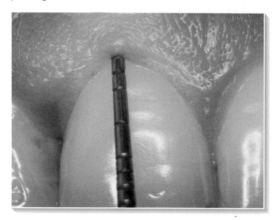

Figure 34.8 Section of gingival tissue stained with haematoxylin and eosin: polymorphonuclear leukocytes, which have migrated from blood vessels into the connective tissue as a response to bacteria on the tooth surface (dental plaque), are present in large numbers as evidenced their darkly stained nuclei, a

Figure 34.7 Histological sections of gum tissue: (a) oral epithelium with deeply stained surface parakeratinised layer; this is a stratified squamous keratinized epithelium on the external surface of the gingiva; (b) junctional epithelium 2–10 cells thick; the enamel has been removed during the preparation of the section leaving the underlying dentine

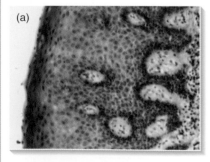

(a)

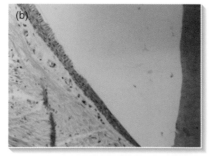

(b)

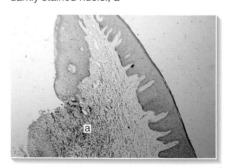

a

Dentistry at a Glance. First Edition. Edited by Elizabeth Kay. © 2016 John Wiley & Sons, Ltd. Published 2016 by John Wiley & Sons, Ltd.
Companion website: www.ataglanceseries.com/dentistryseries/dentistry

The periodontium (Greek *peri*, around; *odontos*, tooth) comprises the tissues that support the teeth. The gingiva is the only one of the periodontal tissues that is visible. The main function of the gingiva is to provide a protective covering tissue, which maintains the integrity of the surface of the masticatory mucosa of the mouth. It is specialised to provide a junction with the tooth surface.

In health the gingiva is pink with no swelling of the gingival margin (Figure 34.1). Small depressions may be visible on the surface, giving it a stippled orange peel appearance. The gingival margin just covers the cement enamel junction (CEJ) of the teeth and runs parallel to it. The gingiva fills the spaces between the teeth, forming interdental papillae which are limited by the contact points or contact areas between the neighbouring teeth. Melanin pigmentation is a normal racial feature but may also occur in response to local irritation from smoking (Figure 34.2). The gingiva is continuous with the other mucosal tissues in the mouth. The mucogingival junction can be identified by the differences in colour and texture between the pink firm-textured gum tissue and the oral mucosa, which is red due to its rich, often visible network of underlying blood vessels, and has a looser texture (Figure 34.1). The width of gum is measured from the gingival margin to the mucogingival junction (range 3–8 mm). Theoretically, a greater width helps to resist tension imposed on the gingival tissues by distension of the labial and buccal mucosae during eating. In the palate the gingival tissues blend with the palatal mucosa. Local anatomical variations, such as frenal attachments, can intrude into the gingival tissue and reduce its width (Figure 34.3). Variations in the gingival tissues, for example how thick or thin they are, reflect genetic mechanisms responsible for the size and shape of the dental and oral tissues. In general, a thin gingival tissue biotype is more likely to be affected by gingival recession in response to traumatic stimulation from vigorous toothbrushing (Figures 34.4 and 34.5).

Between the gingival tissue and the tooth there is a shallow gingival sulcus, which can be measured by inserting a periodontal probe with gentle pressure, no greater than 30 g, which equates to the weight of the probe (Figure 34.6). In the ideal situation this sulcus is about 1 mm in depth; however, there is a normal range of variation and it may be as deep as 3 mm. It should be appreciated that in most 'normal' cases we are examining clinically healthy gingival tissues, reflecting repeated exposure to dental plaque even in those with good oral hygiene.

The cellular structure of the gingiva is a key determinant of its protective function. It is made up of connective tissue covered with a stratified squamous epithelium (Figure 34.7a). The epithelial cells adhere to each other through specialised intracellular structures called desmosomes. One-half of the attachment (hemidesmosome) is contributed by each cell. Cells traverse the epithelium over a 1-month period after division in the basal layer. As the epithelial cells approach the surface keratin forms in those cells, which are exposed to frictional forces from food during mastication. The cells in the basal layer of the epithelium are joined to the underlying connective tissue through a basement membrane. The epithelium can be differentiated into different compartments (oral, sulcular or junctional) depending on its position (see Figure 35.1). The oral epithelium that covers the visible surface of the gum is keratinised (Figure 34.7a). The gingival sulcus in lined by sulcular epithelium, which is not keratinised as it is not exposed to frictional forces. This blends with the junctional epithelium, which is attached via hemidesmosomes to the enamel down to the CEJ (Figure 34.7b).

The connective tissue supports the epithelium and contains a network of blood vessels, nerves and lymphatics. Blood vessels provide nutrition but do not enter the epithelium. They carry circulating inflammatory cells such as polymorphonuclear leukocytes (PMNs) to the gingival tissue (Figures 34.8 and 36.4). Even in clinical health, small numbers of PMNs migrate through the tissues into the gingival crevice and so into the mouth. Lymphocytes in the connective tissue can change into plasma cells, which produce antibodies as a targeted response to bacterial antigens derived from dental plaque.

Many of the mechanical properties of the gingiva depend on the structure of the connective tissue. Within a matrix of ground substance the connective tissue contains fibroblasts, which are responsible for secreting collagen the main structural protein. Collagen is organised into fibres, which are arranged in groups or bundles with a distinct orientation within the gingiva (see Chapter 35). The gingival connective tissue is attached to the surface of the alveolar bone and can be considered a mucoperiosteum.

The relationship between the tooth and the gingiva is unique as it represents the only part of the body in which a hard tissue is partly within the body (tooth root) and outside the body (tooth crown). There is a major challenge to ensure that that there is no break in the integrity of the tissues, which would give bacteria direct access to the tissues with the possibility of recurrent infections. The integrity of the dentogingival junction is maintained by the junctional epithelium attachment to enamel (Figure 34.7b), further supported by the fibre structure in the connective tissue, which holds the gum tissue tightly against the tooth surface. It has been suggested that increased permeability of the junctional epithelium could increase the risk of bacterial toxins gaining access to the underlying connective tissue, leading to inflammation. However, this is only likely to be a factor when bacterial dental plaque has been allowed to accumulate over a period (see Figure 36.3).

35 The periodontal ligament

Figure 35.1 Histological section of a demineralised tooth showing periodontal tissues: a, oral epithelium; b, sulcular epithelium; c, junctional epithelium; d, gingival connective tissue; e, dentine covered by a thin layer of darkly stained cementum; f, alveolar bone which in health is located 1.5–2 mm below the cement–enamel junction; g, periodontal ligament; h, enamel space (enamel is a highly mineralised tissue with virtually no ground substance and so is not seen in histological sections which have been prepared by demineralising a tooth)

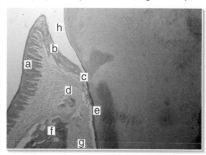

Figure 35.4 Periodontitis has resulted in loss of the attachment of fibres to the root cementum; the junctional epithelium has migrated on to the cementum and is now attached to it. Note also the presence of inflammatory cells, shown by the dark staining which represents their nuclei, in the connective tissue below the epithelium

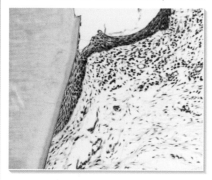

Figure 35.7 Surgical flap raised to show lower first molar: a, prominent distal root with dehiscence of alveolar bone; b, fenestration (window) in alveolar bone over the mesial root

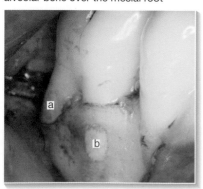

Figure 35.2 Histological section showing: a, alveolar bone margin and b, root surface. The collagen fibres can be seen running into the cementum and the alveolar bone; the orientation of the fibre bundles is evident; Van Gieson stain for collagen

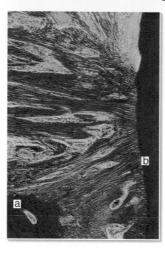

Figure 35.5 Radiograph showing a radio-opaque lamina dura outlining the compact bone forming the wall of the socket

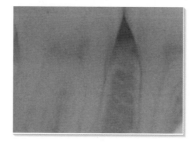

Figure 35.3 Staining to show the collagen fibres which were broken when this carious tooth with a perfectly healthy periodontium was extracted; it is not possible to distinguish where the alveolar bone margin is on this tooth, showing that the collagen fibre attachment is the same in both the extra and intraalveolar portions of the root

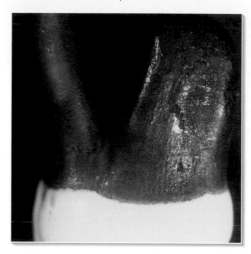

Figure 35.6 Section through the mandible showing the socket of a lower premolar: a, compact bone of socket wall; b, cancellous trabecular bone; c, Volkmann's canals are visible in the socket wall

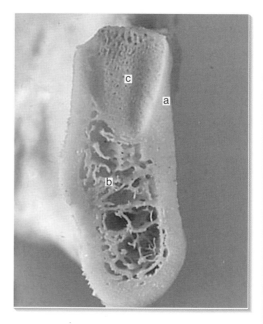

The periodontal tissues include the gingiva, the periodontal ligament, the cementum covering the roots of the teeth and the alveolar bone (Figure 35.1). The major function of the periodontal tissues is to provide an attachment between the teeth and the bone of the jaws to facilitate mastication.

The surface of the roots is covered by a thin layer of cementum, which is a specialised mineralised tissue supported by the underlying dentine. Cementum is made up of collagen fibres in an organic matrix and has a slightly higher mineral content (65%) than bone.

The alveolar bone exists to support the teeth and is maintained by the loading experienced during masticatory function. When teeth are extracted the alveolar bone resorbs, leaving the basal bone of the jaws. In health the alveolar bone does not extend to the cement enamel junction (CEJ) and the margin is located 1.5–2 mm below this landmark leaving an extra-alveolar portion of the root.

The periodontal ligament (PDL) is a highly vascular connective tissue surrounding the roots of teeth, which joins the cementum to the alveolar bone of the socket wall. The PDL contains sensory nerve fibres, lymphatics and isolated epithelial cells (cell rests of Malassez), which are believed to be remnants of the embryonic root sheath. The width of PDL is 0.25 mm (range 0.2–0.4 mm). The collagen fibres of the PDL run into and become indistinguishable from fibre structure of both cementum and alveolar bone (Figure 35.2). The portions of the fibres within the mineralised tissues are called Sharpey fibres. The PDL contains fibre bundles named according to their orientation and position within the socket. The alveolar crest fibres run downwards and outwards from the extra-alveolar cementum to the bone margin; horizontal fibres run just below the alveolar crest; oblique fibres, which are the most numerous, run from cementum in an oblique direction to bone; and apical fibres radiate from cementum around the apex to bone. These fibre bundles allow forces from function or from parafunction, tooth grinding or clenching, to be distributed to the alveolar bone.

Above the alveolar bone margin the PDL is continuous with the connective tissue of the gingival tissues. In this extra-alveolar compartment several groups of fibre bundles can be identified. The dentogingival fibres run from cementum into the connective tissue of the gingiva. There are in addition: dentoperiosteal fibres (cementum to periosteum covering the alveolar bone); alveologingival fibres (alveolar bone into the gingival connective tissue); transeptal fibres (between the necks of neighbouring teeth above the alveolar crest); and circular fibres (encircle the teeth running in the gingival connective tissue). The main function of these extra-alveolar fibres is to strengthen the attachment of the gingiva to the tooth and the alveolar bone and therefore to provide support for the integrity of dentogingival junction. In health there

are collagen fibres inserted into the cement covering the whole surface of the root (Figure 35.3). In periodontitis collagen fibres are lost below the CEJ and the junctional epithelium migrates from enamel onto the root cementum (Figure 35.4).

The walls of the sockets are cortical compact bone and in radiographs a radio-opaque line, termed the lamina dura, may be evident (Figure 35.5). The external surface of the alveolar bone is also compact bone with the area between socket wall and the surface occupied by cancellous spongy bone. The cancellous bone contains a high proportion of vascular connective tissue with bony struts termed trabeculae (Figure 35.6). Blood vessels from cancellous bone run through canals (Volkmann's canals) in the socket wall into the PDL where they anastomose to provide a rich blood supply. The blood vessels are accompanied by sensory and proprioceptive nerve fibres. Proprioceptive mechanisms regulate chewing and protect the teeth from potential damage from sudden contact after biting through a hard component in food. The alveolar bone varies in thickness and is at its thinnest on the buccal of the upper canines and labial of the mandibular incisors. The alveolar bone margin may be deficient (termed a dehiscence) or there may a window in the bone (termed a fenestration) (Figure 35.7). Most often this is genetically determined, resulting in a thin tissue biotype; however, it may be a result of a tooth root being displaced buccally, for example in orthodontic treatment. The overall result is that increased areas of the roots are covered only by gingival tissues, which significantly increases the risk of gingival recession in response to stimuli such as vigorous toothbrushing.

The teeth are subjected to forces in normal function and these are transmitted through the PDL to the alveolar bone. There is constant, rapid turnover in the PDL with breakdown and reformation of the collagen fibres, particularly those adjacent to the alveolar bone. There is also remodelling of the alveolar bone with resorption by specialised multinucleated giant cells (osteoclasts) balanced by new bone formed by osteoblasts (Figure 35.8a). The newly formed bone incorporates collagen fibres from the PDL and thus maintains the attachment to the socket wall. In parafunction there is increased loading due to tooth-to-tooth contacts resulting from grinding and/ or clenching. This results in changes in the PDL with an increased width of the ligament due to bone remodelling, particularly towards the alveolar bone margin, and increased turnover of the collagen with a resulting disordered orientation of the PDL fibres (Figure 35.8b). Clinically, there may be increased tooth mobility; however, there is no loss of collagen fibre attachment to the cementum of the root. The changes that take place in the tissues in response to increased loading are termed occlusal trauma. The remodelling of the alveolar bone in response to increased forces on the teeth is used to facilitate controlled tooth movement in orthodontics.

Figure 35.8 Tooth subjected to increased loading. (a) Resorption of alveolar bone by osteoclasts: a, the extent of the resorption can be visualised by darkly stained reversal lines in the bone, b, and it is on these surfaces that new bone is formed incorporating collagen fibres from the PDL, c. Haematoxylin and eosin staining. (b) Disordered arrangement of collagen fibres: fibres run into alveolar bone, a, and cementum, b. Van Gieson stain for collagen

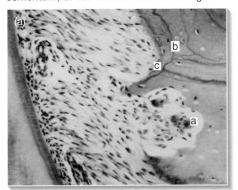
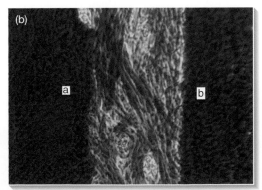

36 Dental plaque and calculus

Figure 36.1 Plaque present on the teeth in a patient with very poor oral hygiene; as the plaque gets thicker it becomes visible on examination

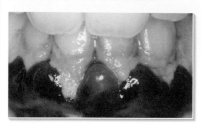

Figure 36.2 Dental plaque biofilm after 3 days of undisturbed growth; clinically, the plaque would not be visible to the eye but can be seen after the application of a disclosing solution

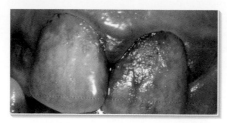

Figure 36.3 Undisturbed plaque accumulation related to the lower incisors for 14 days, in an experimental gingivitis model; there is associated swelling of the gingival margin resulting in the creation of a subgingival environment. Compare to gingival condition related to the upper teeth where there was normal plaque control

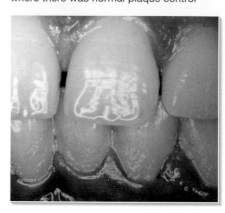

Figure 36.5 Supragingival calculus related to the lingual surfaces of the lower incisor teeth

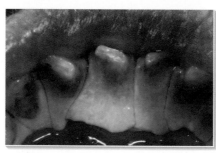

Figure 36.4 Polymorphonuclear leukocytes (PMNs), which have migrated from blood vessels through the connective tissue into the gingival sulcus in response to bacterial plaque: a, a thick layer of PMNs visible by nuclear staining with haematoxylin; b, bacteria in dental plaque; c, gingival tissue

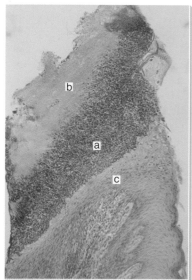

Figure 36.7 Calculus, which was originally formed in a subgingival environment and is dark brown or black in colour; there is a layer of plaque on its surface. There has been gum recession in this patient as their periodontal disease has progressed, exposing the calculus

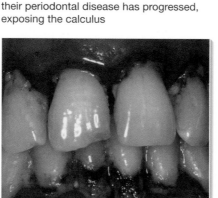

Figure 36.6 Subgingival calculus, which is characteristically dark brown or black in colour and is below the cement enamel junction: a, enamel; b, root surface. It can be tenaciously attached to the root surface interlocking into small irregularities at the sites of former insertion of Sharpey's fibres, which have been exposed by the loss of periodontal attachment fibres

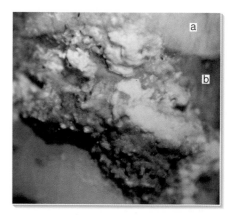

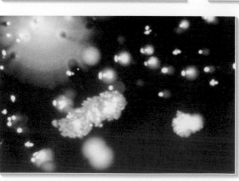

Figure 36.8 Culture of bacteria from a periodontal pocket on blood agar showing black pigmented colonies of *Porphyromonas gingivalis*; this and other species that can produce pigment are responsible for the dark brown or black colour of subgingival calculus

Dentistry at a Glance. First Edition. Edited by Elizabeth Kay. © 2016 John Wiley & Sons, Ltd. Published 2016 by John Wiley & Sons, Ltd.
Companion website: www.ataglanceseries.com/dentistryseries/dentistry

Dental plaque can be defined as a microbial community found on a tooth surface embedded in a matrix of polymers of bacterial and host origin (Figure 36.1). It is a biofilm, which means it is a complex structure containing microorganisms that forms on surfaces immersed in an aqueous environment.

Plaque formation

The tooth surface provides a unique non-shedding environment unlike the soft tissues in the oral cavity. A clean tooth surface is rapidly covered by a layer of protein from saliva, termed the pellicle. Initial colonisation is by single bacterial cells, which have the ability to adhere to the pellicle. These primary colonisers are usually Gram-positive streptococci such as *Streptococcus sanguis*. These bacteria produce carbohydrate polymers, which they export to the extracellular environment as a matrix and acts as an energy store and provides anchoring material for further bacteria. Secondary colonisation occurs between 24 and 48 hours when species such as *Actinomyces naeslundii* attach to the primary colonisers (co-aggregation). In the absence of oral hygiene there is continued increase in the thickness of the plaque biofilm with division of bacteria to form colonies and further formation of extracellular matrix (Figure 36.2). Poor diffusion of oxygen through the biofilm matrix means that it becomes anaerobic in its deeper layers. After a number of days an important step is colonisation by the *Fusobacterium nucleatum*, a key bridging bacterial species, which facilitates co-aggregation to incorporate late colonisers such as the Gram-negative anaerobe *Porphyromonas gingivalis*. Complexity thus increases and with time other Gram-negative anaerobic species can be incorporated into an established stable biofilm. Undisturbed plaque accumulation for 14 days, in an individual with initially healthy gingival tissue, will result in inflammation and provides a model of experimental gingivitis (Figure 36.3).

Tissue changes, which occur as periodontal disease progresses, provide environmental niches that encourage the development of complex biofilms. A subgingival environment such as a periodontal pocket is protected from frictional forces associated with mastication and is inaccessible to plaque control. There will be differences in nutrition, with increased availability of blood serum via the gingival crevicular fluid (GCF) and reduced levels of oxygen. Motile bacteria, such as the spirochaete *Treponema denticola*, will be found in the GCF within a pocket. This organism can co-aggregate with other Gram-negative anaerobes in mature plaque. Biofilms represent the preferred method of growth for bacteria. Advantages include protection from competing microorganisms and from host defence mechanisms such as the influx of polymorphonuclear leukocytes (PMN) (Figure 36.4). Mature intact biofilms are resistant to the effects of antibiotics and antiseptics, which cannot penetrate them to kill bacteria, and the cornerstone of treatment is mechanical disruption.

Calculus can be defined as mineralised bacterial plaque. It forms when bacteria in the deepest layers of plaque die and their cell bodies become mineralised by various crystalline forms of calcium phosphate. Supragingival calculus is creamy whitish to dark yellow in colour and is chalky in consistency (Figure 36.5). It forms in plaque exposed to salivary secretions adjacent to the ducts of salivary glands and is particularly found on the lingual surface of lower incisors. Subgingival calculus is brownish black and provides an ideal surface for bacterial adhesion and further plaque growth (Figure 36.6). Calculus acts as a plaque-retentive factor and subgingival calculus in particular keeps the plaque biofilm in close contact with the soft tissue surface of the wall of the periodontal pocket (Figure 36.7).

Specific bacterial species and periodontitis

About 700 different bacterial species can be identified in the oral cavity and many are commensal bacteria, which exist in harmony with the host. Investigations of mature subgingival plaque biofilms have identified specific groupings of bacterial species. The 'red complex', which consists of *Porphyromonas gingivalis*, *Tannerella forsythia* and *Treponema denticola*, have been found to be strongly associated with each other (co-aggregation) and with diseased sites (Figure 36.8). *Porphyromonas gingivalis* is strongly associated with periodontal disease but is not a potent inducer of inflammation. Experimental studies suggest it is a keystone microorganism, which even in very low numbers can subvert the host response leading to a major increase in commensal microbial load, resulting in periodontal destruction. *Porphyromonas gingivalis* is also present in bacterial biofilms that are not associated with disease. It is possible that pathogenicity may depend on the specific strain of the bacteria; alternatively, the host response may be able to attenuate the capacity of bacteria to cause disease.

Localised aggressive periodontitis (LAP) is a rare type of periodontal disease (see Figure 37.7). The bacterial species *Aggregatibacter actinomycetemcomitans* is almost always recovered from samples taken from affected individuals. A specific clone of this bacteria, the JP2 clone, was identified in populations from Mediterranean Africa. This clone has a genetic mutation and it produces very high levels of leukotoxin, which substantially suppresses PMN function. A prospective 2-year study of teenage schoolchildren in Morocco found that carriers of the JP2 clone of *Aggregatibacter actinomycetemcomitans* at baseline were 18 times more likely to develop LAP and 70% of those with JP2 developed this condition. The study was the first clear demonstration that a specific bacterial species caused periodontal disease, albeit a rare form of the condition.

37 Diseases of the gingivae and periodontium

Figure 37.1 Contained gingivitis: this 72-year-old man presented with pain from a carious upper incisor. He never brushed his teeth as he was too busy with his job running a farming business. He had very obvious gingivitis but little evidence of involvement of the periodontal tissues with loss of periodontal attachment.

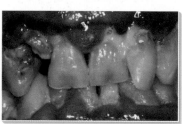

Figure 37.2 Gingivitis in a 22-year-old who was in the third month of her pregnancy. It represents an exaggerated response to dental plaque, which is visible on the teeth: a, localised swelling of the gingival margin related to the upper right central incisor, which is termed a pregnancy epulis

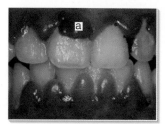

Figure 37.3 Assessment of the periodontal status using the basic periodontal examination: (a) World Health Organisation (WHO) probe in a periodontal pocket; (b) there is bleeding after the probe has been removed showing active inflammation. The band on the probe is between 3.5 and 5.5 mm from the ball-ended tip

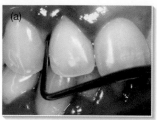
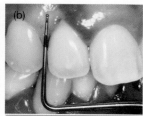

Figure 37.4 Chronic periodontitis in a 45-year-old man with very poor oral hygiene and gross plaque accumulation

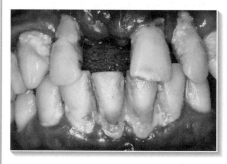

Figure 37.5 A fluctuant swelling of the buccal gingiva in a 50-year-old female related to a periodontal abscess; this represents an infection in a deep pocket on the mesiobuccal surface of the upper right canine. An abscess is defined as a circumscribed collection of pus

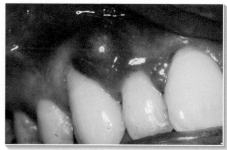

Figure 37.6 This 43-year-old woman was complaining of spacing, which had developed between her upper incisors over the preceding year. She had a good standard of plaque control and no evidence of gingival inflammation. Subgingival calculus deposits are evident on the palatal surfaces of the incisors and there was deep pocketing. The woman had smoked 20 cigarettes per day for over 20 years. Note also the glazed appearance of the palatal tissues

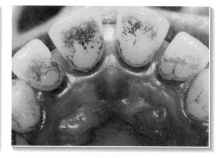

Figure 37.7 Radiograph showing vertical bone loss affecting the first molar and incisor teeth in a 15-year-old boy; the diagnosis was advanced localised aggressive periodontitis

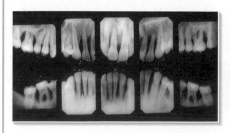

Figure 37.8 Radiographic appearance of a 28-year-old woman with generalised aggressive periodontitis. She presented because a space had developed between her upper central incisors over a 9-month period. Note the generalised advanced bone loss

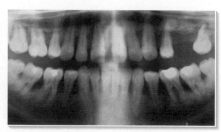

Figure 37.9 Acute ulcerative gingivitis in an 18-year-old female who smoked 15 cigarettes per day. She was complaining of pain in her gums and marked halitosis. Note the loss of the interdental papillae, which is a characteristic presentation of this condition

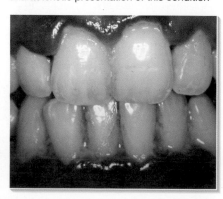

Diseases of the periodontal tissues are among the most common to affect mankind. Gingivitis, a chronic inflammatory condition, represents the response of the gingiva to the accumulation of dental plaque on the surface of the teeth. Those affected will often complain of bleeding gums, particularly in response to toothbrushing or after eating, but the condition is not usually painful (see Figure 36.3). Gingivitis is a reversible condition and the removal of dental plaque and calculus will result in a return to gingival health. Gingival inflammation is a very common and is evident to some degree in virtually all adolescents at puberty, followed by a reduction in its prevalence. It is not the case that all individuals with poor plaque control and persistent gingivitis will progress to periodontitis. Inflammatory changes may be present for many years with limited or no involvement beyond the gingival tissues (contained gingivitis), which fits with the concept that inflammation is a protective response (Figure 37.1). Hormonal influences mean that there is increased expression of gingivitis during pregnancy. There may be localised inflammatory swellings (pregnancy epulis), which regress after childbirth (Figure 37.2). In other cases a definitive diagnosis for a localised swelling of the gingival margin will require a histopathological examination of the excised tissue. Fibrous epulis is the most common diagnosis for such swellings.

Chronic periodontitis can be defined as loss of support of the affected teeth due to loss of connective tissue attachment and alveolar bone. It results in irreversible destruction of components of the periodontal tissues that support the teeth. Chronic periodontitis is not usually painful and often does not become evident to affected individuals until they notice loosening, or a change in the position, of one or more of their teeth. There is considerable variation between different populations with 5–20% of adults suffering from periodontal disease at a level that requires some treatment. As periodontitis develops there are changes in the tissues, which mean that periodontal pockets become deeper and this forms the basis for the basic periodontal examination (BPE) that is used as a screening method to identify periodontal disease and the specific treatment required (www.bsperio.org.uk/publications/index.php) (Figure 37.3). Deepened periodontal pockets provide the ecological niche to support the incorporation of anaerobic Gram-negative microorganisms into the subgingival dental plaque biofilm, increasing the likelihood of progressive periodontal disease. However, ultimately it is loss of periodontal attachment, measured from the cement enamel junction to the bottom of the pocket, which provides a measure of the severity of periodontitis. Chronic periodontitis is often associated with poor oral hygiene, generalised plaque, calculus and obvious inflammatory changes in the gingival tissues (Figure 37.4). Localised infection within a deep periodontal pocket can result in the formation of a periodontal abscess (Figure 37.5). Drainage of pus can usually be established through the pocket. A careful examination is indicated to distinguish this from a periapical abscess.

The absence of obvious signs of inflammation of the gingival margin cannot be used to exclude periodontitis. As periodontitis progresses the inflammatory component is located subgingivally at the bottom of the periodontal pocket and there may be no sign of changes affecting the gingival margin. It is therefore important to examine the periodontal tissues in adults using a screening system, such as the BPE, to exclude periodontitis. There are risk factors that are associated with increased prevalence and severity of periodontitis, in particular smoking which has been implicated in more than 50% of all cases of periodontitis. Smoking suppresses the inflammatory response allowing periodontitis to progress particularly on surfaces where there is direct contact with cigarette smoke. Thus the pattern of periodontal destruction in smokers often includes the anterior teeth and in particular the palatal surfaces of the upper teeth (Figure 37.6).

Aggressive periodontitis is a rare condition representing periodontitis that progresses rapidly and occurs in young individuals. Although uncommon, it has considerable significance as it often affects the very young and may result in tooth loss. Localised aggressive periodontitis is most often reported in adolescents where extensive periodontal destruction typically affects a small number of teeth, including the first molars and incisors (Figure 37.7). Generalised aggressive periodontitis tends to be identified in those aged below 35 years and affects many of the teeth (Figure 37.8). It is generally accepted that there is a strong genetic link in aggressive periodontitis, probably having an effect by suppressing appropriate inflammatory or immune responses to causative bacteria. Alternatively, specific virulent bacteria may suppress the host response (see Chapter 36). Genetic factors may explain the variations worldwide, with a high prevalence in populations from parts of Africa and a very low prevalence in Caucasians.

Acute ulcerative gingivitis (AUG) is a condition that affects young individuals and presents with pain, tenderness, spontaneous gingival bleeding and complaints of halitosis. It often affects the lower incisor region and the loss of gingival contour due to necrosis of interdental papillae is a distinctive feature (Figure 37.9). Smoking is present in virtually all cases and is associated with other risk factors, including poor oral hygiene and stress. There is a specific anaerobic flora in AUG with fusobacteria and spirochaetes. AUG responds rapidly to antibiotics, particularly metronidazole, followed by periodontal treatment; however, rapid recurrence is common if the risk factors persist. Occasionally, particularly if AUG does not respond to treatment, it is associated with systemic diseases that impair immunity such as HIV.

Leukaemias represent the malignant proliferation of white blood cells and can be acute or chronic. These can present as gingival swelling, due to the accumulation of white blood cells in the gingival tissues, or excessive and persistent bleeding, due to secondary thrombocytopenia (decreased platelets) (Figure 37.10). A rapid diagnosis is important and blood tests will identify whether a leukaemia is present.

Figure 37.10 Acute myeloid leukaemia in a 45-year-old man who had been complaining of blood oozing from his gums for a month. He had attended his doctor on two occasions before being referred for a dental opinion. A blood test identified the need for onward referral for specialist management but despite chemotherapy he died 2 months later

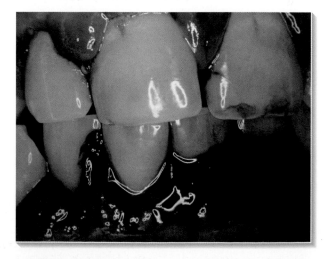

38 Properties of tooth tissue

Figure 38.1 Schematic view of the tooth structure

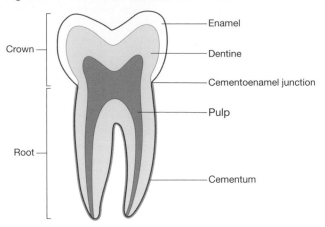

Crown — Enamel
— Dentine
— Cementoenamel junction
— Pulp
Root — Cementum

Figure 38.2 (a) Cross section of the dentinal tubules; (b) when the smear layer is removed, the dentinal tubules can act as passages between the oral environment and the pulp
Source: Reproduced with permission from Dr Nikolas Silikas.

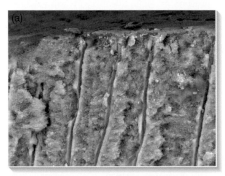

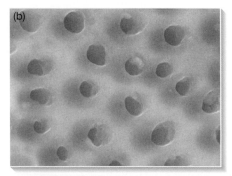

Box 38.1 Enamel properties

Composition (by volume)
Inorganic hydroxyapatite	86%
Water	4–12%
Organic matrix	Trace

Thickness (mm)
Cusp tips	2.5
Incisal edge	2.0
Cervical areas	minimal to nil
Occlusal fissures	minimal to nil

Box 38.2 Dentine properties

Composition (by volume)
Inorganic apatite crystals	45–50%
Organic matrix	30%
Water	25%

Rate of secretion (μm/day)
Primary dentine	4–8
Secondary dentine	1–2

Box 38.3 Types of CEJ

Cementum–enamel relationships
Cementum overlaps enamel	60–65%
Edge-to-edge	30%
Cementum does not meet enamel	5–10%

Box 38.4 Factors causing resorption of cementum

Local factors
- Trauma from occlusion
- Orthodontic movement
- Pressure from malaligned erupting teeth
- Cysts
- Tumours
- Teeth without functional antagonist
- Embedded teeth
- Replanted and transplanted teeth
- Periapical disease
- Periodontal disease

Systemic factors
- Calcium deficiency
- Hypothyroidism
- Hereditary fibrous osteodystrophy
- Paget's disease

Dentistry at a Glance. First Edition. Edited by Elizabeth Kay. © 2016 John Wiley & Sons, Ltd. Published 2016 by John Wiley & Sons, Ltd.
Companion website: www.ataglanceseries.com/dentistryseries/dentistry

A thorough understanding of the anatomy and biology of the tooth is necessary for successful clinical dentistry. Dentistry that violates the physical, chemical and biological parameters of the tooth tissue can lead to premature restoration failure, compromised coronal integrity, recurrent caries, patient discomfort or pulpal necrosis.

Enamel

Enamel provides a hard durable surface to protect the dentine and pulp. Its form and colour also has a major role in aesthetics (Figure 38.1); therefore, the lifelong preservation of the patient's own enamel is one of the goals of modern dentistry.

Permeability: The water in enamel (Box 38.1) is contained within the intercrystalline spaces and in a network of micropores opening to the external surface, which makes enamel a semipermeable material.

Colour: Enamel translucency is directly related to its degree of mineralisation and thickness. The colour of the tooth is determined by the colour of the underlying dentine as well as the translucency of the enamel covering it.

Wear: Enamel is a hard material but it wears when it is opposed by enamel or harder restorative materials (e.g. porcelain).

Acid etching: Enamel is differentially soluble when exposed for a brief time to weak acids. This process is called acid etching and approximately 10 μm of surface enamel (but no rod structures) is removed. If acid exposure continues, the differential dissolution of enamel rod and inter-rod structures forms a three-dimensional macroporous structure, which can be used to attract resin monomer during restorative bonding procedures.

Dentine

The coronal dentine is covered by enamel and forms the bulk of the structure of the tooth. This dentine is responsible for protecting the pulp as well as forming an elastic foundation to support the enamel and dictate the overall tooth shade. The radicular dentine is covered by cementum and forms the roots. Dentine is capable of responding to external thermal, chemical and mechanical stimuli.

Support: The strength, rigidity and integrity of the tooth rely on an intact dentinal structure. When a tooth is prepared for restoration, its resistance to fracture decreases. Removal and replacement of dental restorations result in progressively larger or deeper restorations throughout the patient's life.

Morphology: Dentine is composed of small, thin apatite crystal flakes embedded in a protein matrix of cross-linked collagen fibrils (Box 38.2). Two main types of dentine are present: **intertubular dentine**, which forms the bulk of the dentine structure and is composed of a hydroxyapatite-embedded collagen matrix, and **peritubular dentine**, which is limited to the lining of the dentinal tubule walls. It has little organic matrix and is packed with miniscule apatite crystals.

Permeability: The dentinal tubules have a functional role in forming and maintaining the dentine but, when exposed, they make the dentine permeable (Figure 38.2).

Primary and secondary dentine: Once the odontoblast cells are differentiated from ectomesenchymal cells, they start secreting an organic matrix. This matrix mineralises and forms the **primary dentine**. Approximately 2 to 3 years following tooth eruption, the synthesis of the dentine slows down and continues for as long as the tooth is vital. This dentine is called **secondary dentine** and is responsible for reducing the size of the pulp chamber.

Tertiary dentine: When dentine is lost due to caries or injury, new dentine (**tertiary dentine**) will form at the dentine–pulp interface if the tooth retains its vitality. If the stimulus is low grade, this dentine is made by the odontoblasts and is called **reactionary dentine**. If the stimulus is severe or the thickness of the remaining dentine falls below 0.25 mm, the odontoblasts will die. The stem cells within the vital pulp will form odontoblast-like cells, which will then create a bridge of dentine. This dentine is called **reparative dentine**.

Pulp

Dental pulp is composed of 75% water and 25% organic material, which form a viscous connective tissue of collagen fibres and organic ground substance which supports the cellular, vascular and nerve structures of the tooth.

The dental pulp has several functions:

Formative: Odontolasts within the dental pulp are responsible for generating primary, secondary and tertiary dentine. They also produce growth factors and bioactive signalling molecules, which coordinates the pulpal–dentinal responses for healing and repair. Fibroblasts produce, maintain and remodel pulp matrix and collagen.

Nutritive: The microvascular system of the pulp contains vessels no larger than arterioles and venules. Lymphatic vessels of the pulp return tissue fluid and high-molecular-weight plasma proteins back to the vascular system. The transfer of the oxygen, nutrition and waste materials is done by diffusion within the viscous ground substance of the pulp.

Sensory: The majority of the nerve fibres are either A-δ or unmyelinated C fibres. The A-δ nerves react to hydrodynamic phenomena and their activation results in sharp and intense pain. The C fibres, however, are only activated by a level of stimuli that is capable of creating tissue destruction (i.e. prolonged high temperature or pulpitis). The pain is diffuse in nature and described as burning or throbbing, which maybe difficult to locate. The C fibres are resistant to hypoxia and are not affected by reduction of blood flow or high tissue pressure; therefore, pain may persist in anaesthetised, infected or even non-vital teeth.

Protective: The immunocompetent cells within the pulp consist of macrophages, lymphocytes and dendritic cells. These cells function as a host defence system against foreign bodies and antigens.

Cementum

Cementum is the calcified, avascular mesenchymal tissue that forms the outer covering of the anatomic root. The two main types of cementum are **acellular** (primary) and **cellular** (secondary) and both consist of a calcified interfibrillar matrix and collagen fibrils. The two main sources of collagen fibres in cementum are **Sharpey's fibres** (extrinsic), which are the embedded portion of the principal fibres of the periodontal ligament and are formed by fibroblasts, and fibres that belong to the cementum matrix (intrinsic) and are produced by the cementoblasts.

Permeability: Cementum is very permeable in young teeth but this diminishes with age.

Cementoenamel junction (CEJ): Three types of CEJ may exist (Box 38.3). When there is a gap between enamel and cementum, gingival recession may result in exposed dentine and sensitivity.

Cementum resorption: Primary teeth undergo physiological resorption; however, in adult teeth cementum resorption may occur due to local or systemic factors (Box 38.4) or may occur without apparent aetiology (idiopathic). In rare cases of resorption, cementum and root can be gradually replaced by bone, resulting in **ankylosis**. An ankylosed tooth lacks physiological mobility and makes a metallic sound on percussion.

39 Local anaesthesia for tooth restoration

Figure 39.1 (a) Manually aspirating syringe; (b) the barb of the syringe screws into the bung of a conventional cartridge

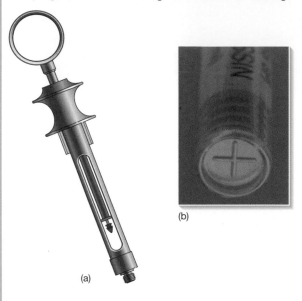

(b)

(a)

Figure 39.2 The Dentsply self-aspirating system: (a) self-aspiration cartridges have a specially adapted bung, needing a different syringe plunger; (b) thin centre of the bung distended when pressure is exerted; (c) when force is stopped, the bung returns to its usual shape – negative pressure (aspiration); (d) the specially adapted bung

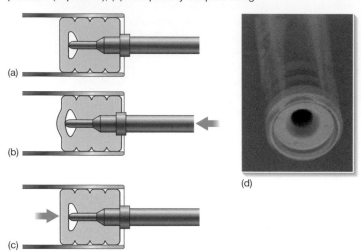

(a)

(b)

(c)

(d)

Figure 39.3 (a–d) Alternative self-aspirating system

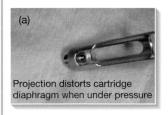

(a)

Projection distorts cartridge diaphragm when under pressure

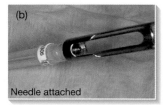

(b)

Needle attached

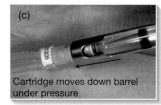

(c)

Cartridge moves down barrel under pressure

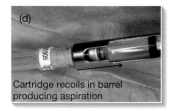

(d)

Cartridge recoils in barrel producing aspiration

Figure 39.4 Stages of the injection technique: (a) the application of topical anaesthetic; (b) needle over puncture site; (c) needle advanced to injection site; (d) buccal approach to palatal anaesthesia; (e) palatal blanching – sign of effective anaesthesia; (f) buccal infiltration in lower jaw; (g) mental (incisive) nerve block; (h) inferior alveolar nerve block

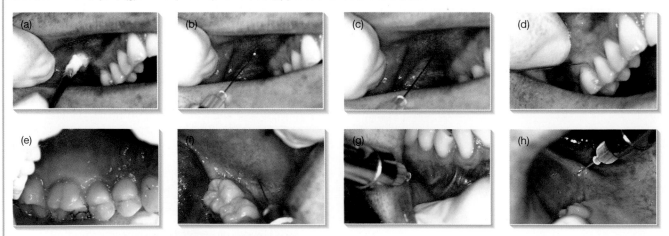

Source: Figures 39.1 and 39.2, reproduced with permission of Dentsply Ltd.

Receiving dental care remains one of the most common fears. The fear of pain is a large part of this fear, with the most common question patients ask being "does it hurt?". Comfortable and effective local anaesthetic (LA) administration is required for successful practice. This chapter provides an introduction to the subject.

Armamentarium

The equipment used must be able to aspirate. Intravascular injection of LA is one of the most common complications of local anaesthesia, which is prevented by aspiration before every injection.

Aspiration involves a negative pressure being created within the cartridge to suck back fluid at the needle tip. If the needle tip is within a blood vessel, blood is aspirated; if it is not, clear interstitial fluid is aspirated. The two main systems are self-aspirating and manually aspirating.

Figure 39.1 shows the manual aspirating system. Aspiration is achieved by pulling the cartridge bung back. There are two main disadvantages:
1 Movement of the needle tip, making false results more likely
2 Difficult for small-handed operators to use.

Figure 39.2 illustrates the Dentsply self-aspirating system that uses a specially designed bung, which is distorted when the plunger is pressed. Releasing the pressure allows the bung to return to the resting state, creating negative pressure.

Self-aspiration is more reliable than manual aspiration because no active movement from the operator is required. The main disadvantage is that once the bung has moved in the cartridge, friction is reduced thus decreasing the efficacy. An alternative self-aspirating system involves distortion of the diaphragm at the needle end of the cartridge (Figure 39.3). SafetyPlus (Dentsply) system utilises this method of aspiration.

A variety of computer-controlled local anaesthetic delivery (CCLAD) systems are available. These systems allow effective aspiration as well as controlled pressure delivery. Although becoming more popular, they are not yet widely used.

Choice of local anaesthetic solution

The properties of LAs are given in Table 39.1. The gold standard and most commonly used LA in the UK is 2% lidocaine with 1 : 80 000 epinephrine in 2.2-mL cartridges. A 3% solution of prilocaine containing 0.03 IU/mL of felypressin has been considered as an alternative for patients who are unable to receive epinephrine. It is rumoured to be less effective than lidocaine and epinephrine, but emerging evidence is that it is slower in producing anaesthesia, not less effective.

Mepivacaine is available as a 3% plain solution or as 2% with epinephrine. As the least vasodilating LA, the plain solution can be used when vasoconstrictors are contraindicated. It is more effective for block anaesthesia than infiltration.

Articaine 4% (with 1 : 100 000 or 1 : 200 000 epinephrine) is a more recent introduction to UK practice, despite having been the first choice in other countries since the 1970s. Evidence is emerging that articaine is more effective than lidocaine. Evidence is also emerging that the reported problems of non-surgical paraesthesia may not be as significant as first thought.

Clinical techniques for anaesthetising teeth for restorative treatment

The main requirement for successful anaesthesia for tooth restoration is that pulpal anaesthesia is achieved. In certain instances, where the gingival tissues are to be incised or manipulated, soft tissue anaesthesia may also be required.

Table 39.1 Properties of local anaesthetics

Local anaesthetic	Vasoconstrictor	Maximum dose		Onset of pulpal anaesthesia (min)	Duration of anaesthesia Pulpal (min)	Duration of anaesthesia Soft tissue (min)
		mg/kg	Absolute			
Lidocaine 2%	Epinephrine 1 : 80 000	4.4	300	2–3 infiltration 5–7 block	60	180–300
Prilocaine 3%	Felypressin	6.0	400	4 infiltration 6–9 block	60	180–300
Prilocaine 4%	Plain solution	6.0	400	4 infiltration 6–9 block	14–40	90–120
Mepivacaine 2%	Epinephrine 1 : 100 000	4.4	300	2 infiltration 5–6 block	45–60	180–300
Mepivacaine 3%	Plain solution	4.4	300	2 infiltration 5–6 block	20–40	120–180
Articaine 4%	Epinephrine 1 : 100 000 or 1 : 200 000	7.0	500	2 infiltration 5–6 block	60–75 45–60	180–360 120–300

General injection technique

Preparation of the surgery: See Table 39.2.

Preparation of the equipment: The correct length needle (see below) should be selected. The syringe and cartridge of the chosen local anaesthetic assembled, after the cartridge has been be checked (Table 39.3).

Table 39.2 Checks on the surgery before administration of local anaesthetic

All the equipment is functional	To avoid having to abort treatment once local has been given
All necessary instruments and materials are present in the surgery	To avoid delays in treatment
All notes and radiographs are present	To ensure correct treatment is provided

Table 39.3 Checks on a local anaesthetic cartridge prior to use

It is the correct local anaesthetic solution	To ensure that the patient is given the appropriate drug for the proposed treatment
The local anaesthetic is in date	Out of date drugs are less effective and may be harmful
The cartridge is undamaged	If the cartridge is damaged there is the potential for the contents not to be sterile
The cartridge is not part used	To prevent transmission of infection
The solution looks as it should appear	The solution should be clear – any loss of clarity might indicate contamination of the contents
There is not an excess of air in the cartridge	This might indicate contamination of the contents

Preparation of the patient: The patient should be checked as in Table 39.4 prior to injection.

Table 39.4 Checks on the patient prior to local anaesthetic

The patients notes are available and the details match the patient	Notes radiographs and treatment plan should be available to ensure correct treatment is provided
There has been no change to the patient's medical history	Ensure there are no contraindications to either the proposed dental treatment or the administration of local anaesthetic
There has been no change to the patient's dental history	To ensure that the proposed treatment is still the next step in the treatment plan
The patient understands the treatment to be carried out	It is important that the patient knows what to expect as part of the consent process
The patient still consents to the dental treatment	Consent is a continuing process – the patient can withdraw it at any stage
Confirm by visual examination that the treatment is still appropriate	To ensure that there have been no changes in the state of the dentition that might require a change of treatment plan

Administration of local anaesthetic

The patient should be positioned for the dental treatment to be performed. As most restorative treatment is carried out with the patient supine, the local anaesthetic should be administered with the patient in this position. The stages in injection technique are given in Table 39.5 and Figure 39.4. These basics apply to all LA injections.

Topical anaesthetics should be used, but in small amounts. Applying too much topical anaesthetic can lead to it spreading to unwanted areas, for example the pharynx.

LA should be administered slowly. There are three reasons for this:

1 It is more comfortable for the patient
2 It makes LA more effective
3 If a portion of the solution is injected intravascularly, it will be detected after a smaller volume has been injected.

Table 39.5 Basic injection technique

Stage	Description
1	Visualise the point of puncture of mucosa
2	Dry the area
3	Apply a small amount of topical anaesthetic and leave to work
4	Stretch the mucosa so that the needle will puncture the tissue without tearing
5	Puncture the mucosa quickly to avoid tearing
6	Slowly advance the tip of the needle until the target area is reached
7	Aspirate twice to ensure that the needle tip is not in a blood vessel
8	Inject the required amount of local anaesthetic at the rate of about 1 mL per minute
9	Remove the needle from the patient's mouth and store for the next injection or dispose of safely
10	Allow LA to take effect prior to commencing treatment

Anaesthesia in the upper jaw

The standard technique for producing anaesthesia in the maxilla is the buccal supraperiosteal infiltration. The technique is described in Table 39.6. It is important to place LA above the apex of the tooth as LA placed too low will be ineffective as it cannot diffuse through tooth tissue to the pulp.

Table 39.6 Maxillary infiltration technique

Stage	Description
1	The right-handed operator sits at the 11 o'clock position, while the left-handed operator sits at the 1 o'clock position relative to the patient
2	The target is above and just distal to the apex of the tooth being treated
3	The operator must visualise the position of the apex taking into account the expected tooth length
4	LA is normally effective after approximately 3 minutes

Patients are normally aware of altered sensation of the lip when upper premolar, canine or incisor teeth are anaesthetised, but may notice little change when molar teeth are anaesthetised. The practice of probing the gingivae or disrupting the junctional epithelium with a probe to test for anaesthesia is to be discouraged.

In restorative cases, local anaesthesia of the palatal mucosa is usually not required. If required, the recommended technique provides anaesthesia from a buccal approach. The technique is described in Table 39.7.

Table 39.7 Chasing technique for palatal anaesthesia

Stage	Description
1	Place the needle horizontally into the interdental papilla distal to the treated tooth, except for the incisor canine and 3rd molar tooth where mesial papilla is used
2	Advance the needle palatally while injecting slowly until the palatal mucosa blanches – it is helpful for the dental nurse to observe this area
3	After blanching has occurred, the needle can be introduced palatally and LA given painlessly

Anaesthesia in the lower jaw

The technique for anaesthesia of the lower teeth depends on the tooth being treated (Table 39.8):

• The technique for the mental (incisive) nerve block is similar to the buccal infiltration. The target area is between the apices of the lower premolars. After administration the solution is massaged into the tissues to encourage spread through the mental foramen. No attempt is made to place the tip of the needle into the mental foramen, as this can cause nerve damage.

Table 39.8 Techniques used to anaesthetise the lower jaw

Teeth	Local anaesthetic technique for different tissues		
	Pulp	Buccal gingivae	Lingual gingivae
Molars	Inferior alveolar nerve block	Buccal infiltration	Lingual nerve anaesthetised by inferior alveolar nerve block injection
Premolars	Mental (incisive nerve block)	Mental (incisive nerve block)	As for palatal injection in upper
Canine and incisor	Buccal infiltration	Buccal infiltration	As for palatal injection in upper

• The technique for inferior alveolar nerve block is given in Table 39.9.
• If buccal soft tissue anaesthesia is required for molar teeth when an inferior alveolar nerve block is used, this is achieved by buccal infiltration as for the upper jaw.

The techniques described in this chapter will provide adequate anaesthesia for the restoration of teeth in the vast majority of cases. Worldwide, millions of local anaesthetic injections are administered daily. The incidence of complications is extremely low; however, it must be remembered, as with all drugs, that local anaesthetics have both beneficial and harmful effects. Their use should be treated with respect. Readers are referred to specialist texts for more detailed information.

Table 39.9 The inferior alveolar nerve block technique

Stage	Description
1	The right-handed operator sits at the 11 o'clock position relative to the patient to administer an injection to the patient's left side and at the 7 o'clock position to administer an injection to the patient's right side The left-handed operator sits at the 1 o'clock position relative to the patient to administer an injection to the patient's right side and at the 5 o'clock position to administer an injection to the patient's left side
2	A 3-cm 27-guage needle is used
3	The puncture point is where the apex of the buccal pad of fat meets the pterygomandibular raphe The syringe is angled so that it passes over the mesial of the contralateral lower first molar parallel to the occlusal plane
4	The needle is advanced until bony contact is achieved at a depth of 2 cm
5	If bony contact is not achieved, or it is too deep, the needle should be withdrawn until about 1 cm is in the tissues and the barrel moved more distally prior to advancing to bony contact If bony contact is achieved too soon, the needle should be withdrawn until only about 1 cm is in the tissues and the barrel moved more mesially prior to advancing to bony contact
6	Local anaesthetic must not be injected without bony contact Follow steps 6–10 of the basic injection technique
7	If local anaesthesia of the lingual nerve is desired, then the last third of the solution can be injected as the needle is withdrawn Usually, sufficient anaesthesia for restorative treatment is achieved without this stage
8	The signs that anaesthesia has been achieved are that there is loss of sensation in the area supplied by the mental nerve – the lower lip on the anaesthetised side This normally takes approximately 5 minutes from the time of injection

40 Tooth isolation

Figure 40.1 (a) High volume suction tip and (b) saliva ejector; saliva ejectors can be moulded for optimal fit

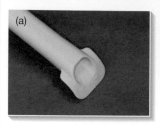
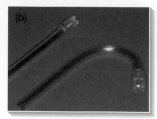

Figure 40.2 (a, b) Svedopter can retract the tongue at the same time as aspirating excess fluids

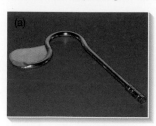
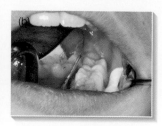

Figure 40.3 Cotton wool roll placed in the buccal sulcus; a mirror can be used to keep the cotton wool roll in place

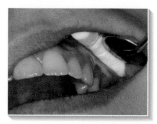

Figure 40.4 (a) Cellulose pad covering the parotid duct and (b) high-volume suction tip aspirating from the lingual side

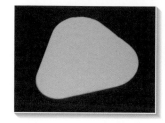
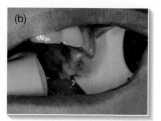

Figure 40.5 Clamps, from left to right: wingless, winged and butterfly

Figure 40.6 Note the wings underneath the dam; this complex can now be delivered into the mouth

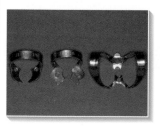
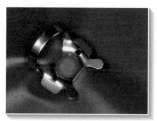

Figure 40.7 Using the punch (a) holes in varying sizes can be created (b), corresponding to the differences in the sizes of the teeth

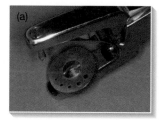
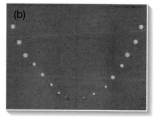

Figure 40.8 If the dam is not inverted (a), oral fluids can push into the operative field; once the dam is inverted (b) the pressure from the fluids seal the dam against the tooth

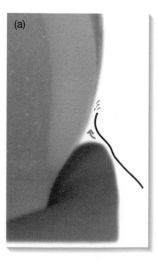
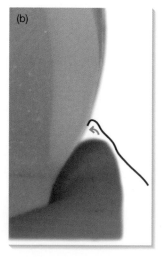

Figure 40.9 The dam is inverted using a flat plastic instrument; note that the assistant can facilitate this by blowing air at high pressure

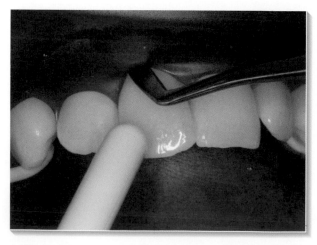

In restorative dentistry teeth are isolated for several reasons:

- **To improve patient's comfort and safety**: Saliva as well as the water produced by handpieces and 3-in-1 syringes can accumulate and cause discomfort. Some of the chemicals and liquids used during operative work can be harmful to the soft tissue and cause irritation or burns. Also small and sharp instruments (for example endodontic files and reamers) can dislodge, putting the patient at the risk of inhaling the implement.
- **To improve access and visibility**: Constant water spray from the handpiece topped up by saliva can reduce visibility dramatically.
- **To prevent the contamination of the restorative procedure**: Several species of microorganisms inhabit the oral cavity. These microorganisms can contaminate the prepared cavities and pulpal tissues and lead to new or persistent infections.
- **To allow proper placement of restorative materials**: Liquid contamination can have a negative effect on the mechanical properties of almost all of the direct restorative materials. When adhesive materials are used, any liquid contamination can cause failure of the restoration.

There are several techniques that can be used to isolate a tooth. Some of the most commonly used are described in this chapter.

Aspiration

A **high-volume suction tip** (Figure 40.1a) can be used by the dental assistant to remove the excess fluid from the operative field. This is an effective device to remove large quantities of fluid quickly.

The **Saliva ejector** is also a useful tool to remove fluids from the oral cavity (Figure 40.1b). It can be a very helpful as an adjunctive tool to be used while a rubber dam is in place to improve the patient's comfort.

A **Svedopter (flange)** is used to isolate the lower teeth (Figure 40.2a). It retracts the tongue and aspirates fluids at the same time. By adding cotton wool rolls on the buccal aspect, enough isolation can be achieved for impression taking or cementation (Figure 40.2b).

Cotton wool rolls and cellulose pads

Cotton wools rolls are used to absorb fluids and retract the lips or cheeks. They can provide an adequate dry field when used in conjunction with effective aspiration. When placed in the buccal or labial sulcus, a mirror can be used to keep the cotton wool roll in place (Figure 40.3).

Cellulose pads are placed on the buccal sulcus and can be used to absorb moisture from the parotid duct (Figure 40.4).

Rubber dam

Rubber dam was introduced to the dental profession in 1864 and has remained the gold standard for tooth isolation. The dam material is available in variety of colours. In restorative dentistry it is important to choose a colour that contrasts with the colour of the teeth. The dam material is also available in several thicknesses or gauges. For restorative work, heavy and extra heavy gauges (0.15–0.35 mm) are recommended. They apply as easily as thinner dams but are less likely to tear. They are available in latex and latex-free forms.

Clamps: Rubber dam clamps are the usual means of securing the dam. There are three basic types of clamps available (Figure 40.5). The dam can be placed on a winged-clamp prior to the application (Figure 40.6). When using a wingless-clamp, rubber dam can be placed in the mouth prior or after placement of the clamp. The butterfly clamp serves as a gingival retractor at the same time as retaining the rubber dam in situ. Clamps are available in different sizes. When choosing a clamp, it is important that only its jaw points contact the tooth. This will create a four-point contact.

Floss ligatures: It is widely recommended that dental floss should be attached to every clamp used in the mouth. This allows retrieval of the clamp if the clamp dislodges or breaks. Certainly it is wise to attach floss to the clamp if it is placed in the mouth prior to the application of the dam; however, the floss can cause leakage and therefore once the rubber dam application is finished, the floss should be removed. Of course if the clamp fractures or dislodges after the application is finished, the dam will prevent dislodgement of the clamp into the oral cavity. When a winged-clamp is attached to the dam prior to placement of the clamp onto a tooth, the use of floss ligature is unnecessary.

Placement: Teeth should be cleaned, if necessary, and contacts should be checked with floss to ensure the dam can pass the contacts with ease. If occlusal restorations are planned, the occlusion should be marked prior to the rubber dam application. A rubber dam stamp can be used to locate the position of the teeth. When doing restorative work on a posterior tooth, usually the most distal tooth in that quadrant is clamped. This will allow exposure of several teeth. Using a rubber dam punch, holes of varying sizes will be created according to the size of the corresponding teeth (Figure 40.7). If a winged-clamp is used, the dam will be attached to the clamp. This combination will then be transferred into the mouth. If a wingless clamp is used, the clamp is placed on the tooth first. The dam is then stretched to pass over the clamp and wraps around the neck of the tooth. A waxed floss is recommended to floss the dam through the interproximal contacts.

Inversion of the dam: The dam should be inverted around the neck of the teeth. If the dam is directed occlusally, fluids will push through to the operative field (Figure 40.8). High-volume air is used to dry the teeth and dam surface to facilitate inversion. A No. 23 explorer or a No. 1–2 plastic instrument can be used to invert the dam (Figure 40.9).

41 Cavity preparation

Figure 41.1 Rounded cavity angles are important to minimise stress concentration

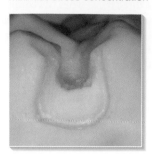

Figure 41.2 A slot preparation showing retentive grooves placed in the line angles between the pulpal wall and the buccal axial wall (a) and palatal axial wall (b)

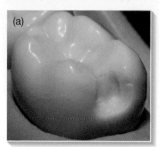
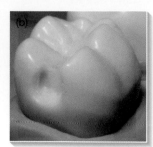

Figure 41.3 Cavity preparations with mechanical retentive features: (a) a pit (yellow arrow) and a groove (blue arrow) placed into dentine; (b) undercut walls which are occlusally convergent

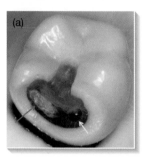
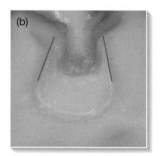

Figure 41.4 When placing amalgam restorations, all cavosurface angles should be 90°, including those on the occlusal (a) and proximal surfaces (b)

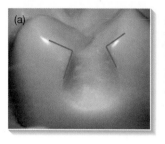
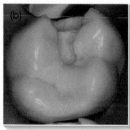

Figure 41.5 When parallel sided burs are used, a cavosurface angle of greater than 90° is created

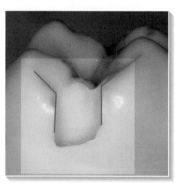

Figure 41.6 An inverted taper bur, which can be useful for amalgam cavity preparations

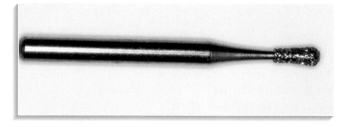

Figure 41.7 Use of a gingival margin trimmer to remove any unsupported enamel in an amalgam cavity; if this cavity were to be restored with composite, this enamel would not be removed

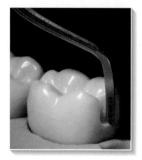

Figure 41.8 (a) Cavity margin suitable for restoration with composite in areas of occlusal loading; (b) bevelled enamel margins on a class V cavity to enhance the available enamel surface area for bonding

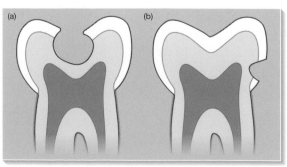

General principles

Optimal cavity preparation is crucial to the long-term success of a restoration. It has been reported that over half of direct restorations placed in general practice are replacement restorations and this, in part, may be due to initial errors when preparing such cavities. Irrespective of the type of cavity and material used to restore it, certain general principles should be followed.

Rounded angles on internal and external cavity walls   Cavity preparation will weaken a tooth. This can be exacerbated by sharp cavity angles, which act as points of stress concentration and ultimately cause cracks to form (Figure 41.1).

Ensure that the remaining tooth tissue has structural durability   Once carious tooth tissue has been removed, the remaining cavity walls need to be assessed as to their durability, as thin walls are prone to fracture. This is often the case in multisurface cavities, especially when replacing large amalgam restorations. In such circumstances, consideration should be given to providing cuspal coverage and protection of the restoration.

Preserve as much tooth tissue as possible   All restorations have a finite lifespan and will ultimately need replacement, a process known as the 'restorative cycle'; each time a restoration is replaced, more tooth tissue is lost. By minimising injudicious tissue removal the lifespan of the tooth can be improved, for example class II cavities should not be extended on the occlusal surface just to provide retention. Instead, grooves should be placed on internal line angles to preserve tooth tissue (Figure 41.2a,b). Large cavities will weaken teeth to a greater extent than smaller cavities.

Consider the location of the restoration margins   The location of the restoration margins are important and can impact upon periodontal health, routine plaque control and bonding procedures. Subgingival restoration margins are harder to clean and can promote plaque retention. Both factors will have a negative effect upon periodontal health. Subgingival margins contraindicate the placement of composite resin as adequate moisture control cannot be maintained, in addition to a lack of enamel available for bonding.

Occlusal harmony   Any restoration must be placed in harmony with the patient's existing occlusion. In order to achieve this, occlusal contacts should be identified before cavity preparation and checked after restoration placement with articulating paper. Occlusal contacts must not be present on the junction of the cavity and the tooth as premature breakdown of the restoration may occur. If this situation is encountered, extension of the cavity is justified so that occlusal contacts are entirely on the restoration.

Provide retention and resistance form   Retention form is those features of the cavity that prevent loss of the restoration in the long axis of the tooth. Resistance form refers to the cavity features that prevent displacement of the restoration due to horizontal or rotational forces. Bonding the restoration to tooth tissue can retain a restoration, but for cavities to be restored conventionally with amalgam, mechanical features must be provided. Such features should have a sharp outline and be placed in dentine, ideally on opposing cavity walls for maximum effect. Such features include:

- pits (Figure 41.3a)
- grooves (Figure 41.3a)
- undercuts (Figure 41.3b)
- peripheral shelf
- slots.

Ensure the restoration will be durable   Make sure that the cavity provides enough space for sufficient thickness of material, for example amalgam requires a minimum thickness of 2 mm. Consider features to minimise stress concentration, such as a groove at the junction of the gingival floor and pulpal wall.

Choice of restorative material   Modify the cavity according the properties of the restorative material to be used (see below).

Preparation techniques

Several methods exist for cavity preparation, but rotary and hand instruments are still the most commonly used. Rotary instruments generate significant amounts of heat, which can damage the pulp. Copious water cooling should be used with both 'fast' and 'slow' hand pieces together with light pressure. It is important to select the correct bur for each part of the preparation. The fast handpiece should be used for accessing the lesion through enamel. Steel burs in the slow handpiece should be used for caries removal and when providing retentive features.

Cavity preparation should occur under a rubber dam. This reduces the risk of bacterial contamination if an inadvertent pulp exposure occurs.

Material-specific cavity features
Amalgam

Amalgam is weak in thin section; therefore all cavosurface angles (CSA) must be 90° to provide sufficient bulk of amalgam so as not to fracture (Figure 41.4a,b). This is often not achieved if the wrong bur is used. Commonly used fissure burs will create a larger CSA, with a thinner edge of amalgam that can fracture off over time (Figure 41.5). To create a 90° CSA, an inverted taper bur should be used in conjunction with gingival margin trimmers to remove any unsupported enamel (Figures 41.6 and 41.7).

Amalgam restorations are usually retained with mechanical features. To provide retention, the cavity should be undercut, having occlusally convergent walls. For more extensive cavities, features such as slots, pits and a peripheral shelf may be required to provide resistance form.

Resin composite

Resin composite can be predictably bonded to enamel and to a lesser extent dentine. Enamel should be present along the entire margin of the cavity (Figure 41.8a). This is often not achieved on the floor of proximal boxes. In this area, every effort should be made to preserve enamel, which will result in a more predictable bond and reduce the risk of failure and resultant microleakage. Unlike amalgam cavities, all unsupported enamel need not be removed during preparation. The enamel can be bevelled to increase the surface area for bonding, although this should not be done in areas of occlusal contact as the thin edge of composite may chip under loading (Figure 41.8b).

Mechanical retention is not usually required, but for large multisurface restorations adjunctive resistance and retention form should be provided to minimise the stresses placed upon the bond. Preparation should be undertaken with small round burs to preserve tooth tissue. A rubber dam should be used during preparation and is mandatory for composite placement.

42 Cavity liners and conditioners

Figure 42.1 (a, b) When greater then 1.5 mm dentine exists, only a sealer is required; this should be applied to all exposed dentinal cavity surfaces (blue)

Figure 42.2 (a, b) When 0.6–1.5 mm of dentine remains overlying the pulp, resin-modified glass ionomer is placed in these areas (green) and sealer placed over the remaining dentine (blue)

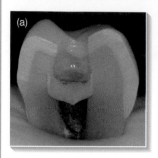

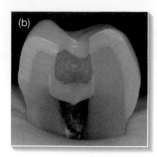

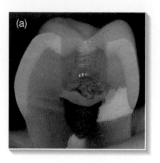

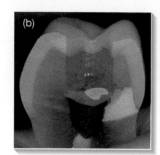

Figure 42.3 (a, b) When less than 0.5 mm of dentine overlies the pulp, calcium hydroxide is placed (yellow); this is covered with resin-modified glass ionomer (green) and a sealer placed over the remaining dentine (blue)

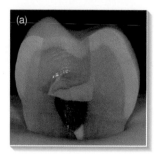

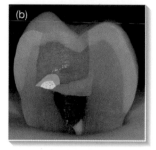

Table 42.1 Materials commonly used for pulp protection

Purpose	Material type	Commercial examples	Indication	Restorative material
Sealer	Dentine bonding agent	Prime and Bond NT (Dentsply International, Philadelphia, USA)	Exposed dentine in a cavity preparation	Use with amalgam or composite restorations
	Desensitiser	Gluma (Heraeus- Kulzer, Hanau, Germany)		Amalgam restorations
Liner	Hard-setting calcium hydroxide	Dycal (Dentsply International, Philadelphia, USA)	In areas where 0.5 mm or less dentine is overlying the pulp	Use with amalgam or composite restorations
	Resin-modified glass ionomer	Vitrebond (3M ESPE Dental Products, Minnesota, USA)	To cover hard setting calcium hydroxide In areas where 0.6–1.5 mm of dentine covers the pulp	Use with amalgam or composite restorations

Dentistry at a Glance. First Edition. Edited by Elizabeth Kay. © 2016 John Wiley & Sons, Ltd. Published 2016 by John Wiley & Sons, Ltd.
Companion website: www.ataglanceseries.com/dentistryseries/dentistry

Pulp protection

The pulp can be damaged prior to, during and after restorative intervention. Preserving pulpal health is a primary goal when undertaking restorative dental procedures. Common causes of pulpal injury associated with procedures include:
• Bacterial contamination
• Excessive heat generation during preparation
• Exposure to noxious chemicals
• Desiccation of tooth tissue during preparation
• Compromised pulpal blood supply due to local anaesthetic vasoconstrictors.

Of these, bacterial contamination is the most significant and occurs commonly. Dentine is permeated by numerous tubules, which communicate directly with the dental pulp. Odontoblast processes and nerve endings also extend into the tubules, which are filled with fluid. Exposure of the dentinal tubules to thermal and chemical stimuli results in fluid movement in the tubules with subsequent deformation and firing of nerve endings, causing patient symptoms. Dentinal tubules also provide a direct pathway for bacteria and their products to enter the pulp, causing inflammation.

Pulp protection materials

Pulp protection materials aim to protect the pulp from thermal, chemical and bacterial insult, in an attempt to maintain pulpal health. Thermal irritation used to be considered an important cause of pulpal inflammation when amalgam was the most widely used direct restorative material, due to it being a conductor of temperature change. Irritant materials may also leach from the restorative material over time and cause pulpal inflammation. Despite this, the main focus of such materials is in preventing microleakage of bacteria (and bacterial products), which are now considered the most important cause of pulpal pathology.

Sealers

Sealers aim to seal the dentinal tubules to prevent ingress of bacteria and fluid movement. The most commonly used sealers include dentine bonding agents and certain desensitising agents, which are aqueous solutions containing 2-hydroxyethylmethacrylate (HEMA) and substances which can occlude dentinal tubules such as glutaraldehyde. Sealers are liquid preparations, which are applied to all the exposed dentine surfaces of a preparation (Figure 42.1a,b).

Liners

Deeper cavities will expose a greater number of tubules, which are larger in diameter, increasing the potential for pulpal inflammation. Liners also seal exposed tubules but often have a therapeutic effect, such as being antibacterial, promoting dentine deposition and releasing fluoride. Liners should be used sparingly, only in the deepest areas of a cavity preparation, in order to retain the maximum area available for bonding. They should be applied in a thickness of 0.5 mm. Materials commonly used as liners include:
• **Hard-setting calcium hydroxide**: This material has a pH of 12 and, as a result, is antibacterial and can induce tertiary dentine formation. The major disadvantages of this material are its inability to bond to tooth tissue and its high solubility. Used on its own, the material will undergo dissolution over time, leaving a void between the restoration and cavity. Microleakage and secondary caries will ensue.
• **Glass ionomer/ resin-modified glass ionomer**: These materials have the advantage of bonding to tooth tissue and the potential to release fluoride, helping to promote remineralisation. Such materials have a lower solubility than calcium hydroxide and are relatively inert to the pulp.

Indications and application techniques

All preparations that result in dentine exposure should be sealed. The type of sealer used will be influenced by the restorative material chosen. For minimal cavities, resin composite will be the material of choice. Placing such a restoration will involve using a dentine bonding agent; therefore, the dentinal tubules will be sealed without an additional clinical procedure. For amalgam cavities, either a dentine bonding agent or desensitising agent can be selected (Table 42.1).

For more extensive cavities, the clinician must assess how much dentine remains over the pulp in the deepest part of the cavity. The depth of dentine remaining in the deepest part of the cavity overlying the pulp should be estimated to fall into one of the three following categories:
• Greater than 1.5 mm (Figure 42.1a,b)
• 0.6–1.5 mm (Figure 42.2a,b)
• 0.5 mm or less (Figure 42.3a,b).

The type of pulp protection required can be seen in Table 42.1.

When less than 0.5 mm of dentine exists over the pulp, every attempt should be made to minimise bacterial load and promote the deposition of tertiary dentine. In such instances, hard-setting calcium hydroxide is the material of choice. Due to its previously mentioned shortcomings, it must be applied sparingly only to the area it is needed. Specific applicators are available, for example the Dycal applicator; however, many clinicians advocate the ball end of a basic periodontal examination (BPE) probe. Resin-modified glass ionomer should be placed over it to prevent dissolution of the calcium hydroxide, again using an applicator. A sealer should then be placed over the remaining exposed dentine (Figure 42.3).

Cavity conditioners

Use of any instrument will leave a residue on the tooth surface, known as the smear layer. Conditioning is a process whereby an acidic substance is applied to the prepared surface to modify/remove this layer and any contaminants such as salivary glycoproteins, making it more conducive to bonding a restoration. This is routinely done when placing composite restorations using 37% orthophosphoric acid, which also demineralises the tooth surface and opens dentinal tubules.

When placing resin-modified and conventional glass ionomer restorations, the tooth surface can also be pretreated using a conditioning agent. Such substances are much weaker acids, which do not cause demineralisation and exposure of tubules. They do remove or modify the smear layer and improve the flow of the restorative material onto the tooth surface by lowering its surface energy. They usually consist of a weak acid such as polyacrylic or polymaleic acid (10–25%). Using such conditioners can improve the bond strength of glass ionomer restorations to tooth tissue when compared to no pretreatment.

43 Cavity preparation for plastic tooth restorations

Figure 43.1 The current clinical practice of mechanical excavation combines a peripheral dentine excavation, carried out using a round burr (a, b), with elimination of the centrally infected tissue using an excavator (c, d). The probe is used to assess clinical consistency, and here dentine that is hard to the touch has not yet been obtained (e). Note that the deeper and soft carious dentine is a fragmented tissue (f). An excavation close to the pulp represents a risk because cracks along the fragments may lead to pulp exposure
Source: Kidd EAM et al. (2008). In: Fejerskov O, Kidd E (eds). *Dental Caries: The Disease and Its Clinical Management*, 2nd edn. Reproduced with permission of John Wiley and Sons, Ltd.

Figure 43.2 Figure 43.2 Partially excavated cavity; note the soft, wet dentine
Source: van Amerongen JP et al. (2008). In: Fejerskov O, Kidd E (eds). *Dental Caries: The Disease and Its Clinical Management*, 2nd edn. Reproduced with permission of John Wiley and Sons, Ltd.

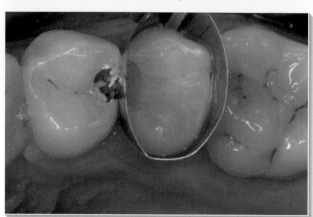

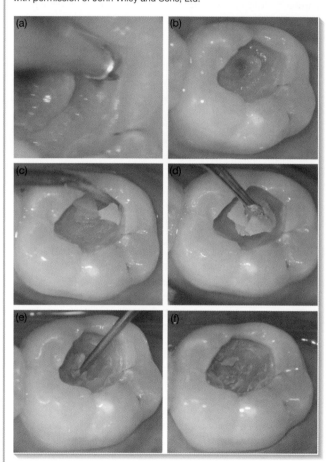

The decision to restore a tooth must be taken carefully, and only when the caries in the tooth has progressed to a stage where remineralisation and repair can no longer be expected. All restorations are 'temporary' in as much as all will fail eventually, with failure rates varying between different types of restorative material. For a summary of published failure rates for different types of plastic restorative material see Figure 44.1.

The principles that underpin cavity preparation were first established by GV Black and are just as valid today as they were in 19th century (Figure 43.1). Essentially, these translate as:

• Gain access to the decay (when the caries is through an enamel surface)
• Remove the caries and resulting unsupported enamel
• Assess which restorative material will give the 'best' outcome bearing in mind the properties of the material
• Modify the residual tooth tissue to make a cavity that will maximise the life expectancy of the restorative material.

Accessing caries

Caries progression through enamel into dentine results in destruction in the dentine that is much 'wider' than the damage to the enamel. Thus it is necessary to remove some of the sound but unsupported enamel to gain adequate access to the underlying carious dentine. Enamel is the hardest of all tissues in the body and requires very powerful cutting tools to remove it. There are a number of options available to the dentist, including air abrasion and lasers, but the most common is a tungsten carbide-tipped or diamond-coated bur in a dental handpiece, most commonly an air rotor. The initial approach into the carious lesion should be sufficient to allow access to the decay whist keeping the cavity small to prevent unnecessary removal of sound tooth tissue.

Once you have exposed the carious you need to remove the carious tissue.

Tip: Make your initial access into a carious lesion with a bur with a cutting tip no more than 2 mm long to reduce the risk of exposing the pulp. You can use the length of the cutting surface of the bur as a depth guide.

Caries removal

We now recognise that there are multiple 'levels' to a carious dentine lesion. The most important distinction from a clinical perspective is the differentiation between caries-infected and caries-affected dentine. Caries is essentially a process of demineralisation driven by acid-producing bacteria. As the caries progresses through dentine the acids cause demineralisation and the demineralised dentine is subsequently colonised by bacteria. So:

• The carious dentine closer to the enamel will be both demineralised and infected with bacteria, this is the **caries-infected dentine** and should be removed.
• The carious dentine closer to the pulp may (depending on the extent of the lesion) be demineralised without infection, this is **caries-affected dentine** and can be left during cavity preparation depending on the choice of restorative material.

Differentiating between infected and affected dentine during cavity preparation can be difficult.

Texture

There are subtle changes in texture between the two; all carious dentine will be relatively soft, wet and crumbly but caries-infected dentine will be softer and wetter than caries-affected tissue. Indeed, caries-affected dentine will become progressively harder as the you progress closer to the advancing margin of the carious lesion. Soft dentine can be removed with a bur, preferably in a slow handpiece or using excavators, but the operator needs considerable experience to differentiate between the subtle texture differences in dentine (Figure 43.2). The most common advice is to remove all wet crumbly (friable) dentine during this process.

Tip: Wherever possible practice removing caries on extracted human teeth to try to develop the sense of feel for carious dentine.

Bacterial presence

A variety of dyes have been advocated to try to differentiate between the presence and absence of bacteria (and hence infected and affected dentine). However, it is now recognised that while these dyes may be an adjunct; they are not selective solely for bacteria, but rather staining the demineralised matrix of carious dentine and other areas of dentine with reduced mineralisation such as the amelodentinal junction and circumpulpal dentine.

Chemomechanical caries removal

A mixture of sodium hypochlorite with lysine, leucine and glutamic acids, and some other amino acids in a carboxymethylcellulose base is commercially available as Carisolv®. Activating this product results in the formation of N-monochloroglycine and N-monochloroaminobutyric acid. When these are applied to carious dentine they dissolve the collagen in the carious lesion making the infected dentine easier to remove. Recent evidence suggests that dentine removal guided by Carisolve is probably the most reliable method for removing infected dentine and leaving the affected dentine that can then remineralise.

Unsupported enamel

Enamel is a brittle material and needs to be supported by dentine to exhibit durability. Where dentine is destroyed by caries, eliminating support for the enamel, consideration needs to be given to removing the enamel.

The decision can be modified by the choice of restorative material, so where a resin composite is being used limited substantial elements of enamel may be retained to be supported by the bonded material. If unsupported enamel is not removed it can fracture during or after restoration of the tooth with resulting marginal discrepancies around an amalgam restoration and marginal gaps round a composite that may result in postoperative sensitivity.

Tip: When in doubt about the support for remaining enamel, push firmly against the enamel with an amalgam plugger in all directions.

Choice of plastic restorative materials

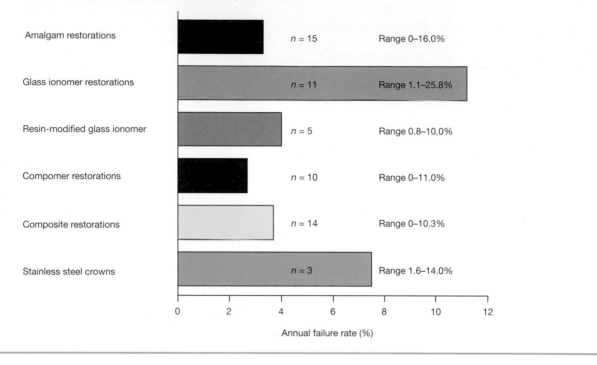

Figure 44.1 Median values and ranges for annual failure rates obtained in longitudinal studies of class I/II restorations in posterior primary teeth using different types of restorative materials; n, number of studies

Source: Qvist V (2008). In: Fejerskov O, Kidd E (eds). *Dental Caries: The Disease and Its Clinical Management*, 2nd edn. Reproduced with permission of John Wiley and Sons, Ltd.

Selection of an appropriate restorative material will depend on a variety of factors:

- The tooth concerned (and hence the need for an aesthetic material) along with the location of the cavity on the tooth
- The extent of destruction of tooth tissue (and hence the physical characteristics of the restorative material in terms of durability)
- The amount of remaining tooth tissue (which can be used to support/retain the 'new' restoration)
- The caries risk status of the individual
- The ability to attain a required level of moisture control to maximise the chances of restoration longevity.

Location of the tooth and extent of the cavity

Generally, teeth in the anterior region of the mouth will be restored using tooth-coloured materials while the options for posterior teeth include metallic restorations where aesthetics may not be so critical.

Anterior teeth

There are two major groups of tooth-coloured direct restorative materials: glass ionomer cements (GICs) and dental composite resins. Their relative longevity can be compared in Figure 44.1.

Generally, the better aesthetic characteristics of composite resins predicate their use for the majority of anterior restorations, particularly extensive restorations involving the incisal edge of teeth. GICs are more likely to be used for small class III and class V restorations, particularly where the patient exhibits high caries risk.

Posterior teeth

The choice of materials for posterior teeth includes not only composite resins and GICs but also includes dental amalgam. Generally, GICs may be used for class V cavities and provisional restorations. The choice between composite resin and dental amalgam for load-bearing restorations on occlusal and proximal surfaces needs to be based on careful consideration of the following variables:

- **Extent of the cavity**: Dental amalgam exhibits greater longevity than composite resins with large restorations where wear of the composite in function becomes a significant problem.
- **Patient choice**: Some patients elect to have tooth coloured restorations rather than metallic.
- **Hypersensitivity**: Some patients manifest a hypersensitivity reaction to dental amalgam with 'lichenoid eruptions' on the cheek mucosa proximate to the restorative material.

It is the responsibility of the dentist/ therapist to obtain informed consent from their patient concerning the choice of restorative material, and particularly when a composite resin is being used in a large cavity to explain that the restoration will exhibit reduced longevity compared with a dental amalgam restoration in the same cavity. There is an impending move to ban the use of dental amalgam to reduce the bio-availability of mercury in the environment. If this happens then the choices will be more stark unless new materials become available.

Quantity and quality of remaining tooth tissue

Restorations need to be both supported and retained by the remaining tooth tissue after cavity preparation. As a consequence, the amount of remaining tooth and its location influences the choice of restorative material. When there are substantial amounts of remaining tooth, there tend to be more options in terms of choice of material. As the amount of remaining tooth diminishes, the options reduce as restorations become bigger, favouring dental amalgam over composite resin in terms of durability. Perversely, with extreme loss of tooth tissue, where an adhesive approach to retention is the only possibility, composite resin may offer the best available alternative, as adhesive options with dental amalgam are not as effective as those for resin composite.

Caries risk

There is limited evidence that GIC restorations are prone to the development of fewer carious lesions associated with the restoration than composite resin in high caries risk patients.

Moisture control

Any restorative technique that is using an adhesive approach to retaining the restoration requires a high level of moisture control during restoration placement. If either a dentine or an enamel surface that has been prepared for bonding is contaminated with saliva or blood a protein film forms on the surface of the tooth, preventing the formation of an acceptable adhesive bond. This applies to both GICs and resin composites. Contamination of the tooth surface will both reduce retention of the restoration and increase the risks of marginal leakage. This is probably the biggest single challenge to finding a replacement for dental amalgam.

Physical (mechanical) retention

Dental amalgam has no intrinsic capacity to bond to tooth tissue. There are some techniques that can result in a bonded amalgam restoration (see Chapter 45) but the majority of amalgam restorations are retained as a result of mechanical retention within a cavity. The nature of the carious process with spread of demineralisation along the amelodentinal junction (ADJ) results in cavities that are wider at the base than at the top, making a naturally undercut shape. The extent of undercut needs to be reassessed once unsupported enamel has been removed to ensure there is adequate mechanical retention present.

Where there is extensive loss of tooth tissue involving the cusps of a tooth, there may be the need to prepare grooves or pits in the remaining dentine to develop mechanical retention for the cavity. These are often used in association with a bonded approach to maximise the retention of the amalgam in a tooth. You need to think about why you are placing a plastic restoration in a tooth in relation to the location of accessory retentive features. So, for example, if you are planning to crown a tooth ultimately the features need to be prepared in such a way that you will not destroy the retention they give when you are cutting your crown preparation.

45 Plastic restorations

Bonding a restoration to a tooth as opposed to relying solely upon mechanical retention is a very significant advantage, and is achievable for dental amalgam, composite resin and glass ionomer cement (GIC) restorations.

Bonding amalgam

The metallic alloy used in dental amalgam has an oxidised metal surface and so can be attached to tooth tissue using any adhesive agent that will bond both enamel and dentine to a metal oxide layer. The concept was originally described in the 1890s as the 'Baldwin' technique. Contemporary practice involves two different groups of materials: either a resin-based agent such as the adhesives RelyX unicem (3M ESPE) or Panavia (Kuraray); or a glass ionomer cement luting agent such as Aquacem (Dentsply). The specific technique will depend on the agent used so the operator needs to follow the manufacturers' instructions for bonding to tooth tissue. However, the principle involved is that a thin film of the relevant agent is applied to a clean, dry dentine and enamel surface of the cavity. The amalgam is then condensed into place on top of the setting bonding agent, producing a thin film of lute at the interface between the amalgam and the tooth. This process is highly technique sensitive, the operator has to work quickly to cover the resin while it is still setting and the process of condensation starts in the middle of the cavity and works towards the periphery to 'squeeze' the lute out along the interface between restorative material and tooth taking care not to incorporate the lute into the amalgam as it is being condensed.

Tip: For bonding to work, a high standard of moisture control is essential. Pellicle that precipitates onto a prepared enamel or dentine surface that is contaminated with saliva will prevent effective bonding.

Bonding composite resins

Bonding composite to tooth has become a routine part of dentistry and there is no difference between posterior and anterior teeth other than the greater challenge of preventing moisture contamination of the bond interface.

Bonding glass ionomer cement

Success in bonding GICs includes removal of the smear layer and any deposited pellicle from the dentine and enamel of the tooth prior to placing the GIC. This is achieved by surface preparation with the same polycarboxylic acid used to manufacture the GIC (most often poly(acrylic) acid). This is washed off the tooth surface prior to drying and applying the GIC.

Matrix techniques

A huge variety of matrices have been developed and described for use with anterior and posterior restorations. Choice depends on the nature of the restorative material and the size and extent of the cavity.

The matrix is used to define the periphery of the restoration. This is important when the caries or cavity preparation has resulted in sufficient destruction of a tooth that the chosen material cannot be placed to restore both form and contact relationships in any other way. It is also used to limit the flow or movement of the material beyond the cavity margins to prevent formation of excess material on the tooth surface, giving an overhanging edge. Overhangs are the most significant variable associated with the development of a new carious lesion around an existing restoration.

Matrices vary in complexity from simple transparent strips held in place with finger pressure, to help shape composite resins, to more complex circumferential or sectional designs for use with composite resin or dental amalgam.

Whenever possible, a matrix should be used to shape a composite resin or GIC restoration. The surface finish of the material formed against a piece of polyester strip is the best that can be achieved in terms of smoothness and gloss.

Matrices for composite restorations have different requirements compared with those for amalgam. They are mostly transparent in nature, to permit light curing of the restorative material and some have a preformed profile to help to reconstruct the natural bulbosity or angles of teeth.

Matrices for amalgam have to be sufficiently robust to be able to withstand the pressures developed during the packing of an amalgam restoration, so are usually made from stainless steel. The matrix also needs to be capable of being held against the surface of the tooth with sufficient 'grip' that amalgam does not get pushed beyond the edge of the cavity to form an overhanging margin. They can be either sectional or circumferential in nature; for both types, there is a need to use a wedge at the base of a box, wherever possible, to hold the band against the tooth to help to prevent ledge formation. Wedging a matrix band also has the benefit of separating the teeth slightly so that when the wedge is removed there is some scope for rebound of the teeth, bringing them back into contact.

Matrices for GICs can either be the same as those for any other material or malleable aluminium foil matrices can be used, which are shaped prior to placing the restoration to reform the curvature of the tooth and then applied to the surface of the restoration after the material has been inserted.

Dentistry at a Glance. First Edition. Edited by Elizabeth Kay. © 2016 John Wiley & Sons, Ltd. Published 2016 by John Wiley & Sons, Ltd.
Companion website: www.ataglanceseries.com/dentistryseries/dentistry

46 Amalgam restorations

Dental amalgam is a brittle material that needs to be used in adequate thickness to have structural integrity. A minimum of 1 mm in depth of amalgam is needed to achieve such structural durability, and the amalgam needs to have a 'but fit' against the adjacent tooth tissue so there are no fine tapered edges of material that can subsequently fracture. Amalgam is packed (or condensed) into the cavity under moderate force, and therefore the floor of the cavity, and particularly the floor of any areas where the cavity comes out onto the surface of the tooth, needs to be perpendicular to the long axis of the tooth and of adequate depth into the tooth to give a restoration with the required structural integrity. Any fine shards of unsupported enamel must be removed prior to placing the restoration and this is particularly important on the vertical walls of a proximal box. Failure to do this will result in the enamel being crushed during matrix placement and rapid breakdown of the margin of the restoration as the crushed fragments are lost.

Once the caries has been removed from the floor of the cavity, modification of the cavity is needed, to both achieve the design principles (outlined above) and to give durability of the material as well as to give adequate mechanical retention. It is at this stage that a decision can be made whether to use accessory grooves or pits cut into the tooth to give mechanical retention and/or to use an adhesive approach.

Once the cavity is finalised, the chosen matrix is selected (if required) and applied around the tooth. Wherever possible, a wedge should be used between teeth to hold the band firmly against the tooth surface below the box of a cavity, and to separate the teeth.

Dental amalgam is mixed in predosed capsules and carried to the tooth in increments using an amalgam 'gun'. It would be best practice only to use non-gamma 2 alloys for amalgam restorations. The first increment should be placed in the least accessible part of the cavity (unless you are using a bonded approach) and the material packed in place using an amalgam condenser. Firm finger pressure is sufficient to produce an homogenous mass of material. During the packing process, the surface of the material becomes mercury rich and as further increments of material are added progressively to the already packed surface this mercury-rich layer moves up the cavity. Packing should continue until the cavity is over filled, allowing the mercury-rich layer to be removed during carving. The speed of the setting reaction of the material can be manipulated by the manufacturer, and so some amalgams set more rapidly than others. You need to practice with a new material to get used to its handling characteristics.

When the material is firm in consistency as part of the setting process, the amalgam can be carved to shape using hand instruments. Carving should initially focus on removing excess material, so that the remaining restoration fills the underlying cavity without extending beyond it and also restores normal functional anatomy. With all restorations there will be an inevitable need to check the functional occlusion once initial carving has been done to ensure that all previous tooth contacts have been restored, with the amalgam also in functional contact with the opposing tooth. During the early stages of the setting reaction, it is necessary to ask the patient to close gently onto the restoration to prevent traumatic damage to the freshly placed material, particularly over the marginal ridge for an interproximal restoration.

The final stage of amalgam placement is to polish the restoration a minimum of 24 hours after placement. This stage is often omitted by dentists but does give benefit in terms of reducing the rate of corrosion of the restoration. Globally there are policy initiatives to reduce the bio-burden of mercury. As part of this process it is likely that there will be a global ban on the use of amalgam for dental purposes in the near future.

Dentistry at a Glance. First Edition. Edited by Elizabeth Kay. © 2016 John Wiley & Sons, Ltd. Published 2016 by John Wiley & Sons, Ltd.
Companion website: www.ataglanceseries.com/dentistryseries/dentistry

Composite resin restorations

Wherever possible, rubber dam should be used to isolate teeth during a bonding procedure. This greatly helps to achieve moisture control through isolation of the tooth. There is little clinical evidence of benefit in terms of longevity of restorations; however, the quality of isolation simply makes it easier to place the relevant restoration. It is not always possible to do so, but in the absence of a dam very careful moisture control with cotton rolls or other agents is essential for success.

Tip: If a surface you want to bond to is consistently being contaminated with blood, saliva or gingival crevicular fluid (GCF) you cannot bond to it and your composite resin is likely to fail quickly as a result.

Composite resin is less brittle than amalgam and so can be left in thinner section at the margins of restorations. However, there is a danger of mechanical failure if these sections are fine and in functional load.

Unsupported enamel should be removed prior to placing a composite material. If this is not done, the fine brittle edges of the cavity will shatter under the strain of curing and shrinkage of the composite material, resulting in a poor seal at the edge of the cavity.

Due consideration needs to be given to the orientation of the enamel to the bond interface. Enamel is an anisotropic material with very different physical characteristics in different bending axes. The majority of bond-strength studies to enamel are done using surfaces prepared perpendicular to the prism axis and this gives the greatest attachment strength. The bond strength to enamel prepared parallel to the prism axis is markedly lower (because the fracture resistance of enamel is lower in this orientation). In the majority of circumstances when bonding an intracoronal restoration, the bond interface to enamel is parallel to the prism axis and not perpendicular.

Furthermore, caries-affected dentine has a different structure compared to dentine that has not been subject to caries, such that the dentine tubules in caries-affected dentine are blocked by substantial plugs of mineral. The dentine preparation processes for bonding does not destroy these mineralised blockages, therefore it is not possible to get plugs of resin extending into the dentine tubules. These plugs produce about 40% of the attachment strength between composite and dentine, and so caries-affected (or sclerotic) dentine is more difficult to bond to. This is the type of surface that dentists are habitually bonding material to during, restorative procedures.

As a consequence, the ability to bond composite resin to a dental cavity is less than might be anticipated on the basis of raw published data about attachment strengths alone.

All composite resins shrink during the setting process to varying extent, with fluid, 'flowable', materials shrinking more and those using ring-opening setting technology shrinking least. Strategies for placing composite restorations are designed to compensate for this shrinkage and also to compensate for the depth of material that can be cured with a dental curing light.

Dentistry at a Glance. First Edition. Edited by Elizabeth Kay. © 2016 John Wiley & Sons, Ltd. Published 2016 by John Wiley & Sons, Ltd.
Companion website: www.ataglanceseries.com/dentistryseries/dentistry

48 Building composite resin restorations

Small interproximal restorations will usually be restored in one increment where the composite is less then 2–3 mm in depth (from any available surface to the maximum depth of cure). Once caries is removed from the cavity and any unsupported enamel removed, the enamel and dentine are prepared for bonding. The matrix most commonly used is a polyester (Mylar®) strip that is wrapped through the contact zone before material is placed in the cavity. With the matrix in place the bonding procedure is performed (specific details of this will vary according to the type of bonding agent used) and the composite is placed from the aspect of the cavity that will give best access for delivery. Then the strip is drawn gently through the cavity away from the direction that the composite was introduced, to maximise material adaptation to the opposite surface of the tooth, before being wrapped round the tooth to form the shape of the restoration. A curing light is then used to set the material. It is important to realise that light travels in straight lines, so the head of the curing tip needs to be perpendicular to the surface of the composite and also as close to the surface of the matrix as possible to optimise cure performance. The curing process takes up to 40 seconds of exposure for each unit area of the curing light (timing will depend on the intensity of the light itself; always follow the manufacturers' instructions).

Once the material is cured in the cavity, the matrix is removed and any excess carefully removed; small amounts can simply be 'flicked off' using a sharp instrument. Larger areas of excess will need to be adjusted with appropriate small-particle diamond finishing burs in a handpiece, before polishing and finishing. The smoothest surface for any composite restoration is that produced by the matrix. However, if the surface needs to be adjusted then it will need to be polished, most commonly using a variety of graded finishing disks.

Tip: Great care is needed when using rotating finishing disks; these can easily lacerate the tongue, lips or cheek if used in a slapdash manner.

Larger restorations

There are three very significant challenges with larger composite resin restorations, to cope with:
- Limitations in terms of depth of cure of individual increments of composite
- Shrinkage of the material during its setting reaction
- Creating a contact between adjacent teeth.

When the composite that is being placed is deeper than the manufacturer's recommended depth of cure and when the composite is in considerable bulk, it is sensible to place the material in a series of increments to optimise the quality of cure and to mitigate the effect of polymerisation shrinkage. Incremental placement does not alter the amount that a composite resin shrinks; that can only be determined by the manufacturer. However, as the material sets, the early stages of shrinkage are accommodated by flow of the material in the cavity. As the material becomes more rigid, the whole bulk of the material starts to contract and this applies forces to the tooth through the bonded interface, potentially damaging the tooth and causing it to distort. Incremental placement allows for a greater proportion of the shrinkage to be accommodated by flow rather than bulk contraction for a given quantity of material.

There have been many different incremental placement techniques described but the most common is the 'herringbone' approach, where the material is placed in opposing diagonal increments against one side of the tooth and then the other.

Creating a contact point is more difficult with composite resin than with dental amalgam; firstly, because the material shrinks during setting, resulting in reduction of the bulk of material and, secondly, because the viscosity and flow characteristics of composite are different from those of amalgam. Amalgam is consolidated into a firm mass during the packing procedure, which pushes the matrix outwards, helping to push the matrix band against the adjacent tooth. Composite is a viscoelastic material and cannot be used to squeeze the matrix band in the same way. Careful use of wedges to separate teeth prior to placement and shaped transparent matrix bands that have the necessary bulge built into the band to form the contact zone can help.

The band is placed on the tooth and wedged in place prior to bonding. Once the tooth has been prepared and the bonding agent placed, the first layer of material can be applied. Some authorities advocate the use of a low-viscosity 'flowable' material in the floor of the cavity and box. This may seem counter intuitive because these materials shrink more than conventional resins, but they also flow more and it has been shown that the set material adapts better to the tooth, creating a better marginal seal. Increments of material are then applied to build the restoration up to full size. It is not necessary to overfill a cavity to the same extent as a dental amalgam; indeed, filling close to the optimal size will both save material and reduce the need for occlusal adjustment after placement.

Once the material has been placed, the rubber dam can be removed and the occlusion of the restoration can be adjusted using small-particle diamond burs in a handpiece and other polishing instruments. Rotating disks are of limited value in the central fissure areas of posterior restorations but may be of value on the outer surfaces of larger restorations. Unlike amalgam, tapping the teeth together alone does not produce marks on the composite and an articulating paper needs to be used from the outset. This needs to be sufficiently thin to detect contacts at the limits of the proprioceptive capacity of the teeth (around 14 μm). Articulating papers that are this thin need to be supported in special forceps to guide them in to place. If a thicker paper is used it will not mark the contacts accurately.

Dentistry at a Glance. First Edition. Edited by Elizabeth Kay. © 2016 John Wiley & Sons, Ltd. Published 2016 by John Wiley & Sons, Ltd.
Companion website: www.ataglanceseries.com/dentistryseries/dentistry

49 Non-plastic intracoronal restorations

Figure 49.1 Illustration of a two-surface inlay in a maxillary posterior tooth

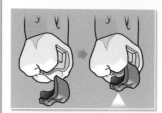

Figure 49.2 Gold inlays in posterior teeth

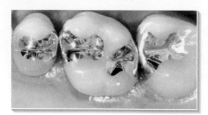
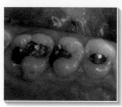

Figure 49.3 Amalgam restorations replaced with resin composite inlays

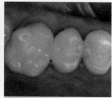

Figure 49.4 Amalgam restorations replaced with ceramic inlays

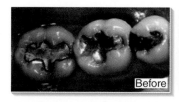
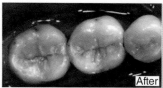

Before

After

Intracoronal restorations are defined as restorations that are placed within the clinical crown of a tooth. Indirect (non-plastic) intracoronal restorations (**inlays**) traditionally were made of cast metal alloys (e.g. gold alloys), but are increasingly made of tooth-coloured materials (e.g. composite resins, ceramics or zirconium).

Onlays are inlays that cover one or more cusps of the tooth, lending strength to the restored tooth unit by providing cuspal reinforcement. Onlays fit 'onto' the tooth (extracoronal restorations) and are not discussed in this chapter.

Unlike plastic restorations, inlays are constructed partly or completely outside the mouth. The construction of inlays is based on an impression taken of the inlay cavity preparation. Subsequently, the inlay is constructed outside the mouth and then cemented into the tooth using a luting cement (Figure 49.1).

Indications: when it is considered that a posterior tooth may not be satisfactorily restored by means of a direct (plastic) restoration and in situations where an indirect approach may be required to successfully restore or, where indicated clinically, modify the form and contacts of a damaged or diseased tooth.

Advantages: There is an opportunity to restore or modify the anatomy, including the contours and contacts of a cavitated tooth outside the mouth. This can be done in a way to facilitate cleaning in clinical service and, in turn, enhance the periodontal response to the restoration.

Disadvantages: More removal of sound tooth tissue is required than for a direct restoration. It is a multiple (at least two) appointment procedure with the need for temporisation between appointments, unless a computer-aided design and computer aided manufacturing (CAD-CAM) technique is used (see below). Other disadvantages are cost and limited opportunity to undertake repairs and refurbishments in clinical service.

Construction techniques:

• The **indirect** technique requires at least two clinical visits with temporisation between visits and laboratory construction of the final restoration. The restoration is constructed on a model cast from a working impression recorded following completion of the cavity preparation.

• The **semidirect** (CAD-CAM) technique (see below) can be performed at chair side with intraoral and extraoral steps during a single visit.

Temporisation: The temporary restoration is intended to temporarily restore, seal and protect the prepared tooth from bacteria, prevent tooth fracture and movement, maintain occlusion, and provide occlusal function until such times as the completed restoration can be fitted.

Gold inlays

Gold inlays, once popular for the restoration of large cavities in posterior teeth (Figure 49.2), are now less commonly used given recent advances in the qualities and durability of direct and indirect tooth-coloured restorative systems and patient preference for 'aesthetic' restorations.

• **Material qualities of gold alloys**
  • High compressive strength
  • High tensile strength
  • Allows thin bevels of metal to be placed over margins to protect fragile enamel walls
  • Does not discolour the tooth nor will it decompose or tarnish
  • As a malleable material, gold can be burnished to adapt to the remaining tooth tissues
  • High wear resistance

• **Key steps of preparation design**
  • All enamel should be supported by sound dentin
  • Undercut-free preparation
  • Isthmus width should be at least 2 mm with a depth of at least 1.5 mm
  • Maximum height of isthmus and walls

- Minimum taper (6° to 15°)
- All internal angles and edges should be rounded to avoid stress and facilitate the construction of the restoration
- Occlusal and proximal bevels
- Single path of insertion.

Tooth-coloured inlays
Composite resin inlays

- **Advantages**
  - Good aesthetics
  - Good control of contact areas
  - Excellent marginal adaptation
  - Readily repairable intraorally
  - Compensation for complete polymerisation shrinkage by curing the material outside the mouth
  - Increased composite resin strength and durability because of laboratory curing processes
- **Advantages over direct placement composites**
  - Polymerisation of fit surface is possible
  - Polymerisation shrinkage takes place on model
  - More efficient overall polymerisation
  - Proximal contours and contacts can be developed outside of the mouth
  - Greater compressive strength (250–450 MPa)
  - Greater tensile strength (60–100 MPa)
  - Greater hardness
  - Less postoperative sensitivity
- **Advantages over ceramic inlays**
  - Less abrasive to opposing tooth structure
  - Repairable
  - Less expensive
- **Disadvantages**
  - Tendency to wear
  - More costly than direct restorations
  - Aesthetic outcome not quite as good as with ceramic inlays
  - More tooth reduction to create path of insertion
- **Indications**
  - Replacement of large direct restorations in premolar and permanent molar teeth (Figure 49.3)
  - Aesthetic management of teeth with extensive cavities or other damage
  - When other composite restorations are present in adjacent and opposing teeth
- **Contraindications**
  - Heavy occlusal forces
  - Inability to maintain dry operative field
  - Deep subgingival cavity margins
  - Small restoration size
  - High-caries-risk patients.
- **Key steps of preparation design**
  - All enamel should be supported by sound dentine
  - Isthmus width should be at least 2 mm with a depth of at least 1.5 mm
  - All internal angles and edges should be rounded to avoid stress and facilitate the fabrication of the restoration
  - All proximal walls should be flared or diverged 5° to 15° (no undercuts)
  - Gingival margins should be prepared to a 90° cavosurface line angle (butt joint)
  - Establish sharp cavosurface margins
  - Occlusal margins should not coincide with an occlusal contact site
  - No feather-edge margins.

Note, as a general guide, when the isthmus preparation exceeds one-half of the distance from the central fossa to the cusp tip, coverage of the cusps should be considered.

Ceramic (porcelain) inlays

- **Advantages**
  - Excellent aesthetics
  - Excellent control of contact areas
  - Excellent marginal adaptation
  - No tendency to wear of restoration
  - Low thermal conductivity
  - Low coefficient of thermal expansion
- **Disadvantages**
  - High cost
  - Construction and cementation processes are technique sensitive
  - Ceramic inlays are brittle and can fracture during try-in or cementation
  - The increased hardness of ceramics can wear the opposing dentition
- **Indications**
  - Replacement of moderate to large existing restoration in premolar and molar teeth (Figure 49.4)
  - Aesthetic management of teeth with extensive cavities or other damage
  - When other all-ceramic restorations are present, in particular, in adjacent and opposing teeth
- **Contraindications**
  - Inability to maintain dry operative field (adhesive bonding problems!)
  - Parafunctional habits like clenching, bruxism
  - Inadequate enamel left for bonding
  - Marked undercuts in the cavity preparation
  - Small restoration size
  - High-caries-risk patients.
- **Key steps of preparation design**
  - All enamel should be supported by sound dentin
  - Isthmus width should be at least 2 mm with a depth of at least 1.5 mm
  - All internal angles and edges should be rounded to avoid stress and facilitate the fabrication of the restoration
  - All proximal walls should be flared or diverged 10° to 15° (no undercuts)
  - Butt-joint margins.

Computer-aided design and manufacture techniques

Computer-aided design and manufacture techniques (CAD-CAM) techniques (e.g. Cerec, Sirona, Germany) are designed to produce ceramic inlays at chair side. An optical impression is captured by placing a small intraoral scanning camera over the prepared tooth. The restoration is designed on the computer screen, using a designated software program, by drawing the position of the finish margin and proximal contacts. Once the restoration has been designed, the digital data is transmitted to a computer-controlled milling machine, which mills the final restoration from a monochromatic ceramic block. The restoration is removed from the milling machine, ready for try-in and cementation. This technique has the advantage of producing a high-quality restoration chair side within minutes and it eliminates the need for a conventional impression, temporary restoration and multiple visits. Disadvantages include high purchasing cost of the system, maintenance, costly upgrades, and the need for extra training.

50 Crowns

Figure 50.1 Example of full coverage gold alloy crowns on a model

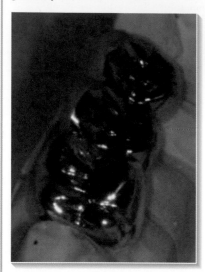

Figure 50.2 Metal–ceramic crown with ceramic occlusal coverage

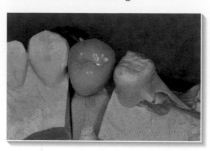

Figure 50.3 Metal–ceramic crowns with metal occlusal coverage

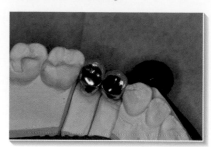

Figure 50.4 Schematic illustration of a post-retained crown

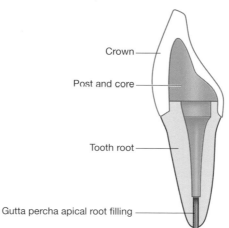

Crown

Post and core

Tooth root

Gutta percha apical root filling

Figure 50.5 Cast gold post and core

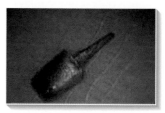

Introduction

Definition: A crown is an extracoronal dental restoration that covers the outer surface of the clinical crown and reproduces the clinical crown of a natural tooth.

The crown is cemented onto the prepared clinical crown to aid in its protection, restore its function and dental appearance.

Types of crowns

• **Full-coverage (= full veneer) crown**: covers all surfaces of the clinical crown of the tooth.

• **Partial-coverage crown**: covers most but not all available surfaces of the clinical crown of the tooth. Typically, most of the buccal surface is left uncovered. Common designs include three-quarter and seven-eighth crowns.

• **Surveyed (= milled) crown**: full-coverage crown for an abutment tooth for a removable partial denture, which incorporates design features intended to aid in the support and retention for the partial denture. Common incorporates design features of surveyed crowns include undercuts, guide planes and one or more rest seat recesses whilst the definitive crown restoration is being constructed.

• **Implant-retained (implant-supported) crown**: a cement or screw-retained crown fitted over an implant abutment. It derives its support from the implant abutment and underlying implant.

• **Temporary crowns**: preformed or customised crowns placed as an interim restoration on prepared teeth. The former are usually made of polycarbonate or aluminium, whereas the latter requires an impression taken prior to tooth preparation. The functions of temporary crowns include: protection of exposed dentine following tooth preparation, maintenance of proximal and occlusal contacts, prevention of overeruption of opposing tooth, and maintenance of function and appearance whilst the definitive crown restoration is being constructed.

General indications for crowns

• Replacement of a large filling when there is not sufficient tooth tissue remaining for an other intracoronal restoration

• Restoration of a fractured or cracked tooth

• Protection of a weak tooth from fracturing

• In situations of heavy occlusal loading where tooth could potentially fracture.

• Cover a (usually posterior) tooth that has had root canal treatment and when an onlay is not indicated (see Chapter 49)

• Cover a severely discoloured or poorly shaped tooth

• Restoration of a single dental implant.

General contraindications

• Evidence of active caries, endodontic or periodontal disease

• Aesthetics (metallic crowns)

• Economic factors

• Where patient management requires short visits and simple procedures.

Dentistry at a Glance. First Edition. Edited by Elizabeth Kay. © 2016 John Wiley & Sons, Ltd. Published 2016 by John Wiley & Sons, Ltd.
Companion website: www.ataglanceseries.com/dentistryseries/dentistry

Types and materials

Metallic crowns

Cast gold alloy crowns are prepared from alloys of various metallic constituents, including but not limited to gold, platinum, palladium, silver, copper and tin (Figure 50.1).

- **Advantages**: Excellent wear resistance, does not cause wear of opposing teeth, anatomy of tooth can readily be reproduced in the wax prior to casting, can be used in thin section, excellent longevity, and less tooth reduction required than for metal–ceramic and all-ceramic restorations.
- **Disadvantages**: Not aesthetic, cost of alloy
- **Preparation features**:
  - 1.5 mm occlusal clearance over functional (supporting) cusps and 1 mm clearance of non-functional cusps
  - Functional cusp bevel
  - 5–16° circumferential taper, 0.8–1 mm chamfer margin removing all undercut areas
  - Should finish supragingivally; this may not always be possible as preparation should extend more gingivally than existing restoration so that the preparation margin finishes on tooth structure.

Metal–ceramic systems

Metal–ceramic crowns (also known as porcelain-fused-to-metal or bonded crowns) combine both the exceptional aesthetic properties of ceramics and the extraordinary mechanical properties of metals. Metal–ceramic crowns have a metal subframe to which the porcelain is added in layers. The inner opaque porcelains are added to mask the metal and over this aesthetic porcelains are added to produce the shape and shade of the crown. Metal–ceramic crowns may have occlusal ceramic coverage (Figure 50.2) or occlusal metal coverage (Figure 50.3). The junction between metal and ceramic should not be in areas of high occlusal stress, as this might result in stress concentration areas with subsequent chipping of the ceramic at the interface.

- **Advantages**: Aesthetics, strength
- **Disadvantages**: Relatively heavy tooth preparation is required to accommodate the metal and ceramic, potentially resulting in weakening the remaining tooth structure. In addition, ceramic occlusal surfaces may result in wear of opposing tooth surfaces, as ceramic is more abrasive than enamel. The aesthetics of metal–ceramic crowns may not match those of all-ceramic crowns.
- **Preparation features**:
  - Minimum 1.5 mm reduction for all porcelain fused to metal surfaces of the crown
  - Functional cusp bevel
  - 1.5 mm axial reduction
  - 5–16° circumferential taper
  - 1.5 mm shoulder (but joint) labially and chamfer margin palatally/ lingually, which need only be shallow if porcelain coverage is partial.

The preparation is more aggressive than for cast gold crowns, but in general less aggressive than for all-ceramic crowns. A less aggressive preparation for metal–ceramic crowns involves full metal coverage of the occlusal surface of the metal–ceramic crown. In addition, unlike with porcelain occlusal coverage, the metal occlusal surface is not abrasive to the opposing natural dentition.

All-ceramic crowns

Although the cores used for all-ceramic crowns are not made of metal, they are usually opaque and require masking. Thus, the bright and opaque ceramic coping, like metal copings, need masking by the addition of porcelain layers to produce the shape and shade of the final crown. Because there is no metal to block light transmission, all-ceramic crowns can resemble natural tooth structure better in terms of shade and translucency than any other restorative option. As a result, these crowns are increasingly popular with dentists and patients to provide the most pleasing aesthetic restoration.

All-ceramic materials can be classified as follows:

Conventional ceramics: This type of crown (e.g. Inceram®, Vita Zahnfabrik, Bad Säckingen, Germany) consists of two distinct layers. The strength of the crown is derived from its inner core, which is made from zirconium and aluminium oxide. Conventional low-fusing porcelains are fired onto the core to create an aesthetically pleasing high-compressive-strength restoration.

Pressed ceramics: An example of a pressed glass ceramic is IPS Empress (Ivoclar®, Vivadent, Schaan, Liechtenstein). It comprises two layers: an inner core material made of lithium disilicate (the ingot) and an outer layer made from fluouroapatite ceramic. The core is made using the lost wax technique. Wax is invested in a phosphate-bonded investment material and, following burn-out, the leucite reinforced glass ceramic is pressed under pressure into the space left by the wax.

CAD/CAM without coping: This type of crown (e.g. Cerec III system) is manufactured by capturing a digital image of the preparation and opposing dentition, using a special digital scanning camera to capture a 3D image. The software program of the system allows for the preparation margins to be outlined. Subsequently, the digital data is transmitted to a computer-controlled milling machine, which mills the final restoration from a monochromatic ceramic block. The ceramic crown is milled within 20 minutes. Disadvantages of this system include the relatively high cost of the equipment and that the restorations is limited to one shade only. This can restrict the aesthetic outcome of the all-ceramic crown. Reservations have also been expressed about the accuracy of marginal fit of the restorations made from digital impressions. Although the newer Cerec system has addressed this limitation, further developments are to be expected.

CAD/CAM with coping: An example of a CAD/CAM system with coping is the Procera® crown (NobelBiocare, Gothenburg, Sweden). The coping is produced by the Procera® machine, a computer-driven ruby sapphire probe scanner, which digitises the master die in the local laboratory. The collected and digitised data is then sent, via e-mail, to a central laboratory in either Sweden or the USA. An alumina coping is then returned to the local technician to complete the crown by veneering it with additional layers of conventional porcelain to create the final restoration.

Luting of all-ceramic crowns usually consists of bonding the ceramic restoration to the prepared tooth using the acid etch technique and the use of a resin luting cement. Bonding to ceramic is achieved by etching the fit surface with hydrofluoric acid and the use of a silane coupling agent.

- **Advantages**: superior aesthetics, excellent translucency, high compressive strength, good soft tissue response, i.e. high biocompatibility.
- **Disadvantages**: brittle low-tensile strength, shoulder-type margin preparation circumferentially results in significantly more tooth preparation on the palatal/lingual and proximal surfaces than for metal–ceramic crowns.
- **Indications**: areas with high aesthetic requirement where a more conservative restoration would be inadequate.
- **Contraindications**: when more conservative restorations can be used. All-ceramic crowns are rarely indicated for molars because of the increased occlusal load and reduced aesthetic demand.

Post-retained crowns

Posts are used to retain restorations or cores for extracoronal restorations in endodontically treated teeth when there is insufficient tooth tissue to provide retention and support for a restoration. It is important to note that posts do not reinforce roots of weakened, endodontically treated teeth. On the contrary, preparation for a post results in further weakening of the root, potentially predisposing it to root fracture.

Components

- **Post:** The component that extends into the root canal. Its length should be at least equal to the height of the clinical crown. At least 5 mm of gutta percha must remain apical to the post in order to maintain an adequate apical seal (Figure 50.4).
- **Core:** The structure connected to the post that supports and retains the crown.
- **Crown:** The component that fits over the core to restore the function and appearance of the tooth.

Indications

- **Endodontic factors:**
  - Good-quality, symptom-free root filling
  - Evidence or prospect of periapical healing
- **Periodontal factors:**
  - Absence of progressive periodontal disease
  - Alveolar bone sufficient to support the restored tooth in clinical service
- **Restorative and occlusal factors:**
  - Sufficient (radicular) tooth tissue remaining to support and retain a post crown
  - Favourable location and angulation of endodontically treated root relative to the adjacent and opposing teeth
  - Favourable occlusal relationship to limit loading of the post crown in function.

The success of a post-retained restoration is greatly increased if sufficient coronal tooth tissue remains supragingivally for the availability of a ferrule. The ferrule effect has been described as an encircling band of the cast restoration around the coronal surface of the tooth, which provides bracing and retention.

The presence of a ferrule reduces the stresses at the end of the post, thus reducing the risk of root fracture. The additional support and retention gained by a ferrule reduces the risk of de-bonding of the restoration. Whilst at least 1 mm in height improves fracture resistance, at least 2 mm is considered optimal. The thickness of the axial walls must be at least 1 mm to contribute to the ferrule.

Careful assessment of the endodontically treated tooth is made for the following:
- Good apical seal
- No sensitivity to pressure
- No exudates
- No fistula
- No apical sensitivity
- No active inflammation.

Note that an inadequately root filled tooth should be retreated prior to the placement of a new post core.

Contraindications

- Carious root surface
- Evidence of apical periodontitis
- Active periodontal disease
- Inadequate alveolar bone support
- Root perforations, cracks and fractures
- Deep subgingival margins – consider crown lengthening or extrusion
- Crown length will exceed remaining root length
- Failed endodontic treatment
- Insufficient space for final restoration.

Types of posts

Active and passive posts: Active posts are usually prefabricated and threaded in design, and can either be self-threading or pre-tapped. When placing a self-threading post, the thread of the post cuts the counter thread into the walls of the dentine. The use of active, threaded posts, such as the Dentatus screw, is associated with increased stresses and root fracture; particularly with a tapered design resulting in an additional 'wedging' effect into the post space. Pretapped post systems use a pretapping device to cut the counter thread into the dentine walls prior to post cementation.

Whilst active posts are more retentive than passive posts of similar dimensions, the latter are often preferred, as less strain is introduced into the root, thus reducing the risk of root fracture. Passive posts can either be custom-made (i.e. cast post and core) or prefabricated. Their surface is usually either smooth or serrated and their shape can be either tapered or parallel. In general, parallel-sided, serrated posts are the most retentive types of passive posts.

Metallic and non-metal posts: Custom-made cast posts and cores (indirect, laboratory made) are most commonly made from precious metal alloys (Figure 50.5), whilst prefabricated metallic posts are commonly made from stainless steel, titanium alloy, nickel–chrome or other non-precious metal alloys. An advantage of metallic posts is their strength and radiopacity (Table 50.1). A potential disadvantage of using non-precious metal alloy posts is their tendency to undergo corrosion.

The more recent, non-metallic posts are made out of either carbon, silica or quartz fibres embedded longitudinally in an epoxy resin, or zirconia. These are more radiolucent than the metal alternatives and rely on resin based luting cements.

Table 50.1 Comparison of metallic and non-metallic posts

Metallic posts		Non-metallic posts	
Advantages	**Disadvantages**	**Advantages**	**Disadvantages**
Radiopaque	Increased risk of vertical root fracture (due to direct transmission of occlusal forces to root dentine)	Microscopic flexure (modulus of elasticity is similar to dentine)	Radiolucent
Good strength	Corrosion (only non-precious alloys)	Aesthetics (posts are translucent, white or tooth-coloured)	If resin luting cement failure occurs then it is usually partial and does not result in complete debonding (decementation) of the post; thus allowing ingress of saliva and bacteria into radicular dentine (where partial debonding has occurred) resulting in extensive decay and catastrophic failure of the remaining tooth.

51 Glass ionomer cements and provisional restorations

Glass ionomer cements (GICs) are inherently weak in thin section and cavity margin depth should be of the order of 1 mm with a perpendicular cavosurface margin. GIc's are most commonly used to restore cavities on the gingival surface of the tooth as their aesthetics are adequate as dentine replacements but inadequate to replace or simulate enamel.

There are two forms of matrix that are commonly used: either the same polyester strips that are used with composite or malleable aluminium matrices, which can be preshaped to the surface of the tooth and then applied to the material after placement. Obviously, if a light-curing GIC is being used then an aluminium matrix is not practical.

GICs are inherently self-adhesive to both enamel and dentine and so are placed directly onto prepared tooth tissue without a conditioning step, unless the prepared tooth surface has been exposed to saliva when the pellicle will interfere with bond formation and a conditioning step should be employed. The conditioner used is a solution of the same poly(alkenoic) acid used by the manufacturer to form the cement, most commonly poly(acrylic) acid.

GICs are most commonly delivered in an encapsulated form, which has the advantage of giving a powder : liquid ratio which maintains a consistency in the material so that it can be handled easily. The capsules usually incorporate a delivery tip so the material can be dispensed directly into the cavity, and then the matrix is applied for buccal restorations or in a similar fashion to composite resins for proximal restorations using a wrap-around polyester matrix. The matrix needs to be left or held in place for the duration of the setting reaction for chemically setting materials or a light-curing unit is used to set the material for the light-activated products.

Chemically setting GICs are susceptible to either moisture contamination or desiccation during the early stage after set; therefore, the surface of the material needs to be protected using a varnish or unfilled resin. This should be applied to the material immediately after the matrix is removed and before any adjustment. It is good practice not to adjust the margins of a GIC until the material is fully set (about 24 hours after placement) unless there is gross excess that needs to be removed. Finishing needs to be done with care to minimise the risk of desiccation of the surface, particularly when rotating disks or rubber-mounted abrasives are used.

Provisional restoration

Provisional restorations are used in two circumstances during operative procedures:
• To seal an endodontic access cavity between visits where a single-visit procedure is not possible
• To seal a cavity during caries management as part of a step-wise caries excavation approach.

For both options, similar characteristics are required of the material chosen. It needs to have adequate structural durability to withstand biting and guidance forces that may affect the restoration, and it needs to provide an acceptable seal at the interface between the material and the cavity margins to prevent ingress of bacteria or sugars.

There are two groups of materials that are commonly used for provisional restorations: zinc oxide/ eugenol (ZnO/E) cements and GICs. Both can establish an adequate seal with tooth tissue; furthermore, ZnO/E materials have significant antimicrobial characteristics in their own right. ZnO/E materials are relatively soft and there are a number of materials available where acrylic resin is incorporated into the powder to give improved physical properties. However, the structural characteristics of GICs make them the material of choice for use with a step-wise approach to caries removal as the cavities involved are likely to be relatively large. Both materials can be used to seal a relatively small access cavity in a tooth. If the access cavity is large, a GIC is the appropriate choice of material.

Cavity preparation

The most important part of preparation prior to placing a provisional restoration is to remove unsupported enamel from the peripheral margins and to ensure that caries is removed from the amelodentinal junction (ADJ). This will help to ensure that the all-important seal is established and maintained for the life of the restoration. It would be anticipated that a ZnO/E restoration could function for a few weeks without significant detriment, whilst a GIC could last months.

Other considerations

Where the restoration is being used to seal an endodontic access cavity, it will be important to ensure that a plug of cotton wool is placed in the cavity before placing the provisional restoration to ensure that the restorative material is not pushed into the canal system, interfering with access to the canals on future visits.

Where a restoration is being placed in a cavity that involves a proximal surface, an appropriate matrix system should be used to help to shape the restoration and prevent excess material causing gingival irritation. There is no hard and fast rule about which matrix is the best for this purpose; again, the principal objective here is to seal the cavity rather than, necessarily, reproducing anatomical accuracy. However, it is also important to ensure that the restoration does not encroach on the proximal gingival tissues as this will result in increased gingival inflammation and bleeding when the definitive restoration is placed.

Material placement

ZnO/E materials are hand mixed on a glass or paper slab until the mix is 'stiff' and can be readily shaped into a ball or sausage. Handling of the material can be easier if the surface is rolled in fresh ZnO powder to dry its surface. The material is then packed into the cavity using a flat plastic instrument and the occlusal surface shaped to conform to the tooth anatomy.

GICs tend to be capsule mixed as this mechanical mixing is more efficient, allowing a greater powder : liquid ratio to be used for a given consistency of material. The capsules usually have a syringe-type nozzle that allows the material to be placed directly into the cavity.

Once the provisional restoration has been placed, the occlusion must be checked to ensure that the provisional restoration does not cause an occlusal interference. It is not necessary to varnish or surface treat the GIC material in this circumstance as it is not the intention that such restorations are designed to exhibit long-term durability.

52 Resin-retained bridges

Figure 52.1 Excellent aesthetics give high patient satisfaction levels

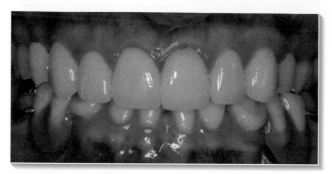

Figure 52.2 (a) Abutment teeth must be restored; (b) restoration and retainers may be combined

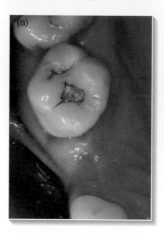 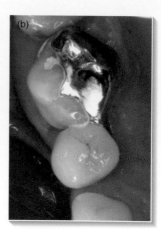

(a)

(b)

Figure 52.3 Retainers on posterior teeth should have occlusal coverage

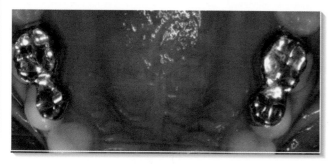

Figure 52.4 Anteriorly the framework should extend up to the incisal edge

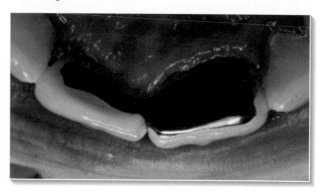

Figure 52.5 The cervical anatomy around the pontic must be good

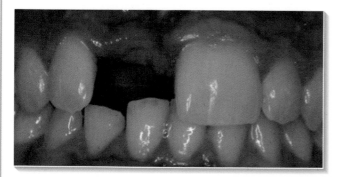

Figure 52.6 Resin retained bridges can be cemented slightly high in the bite

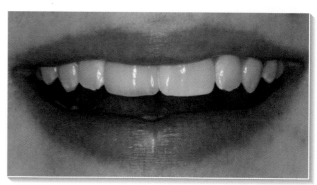

Resin-retained bridges (RRBs) are a minimally invasive and cost effective means of replacing lost teeth and can give patients high levels of comfort, function and satisfaction for considerable lengths of time. RRBs give excellent aesthetic results, which accounts for the high levels of patient satisfaction (Figure 52.1). They have been in use since the 1970s, since when the design, and consequently the success rate, have improved significantly. Even relatively inexperienced operators can carry out the procedure reliably and successfully. A number of criteria need to be kept in mind in order for a RRB to be successful and give the best possible aesthetic result.

Case selection

Among the factors influencing the performance of RRBs, careful case selection is crucial for high rates of success. The patients' health, age and expectations all need to be taken into account and overall oral health, as well as the tooth to be replaced, must be carefully considered. A most important issue is the prognosis of the abutment teeth (Figure 52.2a). The endodontic condition, overall restorability and periodontal health of the abutment teeth all need to be good. Abutment teeth must be free from active disease and it is essential that there is enough sound enamel for bonding. The aim is to achieve the maximum surface area for bonding as the larger the bond area, the greater the strength of the bond.

Design considerations

The design of the bridge is crucial to success, and good communication between dentist and laboratory technician is essential in order to maximise understanding of what is required and what will work.

The framework should give 180° wraparound if at all possible. The exception to this is if aesthetics are affected. Retainers on posterior teeth should be extended onto the palatal or lingual cusps and as much of the occlusal surface as possible (Figure52.2b and 52.3), whilst anteriorly the framework should extend up to the incisal edge (Figure 52.4). The framework should be thick enough to allow sufficient rigidity to prevent flexing, as flex increases the likelihood of debonding because it increases the stress on the luting cement. The connector onto the pontic should extend onto the palatal or lingual aspect. This will aid the overall aesthetics of the porcelain work on the pontic. Achieving the correct cervical anatomy and apparent emergence angle from the soft tissues will give the illusion that the tooth is natural (Figure 52.5).

The restoration may be cemented high in the bite (Figure 52.6). The restoration will adapt into the occlusal plane, due to a combination of extrusion of non-contact teeth and intrusion of the bridge abutment and retainer. This process has been described as the Dahl concept.

The clinical technique

One area that creates debate is whether there is a need to prepare the teeth for RRBs. Extensive preparations are destructive and may be unnecessary. Existing restorations that are present in the abutment teeth should be replaced, ideally with composite resin. If the tooth is to be prepared, the preparation should remain in the enamel and limited to removing undercuts and creating guide planes. In the anterior teeth the incisal edge can be bevelled to allow for the framework thickness.

Procedures

An impression should record the fine detail of the tooth anatomy and the soft tissue. A working model is then created on which the framework is constructed. The working model may need to be adjusted by creating a small ovate concavity in the stone in order to accommodate the pontic in an aesthetic position.

The shade of tooth should be carefully chosen using a recommended shade guide. The shade should take account of the metal work and the use of an opaque resin cement at the incisal edge can help to recreate the effect of a reduced translucent edge.

The RRB should be tried in and assessed for fit and accuracy prior to cementing. To simulate the cement white Plasticine can be used.

Adjustments to the RRB can then be made; this can be adjustment to the porcelain to improve the aesthetics or to the metalwork to improve the fit. New instructions can then be communicated to the technician or if no adjustments are required then the RRB can be cemented.

The RRB cementation process requires the tooth to be uncontaminated, etched and primed to generate maximum bond strength, and so after try-in of the RRB the tooth will need to be prepared for the process of cementation and sandblasted to create micromechanical retention and enhance the bond strength. A resin-based cement should be used and the recommendations of the system followed carefully. Isolation of the tooth during cementation is essential and where moisture control is difficult to achieve a rubber dam should be used.

Following the cementation process, the excess cement should be removed and careful instructions given to the patient about the maintenance and care of the RRB. Any instructions should be communicated verbally and in writing and also documented in the clinical notes.

Dealing with failure

The most common reason for failure is debonding and this leaves the clinician with the dilemma of either recementing the initial RRB or remaking the prosthesis. The correct diagnosis of the reason for the debond will aid this decision-making process. The design features of the bridge and the patient suitability should be reassessed.

53 Bridges

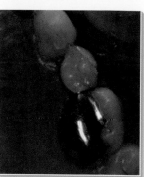

Figure 53.3 Example of a posterior cantilever resin-retained bridge

Figure 53.1 Example of a conventional fixed–fixed three-unit bridge replacing UL2

Figure 53.2 Example of an anterior cantilever resin-retained bridge: (a) frontal view and (b) palatal view

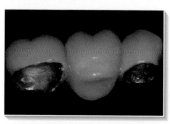

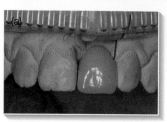

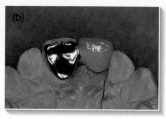

Figure 53.4 (a) UL1 and UL2 missing. Note: UR1 has been previously prepared for a PFM retainer and UL3 is sound. (b) Hybrid bridge with conventional retainer UR1 and adhesive retainer wing on UL3. (c) Movable joint connector between UR1 conventional retainer and UL1 pontic. (d) Hybrid bridge *in situ*

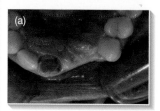

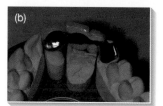

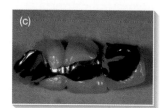

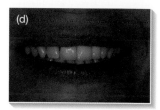

Introduction

Definition: A bridge is a dental prosthesis used to replace a missing tooth or teeth. It typically cannot be removed by the patient.

The components of a bridge include:

Retainer: part of bridge that is fitted to the abutment tooth

Pontic: artificial tooth that replaces the missing natural tooth or teeth

Connector: the element of the bridge that joins the pontic to the retainer; the connector may be rigid or movable.

Further relevant terms include:

Unit: a term used to indicate the number of pontics and retainers associated with the bridge; for example, a three-unit bridge = two retainers + one pontic

Pier abutment: a non-terminal abutment tooth incorporated in the bridge design; it usually acts as a point of rotation of the bridge and is commonly the weak link in the bridge design, particularly with long bridges.

Bridges can be broadly classified as follows:

- Conventional
- Resin-bonded (=resin retained or adhesive)
- Hybrid.

Conventional bridges

Fixed–fixed design

A retainer is at both ends of the edentulous span; pontic(s) lie between retainers; rigid connector joins pontic to retainers; three or more units (Figure 53.1).

Advantages:

- Robust design for maximum strength and retention
- Splinting of abutment teeth may be advantageous in a patient with stable periodontal disease
- Laboratory construction is relatively uncomplicated

Disadvantages:

- Extensive tooth preparation of abutment teeth is required
- Paralleling the preparations can be difficult if they are widely separated
- May experience cementation difficulties as the bridge must be inserted in one piece
- Design is not suitable for abutment teeth that are markedly tilted.

Fixed–movable design

Utilises a custom-made or proprietary precision attachment to allow a degree of movement between two component parts of the bridge. Typically, on its mesial aspect the pontic is connected,

Dentistry at a Glance. First Edition. Edited by Elizabeth Kay. © 2016 John Wiley & Sons, Ltd. Published 2016 by John Wiley & Sons, Ltd.
Companion website: www.ataglanceseries.com/dentistryseries/dentistry

via a movable connector, to the distal end of the mesial retainer. On its distal aspect the pontic is usually connected rigidly to the distal retainer; thereby allowing limited predominantly vertical movement between the pontic and the retainer to which it is linked via the movable connector.

Advantages:
- Can be used when abutment teeth are divergent
- Allows a limited degree of tooth movement
- Allows cementation of the bridge in two stages

Disadvantages:
- Length of the span is limited to one or two pontics, especially if teeth have some mobility
- Laboratory construction is complicated and costly due to incorporation of intracoronal movable component
- Difficult to construct a temporary bridge.

Cantilever design

The pontic is connected to the retainer(s) at one end only.

Advantages:
- Preparation of only one abutment tooth is required
- Involves one retainer only
- No need for paralleling of multiple abutments
- Laboratory construction is relatively uncomplicated

Disadvantages:
- Leverage forces on the abutment tooth
- Torquing forces must not act on the pontic.

Resin-bonded bridge

A fixed prosthesis that is adhesively bonded to one or more unprepared (or minimally prepared) natural teeth and which replaces one or more missing teeth. Resin-bonded bridges are useful for tooth replacement anteriorly (Figure 53.2) and posteriorly (Figure 53.3).

Advantages:
- Fixed prosthesis
- Conservative of tooth structure
- Suitable for use in adolescent patients
- Usually does not require local anaesthesia
- Limited clinical time required to complete
- Relatively inexpensive
- Potentially reversible
- Good longevity (>80% survival over 10 years)
- Possible diagnostic precursor to conventional bridgework

Disadvantages:
- Sometimes 'greying' shine through appearance of abutment tooth/teeth may be seen from frontal view. However, this can be usually overcome by the use of an opaque luting cement
- Risk of debonding (but recementation is usually possible)
- Longevity is less than for conventional bridgework
- Risk of caries is greater in the case of partial debond in the fixed–fixed design (note: a cantilever design overcomes this problem and is the preferred option, whenever possible)

Indications:
- Ideally, single-tooth replacement using cantilever design (note: fixed–fixed resin-bonded bridges with several pontics have been shown to have a significantly increased debond rate)
- Sound or minimally restored abutment teeth with sufficient, good-quality enamel for bonding
- Intermediate prostheses in young patients during growth phase and prior to implant placement

Contraindications:
- Heavily restored abutment teeth
- Teeth with short clinical crowns

- Abutment teeth damaged by wear
- Presence of unstable periodontal disease
- Occlusal parafunction
- Difficulty in achieving a dry operating field for cementation
- Very translucent incisal edges (anterior teeth) because of likelihood of metal shine through appearance. However, this can be counteracted by the application of composite resin restorative materials.

Note: when designing posterior resin-bonded bridges it is essential to wrap the metal wing retainer at least half-way onto the occlusal surface of the abutment tooth for the bridge to adequately withstand shear forces.

Hybrid bridge

Hybrid bridges consist of a combination of a conventional retainer and an adhesive retainer on the terminal abutment teeth. It is advisable to incorporate a movable joint into the design to allow for differential movement between the component of the bridge attached via the conventional retainer on one side and the component attached via the adhesive metal wing retainer on the other side (Figure 53.4a–d). Cementation of the bridge involves the use of conventional cement for the conventional retainer and an adhesive resin-based cement for the adhesive retainer.

Advantages:
- Fixed prosthesis
- Preserves tooth tissue by using an adhesive wing retainer for one of the abutments

Disadvantages:
- Failure rate is higher than conventional bridgework
- Risk of caries is greater in the case of partial debond.

Pontic design for bridges

Bridge pontic designs include:
- Ridge lap pontic
- Modified ridge lap pontic
- Ovate pontics
- Bullet-nose pontic
- Sanitary pontic.

The ridge lap pontic closely adapts to, and covers a relatively wide area of, the underlying alveolar ridge. This extensive coverage makes it difficult to clean under the pontic and often leads to inflammation of the area in contact with the pontic. Hence, this type of pontic is unfavourable and should be avoided.

The modified ridge lap pontic was designed to further reduce tissue contact with the underlying ridge. Tissue contact is limited to the labial/buccal surface of the ridge crest, resulting in less tissue irritation than ridge lap pontics. A modified ridge lap pontic allows good cleaning with maximum aesthetics by overlying part of the ridge to mimic emergence of the pontic from the gingival tissues in a similar way to the natural tooth.

Ovate pontics may be used in cases where the residual ridge has a localised defect or has incompletely healed. They can also be used in broad and flat ridges. The design of the pontic is such that its cervical end extends into the defect of the edentulous alveolar ridge. The ovate pontic provides an aesthetically pleasing appearance, as it appears to emerge from the ridge like a natural tooth.

Sanitary and bullet-nose pontics are preferred posteriorly where aesthetics is of less concern. This pontic has no tissue contact with the underlying alveolar ridge, which facilitates cleaning under the pontic.

54 Implant-retained options

Figure 54.1 Reduced bone volume, augmented with an onlay bone graft

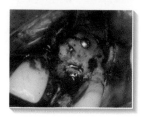

Figure 54.2 Exposed implant threads covered with autogenous bone chips and a membrane

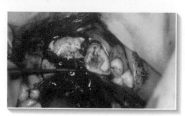

Figure 54.3 High smile line, which would present complex aesthetic management problems

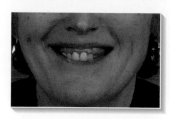

Figure 54.4 Maxillary anterior teeth lost to trauma, long span, surrounding dentition unrestored: (a) occlusal view; (b) labial view

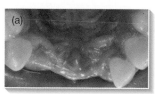
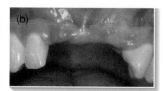

Figure 54.5 Diastema adjacent to missing tooth currently restored with an RPD; note also the significant soft and hard tissue deficit causing poor appearance

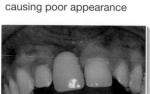

Figure 54.6 Patient with congenital absence of teeth (hypodontia); note narrow alveolar ridge in area of missing teeth

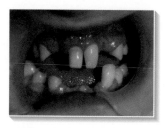

Figure 54.7 Diagnostic wax-up cast

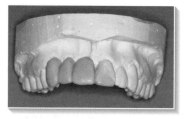

Figure 54.8 Surgical stent based on diagnostic wax-up used to guide placement of implant

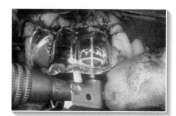

Figure 54.9 Customised abutments connected to implants: (a) titanium; (b) zirconia

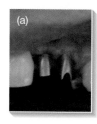
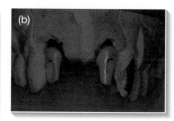

Figure 54.10 Provisional restoration used to shape the papillae postsurgery; note blanching of tissues around restorations

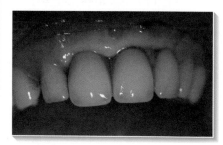

Figure 54.11 (a) Cement-retained restoration replacing maxillary central incisors; (b) screw-retained restoration replacing lower left second premolar

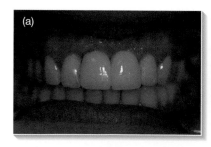
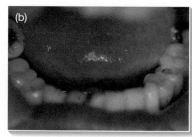

Dentistry at a Glance. First Edition. Edited by Elizabeth Kay. © 2016 John Wiley & Sons, Ltd. Published 2016 by John Wiley & Sons, Ltd.
Companion website: www.ataglanceseries.com/dentistryseries/dentistry

Indications for implant-retained prostheses

Replacement of missing teeth can be challenging, as bone is lost both immediately and gradually following tooth loss. Implants provide a means by which a prosthesis can be attached directly to bone without the involvement of adjacent teeth. A successful outcome for this treatment is contingent upon the prognosis for the surrounding dentition, the presence of favourable healing conditions to facilitate osseointegration and favourable bone volume. There are very few absolute contraindications to implant surgery, but any factor that compromises good healing is a relative contraindication. This would include poorly controlled diabetes mellitus and prolonged use of bisphosphonate medication (particularly IV bisphosphonates). Smoking is not a contraindication per se, but cigarette smoking adversely influences treatment outcomes.

When anterior teeth are missing, particularly those in the aesthetic zone, it is vital that the clinician fully understands the patient's expectations for treatment in advance of placing dental implants. It is important to remember that a prosthesis is required to replace teeth and associated bone, and this is not always straightforward when a fixed prosthesis is planned. On the other hand, a removable partial denture (RPD), by virtue of having teeth and a flange, presents a means of replacing lost teeth and bone more readily. In an ideal world, teeth would be replaced as soon as they were lost. However, this is highly unusual and the longer the delay in replacing teeth with implant-retained restorations, the more complex the replacement challenge becomes. Ideally, implants would be placed within 8 weeks of tooth loss. Where there is congenital absence of permanent teeth, the alveolar ridge in the area of absent teeth is very narrow. In these situations, the alveolar ridge has to be augmented prior to placing implants (Figure 54.1) or at the time of implant placement (Figure 54.2). A further consideration is the condition of the soft tissues at the implant site and the gingival biotype. If the patient has a thin biotype with a high smile line, it is very challenging. A thick tissue biotype with a low smile line is far less problematic (Figure 54.3).

The specific indications for implant-retained prostheses in partially dentate patients include:
- A healthy dentition where teeth have been lost to trauma (Figure 54.4)
- Missing teeth with unrestored teeth adjacent to the space
- Diastema present in the area where the tooth has been lost (Figure 54.5)
- Unfavourable span for conventional fixed prosthodontics
- Patients with congenital absence of teeth (Figure 54.6).

Planning procedures

When planning tooth replacement, it important to ensure that pathology and unfavourable occlusal forces are controlled. If the patient exhibits signs of parafunction, this can cause delayed failure of implants. It is also important to ensure that heavy excursive forces are not introduced into an implant-retained crown or bridge restoration. Further examination requirements include:
- Assessment of alveolar bone width and height (clinical and radiographic examination)
- Mesiodistal distance between teeth (approximately 7 mm mesiodistal width per implant is required)
- Interocclusal space assessment (particularly relevant posteriorly)
- Assessment of soft tissues and presence or absence of papilla
- Height of smile line (very high lip line is challenging).

Aids to planning include the use of plain film radiographs and good-quality mounted study casts. Three-dimensional imaging is advisable when teeth are lost either due to trauma or chronic infection, as significant bone volume deficit is likely in these cases.

The positioning and placement of implants must be related to the desired cosmetic outcome. A diagnostic wax-up cast is essential to help simulate the appearance of the final restoration and evaluate whether it is acceptable to the patient. The wax-up can be based on a previously satisfactory restoration (e.g. a failed conventional bridge or RPD). Alternatively, it can be done de novo and altered until the patient is satisfied (Figure 54.7). In addition to establishing what the patient expects in terms of appearance, the wax-up can also help determine if sufficient tissue is available to achieve this appearance at the end of treatment. In conjunction with the radiographic information, the need for bony ridge augmentation and connective tissue grafting can be decided.

The final wax-up is then used to fabricate a surgical stent to guide implant placement (Figure 54.8). It is essential that the operator placing the implants uses the surgical guide to ensure optimal placement.

Surgical phase

A standardised protocol is use to place implants, and it is important that there is careful handling of soft and hard tissues. Good irrigation is essential, and controlled drill speed is used to avoid damaging bone. With the aid of the surgical stent, pilot holes are used to check the orientation of the implant site as it is being prepared. Any granulation tissue or foreign body material in the implant site should be completely debrided. The implant site should be gradually widened to the predetermined length and diameter, and the implant itself then placed. It is important to get good primary stability of the implant in the bone. Where implant threads are exposed, these should be covered with an autogenous bone graft material with a membrane to facilitate bone regeneration over the exposed threads (Figure 54.2). Depending on the stability of the implant, it can then be covered with a healing cap and the mucoperiosteal flap sutured around this, or covered with the flap for a period of 4–6 months to facilitate osseointegration.

Restorative phase

Once initial healing has occurred, the restorative treatment can commence. Implants have successfully osseointegrated when there a torque force exerted on the implant elicits neither movement nor pain. The normal treatment sequence is as follows:

1 Primary impression, followed by a 'pick-up' impression in a customised impression tray using premachined impression copings. An interocclusal record should be sent with this and an opposing cast to the laboratory.

2 Once cast, either premachined or customised transmucosal abutment components are used to retain the crown or bridgework (Figure 54.9). In the aesthetic zone, use of provisional restorations to shape soft tissues is recommended (Figure 54.10). These are made of heat-cured acrylic or composite resin materials, which are easy to adjust as required.

3 Once the final shape of soft tissues has been achieved and any occlusal adjustments have been made, the final restoration can be made. A new impression is made, and the crown or bridge is fabricated. This can be cement or screw retained, depending on the position of the implant and the need for retrievability (Figure 54.11).

The long-term prognosis for implant-retained restorations is very good, but there is a degree of maintenance required. It is important that the patient maintains a good standard of oral hygiene to avoid peri-implant soft tissue inflammation.

55 Partial dentures

Figure 55.1 Spaces (actual and that caused by decoronation) require consideration for restoration

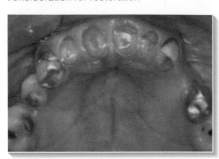

Figure 55.2 Articulated casts help visualise spaces available and permit surveying

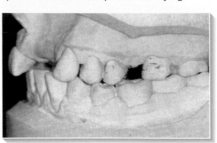

Figure 55.3 The retention here is provided by silicone rubber added to the poly (methyl) methacrylate denture base postcuring (arrowed)

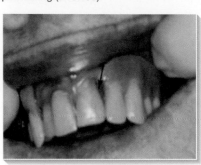

Table 55.1 Types of RPD

Option	Clinical indications
Immediate RPD	To preserve interdental (and interarch space following loss of a tooth or teeth To preserve appearance and phonetics for social reasons
Transitional RPD	May be used in an attempt to raise overdenture or to improve interarch relationships or postinsertion of an implant and prior to integration
Occlusal splint	As used to treat a temporomandibular problem
Definitive RPD	As a planned option to replace missing teeth

Table 55.2 Possible sources of support

Source	Descriptor
Mucosa	Least desired as this will tend to accelerate bone loss
Tooth and mucosa	Better than above, but may necessitate planning for antirotational component; the mucosal supporting portion will still promote bone loss, however
Tooth	Best of the 3 conventional options owing to forces being transferred (ideally) down long axes of the teeth May involve tooth via crown or via a root (overdenture)
Implant	Unlikely to have RPD option, but this is possible
Implant and tooth	Popular and better than any option involving mucosal support
Implant and mucosa	Currently popular but rotational movements still possible and therefore a minimum of 3 well-spaced implants will be required

Table 55.3 Possible sources of retention of RPDs

Means of retention	Comments
Clasps	Gingivally approaching Occlusally approaching Note, in order to find undercuts into which to direct the clasp tips, surveying is necessary as is a knowledge of the properties of the material chosen
Guide planes	May be used in Kennedy I, II or IV denture designs
Precision attachments	Intracoronal Extracoronal Studs Bars Ancillary
Indirect retainers	For use in tooth and mucosal or implant and mucosal supported RPDs
Other	Silicone rubber to engage undercuts interdentally Denture adhesives

Table 55.4 Types of major connector

Maxillary	Mandibular
Full palatal coverage	Lingual plate
Palatal plate	Lingual bar
Palatal bar	Sublingual bar
Skeletal design (anterior and posterior palatal bars	Kennedy bar
Labial bar	Labial bar
Horseshoe	

Dentistry at a Glance. First Edition. Edited by Elizabeth Kay. © 2016 John Wiley & Sons, Ltd. Published 2016 by John Wiley & Sons, Ltd.
Companion website: www.ataglanceseries.com/dentistryseries/dentistry

Introduction

When teeth are lost, there are a variety of options available to the clinician (Figure 55.1); some of these depend on the patient's oral status, some on her/ his motivation and the others depend on ability to meet the potential cost. These options are:

- Do nothing; leave the space or spaces unrestored
- Provide a fixed prosthesis
- Provide an implant-supported fixed prosthesis
- Provide an implant-supported plus removable partial denture (RPD)
- Provide a (conventional) RPD
- Provide complete denture/s.

This section will deal with RPDs. There are several types of RPD that may be prescribed and these are listed in Table 55.1, along with some indications for their use. Always remember, however, that RPDs will inevitably serve as plaque-retaining agents and sound advice should be given to the patient on oral hygiene and aftercare.

Planning partial dentures

The stages involved in planning and designing RPDs are listed in Box 55.1. Following a thorough clinical examination, and after due consultation with the patient, primary impressions should be taken. Depending on the reproducibility and positivity of the retruded contact position (RCP), a primary occlusal registration may also be required. An adequate cast analysis (Figure 55.2.) should be undertaken so that space between the arches for the RPD can be assessed for undercuts and possible guide planes (see below).

Box 55.1 Stages in the design of a RPD

1 Identify and analyse saddles
2 Determine which ones to restore
3 Determine support
4 Join up saddles (major connector)
5 Join supporting elements/ retaining elements to major connector
6 Consider indirect retention (Kennedy I, II or IV cases)
7 Reconsider with prevention/ maintenance in mind

Sources of support

Sources of support are listed in Table 55.2. Where only a few teeth remain, mucosal support may well be the only option available. Clinicians should appreciate that, ultimately, such a denture, under occlusal forces, will cause more resorption of the underlying bone and therefore long-term viability and maintenance must be considered. Tooth support is theoretically the optimal option as occlusal forces are directed down the long axes of the teeth, thereby stimulating the periodontal membranes optimally. However, some tooth preparation

is likely, for occlusal rests or retaining elements, for example addition of (composite resin) undercuts to retain the denture or to shape guiding surfaces.

Retention of dentures

It is incumbent on the clinician to ensure that the denture provided has a retaining element to prevent easy dislodgement from the mouth. There are several ways that this may be provided and these are listed in Table 55.3.

The most common means of retention of a RPD is via a metallic component called a clasp. Basically, this component should engage an undercut and have rigidity to resist distortion yet be sufficient flexibility to slide over the undercut during removal and insertion. A knowledge of the properties of dental alloys is therefore required. Guide planes are surfaces adjacent to saddles, which may be used (and created by selective grinding if required) to resist vertical removal from the mouth. Precision attachments are becoming very popular with implant-supported cases but an awareness of space requirements and aftercare is essential. Indirect retainers are supporting elements that act on the opposite end of the axis of rotation of the denture from the saddle to oppose and hinder rotation. More-flexible materials may be applied to the (freshly cured) denture to engage undercuts between the few remaining teeth and the denture when conventional means of retention is not feasible (Figure 55.3).

Joining the saddles

This is achieved via major connectors. What we term 'pontics' in fixed bridgework, we term 'major connectors' in RPDs. As can be seen in Table 55.4, there are six types of maxillary major connector and five mandibular types. The type of major connector selected will depend on clinical factors (e.g. status and number of the remaining teeth) , anatomical factors (e.g. at least 7.5 mm space is required between the floor of the mouth and the lingual gingival margins of mandibular incisors for a lingual bar and 10.5 mm for a sublingual bar), aesthetic factors (e.g. labial bar may be perceived as unsightly and incisal spacing may preclude metallic anterior bars) and social factors (e.g. anterior bars may affect speech).

Completing the design

Consideration should then be given as to how the supporting and retaining elements are added to the major connector (these are called minor connectors). In simple RPDs they will be incorporated in the acrylic resin denture base. In cobalt chromium dentures, the minor connections will be part of the casting. Thereafter, the denture should be reconsidered along with oral hygiene and patient-related factors, such as the patient's manual dexterity to remove and insert the denture. Always give the patient a leaflet to explain denture care and maintenance.

56 Implant overdentures

Figure 56.1 (a) Ball attachments on two mandibular implants; (b) gold cap components, which connect to ball attachments shown in a; (c) customised cast gold bar linking two mandibular implants; (d) clip attachment, which connects to gold bar shown in c

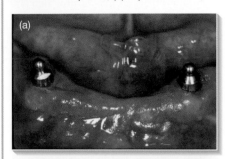

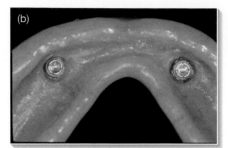

Figure 56.2 Customised gold bar on three implants to provide support and retention for a mandibular overdenture

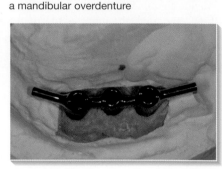

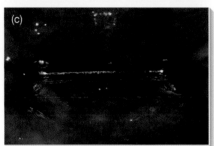

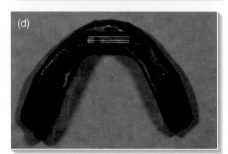

Figure 56.3 Panoramic radiograph showing two implants in the anterior maxilla; note the size of the maxillary sinuses and lack of bone in these regions

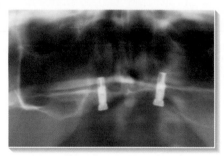

Table 56.1 Circumstances where prognosis for complete replacement dentures is poor

Case presentation	Indicators of problem
Terminal natural dentition	Patient resistant to the idea of removable denture
Maladaptive	Multiple attempts made at making complete replacement dentures, none successful; indicates that patient has not developed the necessary skills to control denture
Problems of recent onset	Alveolar resorption has advanced to such an extent that denture control difficult; recurrent pain indicated deteriorating support for denture
Loss of neuromuscular control	Recent stroke or neuromuscular disease, e.g. Parkinson disease
Damage to denture bearing tissues	Surgical resection of denture bearing tissues following surgical removal of intraoral tumour

The goal of treatment for the edentulous patient is to restore oral function and satisfactory aesthetics using prostheses that are comfortable to wear. For many patients, this is achieved using complete replacement dentures. If the patient has developed the reflexes required to control tissue-supported complete dentures, then the prognosis for treatment is good. However, a proportion of edentate patients do not develop the skills necessary to control complete replacement dentures and require a different form of prosthesis. Examples of patients likely to require alternative treatment are shown in Table 56.1.

Implant overdentures and retention considerations

Implant-retained overdentures, in either or both jaws, are an alternative to replacement dentures in these cases. The process involves the use of endosseous implants to provide a means of

Dentistry at a Glance. First Edition. Edited by Elizabeth Kay. © 2016 John Wiley & Sons, Ltd. Published 2016 by John Wiley & Sons, Ltd.
Companion website: www.ataglanceseries.com/dentistryseries/dentistry

retaining the denture. At its simplest level, this can be achieved using one implant in the midline of the lower jaw. However, it is much more common to use two symmetrically placed implants, connect a suitable abutment to each implant and incorporate a retentive component in the fitting surface of the denture which connects to the abutment (Figure 56.1a–d). The use of retentive components reduces the reliance on the patient's ability to control the denture during function and provides a positive form of retention.

Implant overdentures and support considerations

In addition to retention difficulties, some patients report recurrent discomfort in the denture-bearing tissues, which is not related to denture periphery extension. Support for the denture is still primarily provided by the denture-bearing tissues, but further support may be achieved using a bar-design retainer. In cases of advanced resorption, bony irregularities (exostoses) may be covered by poorly keratinsed mucosa. These tissues are poorly resistant to trauma and can ulcerate, causing discomfort during chewing movements. A further manifestation of this problem may be mental nerve paraesthesia, which arises when the mental nerve is traumatised by the overlying denture. In these cases, the problem can be alleviated by using the transmucosal component of the implants to provide support for the denture. This requires three or four implants in the lower jaw and a bar-design retainer (Figure 56.2).

Implant overdentures – planning considerations

It is important to take a thorough history from the patient and undertake an examination of the patient's denture-bearing tissues and the existing dentures. The clinician needs to clearly understand the patient's complaint and what the patient expects at the end of treatment. When considering implant overdentures, it is important to examine bone volume to ensure there is sufficient bone into which implants can be placed. This can be estimated by clinical examination, but should be supplemented by radiographic examination. Panoramic views ordinarily suffice (Figure 56.3) but three-dimensional imaging may also be used. There is a trend towards the use of computer-aided surgical planning, which requires computed tomography scanning, but this increases the exposure of the patient to further radiation and should be used judiciously. The quality of the soft tissues should be assessed and areas of poorly keratinised tissues noted. This will influence the design of the final prosthesis, as described earlier. In terms of the prosthetic treatment planning, this involves basic principles; use the existing dentures as a guide to polished surface shape, appearance and the amount of freeway space planned for the final prosthesis. It is important to make a surgical guide for implant placement and this is based on the planned appearance of the final denture.

Implant overdentures – prosthetic phase of treatment

When planning the prosthetic phase of care, a decision has to made about how soon after surgery the implants should be loaded. For many years, the protocol was to 'bury' the implants at the first-stage surgery and to allow 4–6 months for osseointegration to occur. A second surgical procedure was then required to uncover the implants prior to commencing the prosthetic phase of treatment. More recently, the trend has been to commence the prosthetic phase either immediately, or more commonly, at an early stage (3–4 weeks) following the surgical placement of the implants. Delayed loading, as per the earlier protocol, tends to be reserved for cases where initial implant stability is poor or in fragile bone in the maxilla. The prosthetic phase of care follows a similar series of steps to conventional dentures, namely:

1 A primary impression using a stock tray and a suitably rigid impression material.

2 A master impression using a 'pick-up' technique and a customised impression tray. Impression copings are screwed onto the implants and picked up with the set impression material. The material should be rigid enough to stabilise and lock the impression copings in the impression.

3 A jaw relationship record is made on the master cast and trimmed chairside, and the jaw relationship recorded.

4 A trial denture is used to establish satisfactory appearance and occlusion.

5 Once this is returned to the laboratory, the retention mechanism can be finalised. If a bar mechanism is planned, this can now be made to ensure it fits beneath the denture without compromising strength of the denture or appearance. If ball attachments, locator or magnet attachments are planned, the height of these abutments can be checked relative to the planned appearance and a suitable size component chosen for use.

6 Processing of dentures and delivery to the patient: if the retentive components are finalised chairside, these can be incorporated into the denture using self-cure acrylic resin. Alternatively, the bar or abutments can be screwed into place and a wash impression recorded in the denture base. This is then sent back to the laboratory for a permanent reline to incorporate the retentive components.

Implant overdenture maintenance

It is important that the patient is shown how to control plaque around the abutments using a soft brush. They should also be advised that there may be a requirement to replace or adjust retentive components over time.

57 Precision attachments

Figure 57.1 Ball attachments soldered onto cast gold post-retained diaphragms on two mandibular canine teeth; reciprocal components will be in fitting surface of the overlying denture

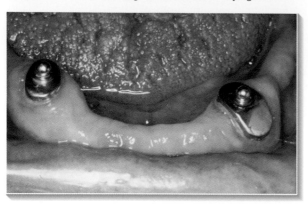

Figure 57.2 Cast gold bar retained on three retained natural teeth in a patient with guarded prognosis for wearing a complete removable maxillary denture

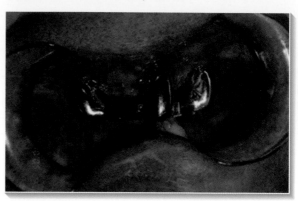

Figure 57.3 (a) Magnetic keepers on the mandibular canine teeth; (b) magnets in fitting surface of mandibular denture which are attracted to the keepers shown in (a)

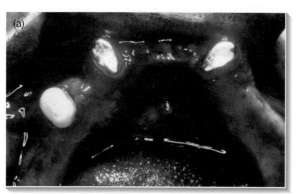

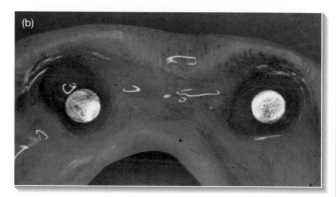

Figure 57.4 Cast framework for removable partial denture with intracoronal sliding attachment connecting it to metal castings for anterior full-veneer crownwork

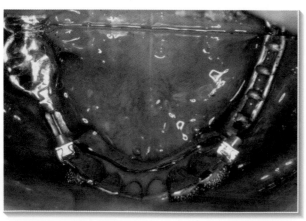

Figure 57.5 Extracoronal attachment mechanism, with patrix on the distal surfaces of anterior bridgework and matrix component embedded in the removable partial denture

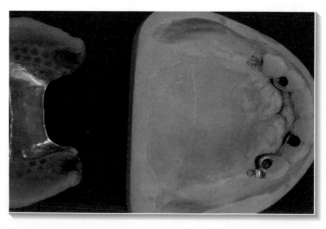

A precision attachment can be defined as: 'An interlocking device, one component of which is fixed to an abutment, while the other is incorporated into a denture or bridge' (British Society for the Study of Prosthetic Dentistry Guidelines, 1996).

Precision attachments and complete dentures

In cases where retention of complete dentures is likely to be severely compromised, the clinician can consider retaining some natural teeth and using precision attachments to enhance denture retention. Situations where this is likely to arise include:
• Elderly adults with a failing dentition where it is planned to provide them with a complete denture for the first time
• Patients likely to have poor muscular control, such as those with Parkinson disease or following cerebrovascular accident (stroke)
• Patients with a history of oral cancer, following tumour resection and substantial compromise of the denture bearing tissues.

In these cases, the clinician needs to anticipate where successful adaptation to edentulousness is unlikely. In a compromised dentition, where possible, natural teeth should be lost on a phased basis and some natural teeth need to be preserved with a view to providing precision attachments to aid denture retention. This type of prosthesis is known as an overdenture, whereby natural teeth are used to retain and support a removable complete denture. A minimum of two symmetrically distributed teeth are required, and it should be possible to restore these with cast post-retained restorations with a supracrestal diaphragm. Abutment teeth should also have a minimum of 50% alveolar bone support.

The possible attachment mechanisms are:
• Ball attachments/ press studs (Figure 57.1)
• Bar and clips (Figure 57.2).

Examples of precision attachment ball attachment/ stud systems include the CEKA (Preat Corporation), Rothermann (Preat Corporation) and Dalbo (Cendres + Metaux USA Inc.) systems. They generally comprise matrix and patrix components that clip together. One component is placed in the abutment tooth (usually the patrix) and a reciprocal component is housed in the denture (usually the matrix).

Having selected abutment teeth, these teeth must have endodontic treatment using conventional endodontic treatment guidelines. The root canal should be prepared for a cast post restoration. The attachment component is soldered to a cast post-retained diaphragm and the reciprocal component incorporated into the denture. Bar systems involve soldering a preformed bar (e.g. Hader or Dolder bar) to castings retained on the abutment teeth. A clip retained in the fitting surface of the denture is used to attach the denture to the bar.

When contemplating the use of precision attachments, the clinician should be certain that they are necessary and likely to be of benefit to the patient. They are expensive in terms of financial cost and increase the length of treatment time. They also increase maintenance requirements. Finally, they exert significant stresses on the abutment teeth. There is no evidence to indicate that any one of these mechanisms is better than another and the choice is often one of clinician's preference.

Magnets can be considered as an alternative to precision attachments for enhancing denture retention, as these exert little force on the periodontal ligament of abutment teeth. Magnet-retained dentures are easier to remove from the mouth than precision attachment-retained dentures, and this may be a factor influencing choice for patients with reduced manual dexterity. In dentistry, rare earth alloy magnets (e.g. neodymium/boron/iron alloy) are used, as these have significant attraction force in the relatively small diameter suitable for use in the mouth. The magnet itself is housed in the denture, and the metal to which it is attracted is contained within the abutment tooth, known as the 'keeper' (Figure 57.3a,b). They are an 'open field' design, which facilitates continued magnetic attraction even when the components are moved apart by functional movements. In the past, corrosion of the metal casing containing the magnets was a problem, but this has diminished considerably with the development of durable stainless steel alloy materials. Magnets come in different heights, and it is important to bear this in mind to ensure sufficient space is available for containing the magnet chosen within the denture. Commercially available dental magnet systems include the Dyna™ (Dyna Dental) and Magfit™ (Aichi Corporation) systems.

Precision attachments are also used to retain implant overdentures, as described in Chapter 56.

Precision attachments and removable partial dentures

Precision attachments can be used as an alternative to conventional clasp retention, particularly when clasps on anterior teeth are likely to be unaesthetic. Attachment mechanisms are described as intracoronal or extracoronal. Both require the provision of full veneer crowns on abutment teeth. In the case of intracoronal attachments, a slot is incorporated into the distal surface of the cast crown (Figure 57.4). This accommodates a 'dovetail' in the metal framework of the removable partial denture (RPD). This mechanism provides a precise path of insertion for the denture, but no friction grip per se. It also requires the clinician to undertake an extensive preparation on the proximal surface to incorporate the slot in the crown. The extracoronal mechanism incorporates a patrix component on the proximal surface of the crown with a matrix component in the denture (Figure 57.5). This provides a friction fit with positive retention, but it is difficult for the patient to maintain good plaque control in this area.

In planning the use of precision attachments for RPDs, it is important to ensure that there is sufficient interocclusal height to incorporate the attachment mechanism within the denture at the planned occlusal vertical dimension. This should be checked prior to any tooth preparation for full veneer crowns using mounted study casts. As per standard RPD principles, a planned path of insertion for the denture is required and the precision attachments are aligned parallel with this path. It is essential that the full veneer crowns and RPD are constructed with this in mind to ensure that both parts fit together accurately. Finally, it is important to remember that precision attachments exert considerable lateral forces on abutment teeth. If they are already periodontally compromised, then it is not wise to use teeth as retainers for precision attachments.

58 Immediate insertion dentures

Figure 58.1 This extraction socket (plus bulbous ridges) would result in discomfort in insertion/removal of the IID in addition to discomfort in eating

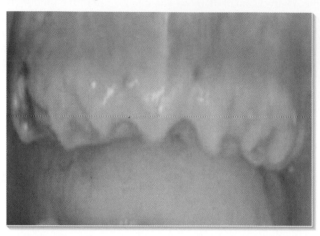

Table 58.1 Types of immediate insertion denture

Addition to current denture (RPD or C/C)	Requires an impression to be made with the present denture in situ and the addition made (this will generally the patient being without the denture for a period of time, which may not be convenient for the patient)
RPD II	This means that the denture is fabricated prior to the extraction or decoration of a tooth
Complete denture/s	As above only there will be no remaining crowns of teeth to facilitate support or retention

Figure 58.2 (a) A flanged IID; (b) an IID that is ridge-lapped (arrowed)

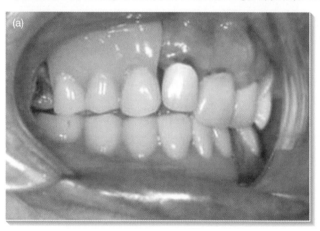

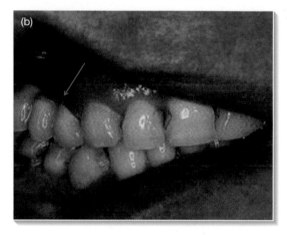

Table 58.2 Clinical stages in the provision of IIDs

Clinical stage	Details
History and examination	Should be thorough, as with RPDs and C/Cs
Informed consent – make patient aware of options and of residual ridge resorption (RRR)	Conventional IIDs will cease to fit almost on insertion Their short-term nature should be explained
Primary impressions	In some cases, standard trays may need to be customised (e.g. with impression compound or PVS putty)
Definitive impressions	In customised tray
Registration	Form of registration will depend on the number of teeth present and their situation in the mouth
Try-in (not always possible)	Not always feasible (e.g. if adding to present denture or providing an overdenture)
Insertion	Not always straightforward!
Maintenance	Essential
Replacement	Patient should be informed of the need for replacement RPD or other restorative option

Dentistry at a Glance. First Edition. Edited by Elizabeth Kay. © 2016 John Wiley & Sons, Ltd. Published 2016 by John Wiley & Sons, Ltd.
Companion website: www.ataglanceseries.com/dentistryseries/dentistry

Introduction

Originally, immediate insertion dentures (IIDs) were intended to ensure that immediately following extraction of teeth, the patient was provided with a denture to restore/ improve appearance and also so that they could function socially. Complete functional replacement was not always feasible because of discomfort in the extraction socket (Figure 58.1). From the 1960s, immediate overdentures became acceptable and, with this form of denture restoration of masticatory function was more feasible. As listed in Table 58.1, there are several forms of immediate insertion denture. Some dentures are provided with a full flange while others merely touch the curvature of the socket/ gingivae adjacent to the root. These are called ridge-lapping dentures and are usually required when bulbous ridges are present or where the smile line discourages the provision of a flange (Figure 58.2).

Clinical stages involved in immediate insertion dentures

History and examination: As with all aspects of dentistry, a thorough history and examination is essential, particularly when exodontia is involved. Further information such as radiographic imaging will be required in the case of overdentures (Table 58.2).

Informed consent: In addition to the obvious, patients receiving an IID need to be informed that the denture may well not be a perfect 'fit'. The same will probably hold true when an addition is made to an existing denture, especially if is several years old and of a mucosal-supported type. The patient needs to be informed that IIDs are not definitive prostheses and a replacement denture will be recommended within 3–6 months. This will clearly have a cost implication. The patient should also be made aware of any potential postextraction problems.

Primary impressions: These are required in all cases and may serve as definitive impressions if the IID is created by adding to an existing denture, or when the arches are otherwise intact and only one or two teeth are to be replaced. Only one impression of each arch may be required in such cases, where the intercuspal position (ICP) is unambiguous. Not all clinical situations lend themselves to stock trays and alginate impressions; however, sometimes (e.g. when there are large edentulous areas in several areas of the arch) it is sensible to customise the stock tray by adding impression compound or polyvinyl siloxane (PVS) putty to the tray to record the edentulous areas (including the palate) and this will mean a more comfortable impression visit for patients, particularly those with a history of gagging.

Definitive impressions: These should be recorded in a perforated tray with spacing commensurate to the impression material being used. Note, if the remaining teeth are loose or if a fixed bridge is present, it may not be a sound idea to use a rigid impression material (e.g. polyether).

Registration: As mentioned above, a cast of the arch being restored is essential as is one of the opposing arch. Where the retruded contact position (RCP) is unambiguous, it may not always be necessary to actively record the registration as long as the clinician marks on the casts where interdigitation occurs. Where this is not obvious, however, conventional wax rims are recommended. Included in the instructions to the dental technician should be tooth shade and mould. Clinical photographs may also be useful.

Trial insertion visit: Clearly this will not be an option when there is to be an extraction/ decoronation and there will be an addition to the existing denture.

Insertion visit: This may well be a straightforward visit where an addition to an existing denture has occurred. In other cases, the clinician is advised to ask the laboratory to return the completed denture on a duplicate of the master cast to ensure that no undercuts to prevent insertion and subsequent removal into or from the mouth. Particular care is required when a complete overdenture IID is provided and no denture has been worn previously; in such instances, the mucosa should be inherently healthy and the denture will take some time to depress the soft tissues of the denture-bearing area.

Maintenance: Clinicians should plan for maintenance visits in all denture cases. Complete dentures (C/C) or removable partial denture (RPD) cases often need little maintenance, but IID cases inevitably will. There is a strong likelihood that chairside relines will be required until residual ridge resorption (RRR) has reached its maximum phase (3–6 months), at which point restoration of the arch with definitive prosthesis will usually be required.

59 Complete dentures

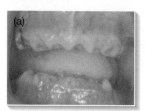

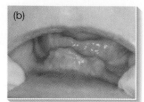

Figure 59.1 Examples of support problems: (a,b) these healing sockets will present support problems; (c) neither the image nor a study cast will reflect that the anterior ridge is flabby

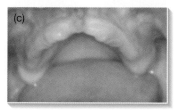

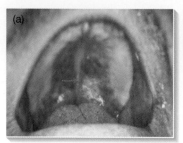

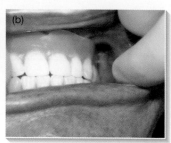

Figure 59.2 Examples of retention problems: (a) a palatal fissure in the post dam area (arrowed); (b) denture flange on the patient's left which, although impinging slightly on the muscle attachment, does not fill the peripheral roll

Edentulousness

This clinical condition may arise from neglect, accident or may be hereditary, resulting in anodontia. According to the World Health Organisation, edentulous patients are classified as handicapped and therefore the provision of complete dentures requires an understanding of the underlying science, an appreciation of patient factors and a sound understanding of basic prosthodontic principles.

Table 59.1 lists some of the common features and changes associated with (complete) tooth loss. Resorption affects the residual ridges and this in turn affects extraoral and facial appearance. Clinicians ought to utilise their knowledge of facial types when prescribing replacement dentures and, further, be aware of the fact that some types; for example Angle's Class 2 div. ii types will tend to lose more bone postextraction, (especially in the mandible) than other types owing to their 90° mandibular angles and a tendency for more prominent masseter muscles.

Assessing the patient

When contemplating prescribing replacement dentures, the clinician should be aware of the basic prosthodontic parameters involved, in addition to assessing the patient's wishes and perceptions; if such expectations are unrealistic or beyond your (current) clinical expertise, then common sense should prevail and the patient should be referred to a more senior and experienced colleague. These factors are listed in Table 59.2.

Prosthodontic factors

Support: It is essential that the clinician assesses, thoroughly, the denture bearing tissues (DBTs) to determine areas that are unlikely to withstand occlusal loading (e.g. flabby ridges) and which are vulnerable to pressure (e.g. atrophic mucosa, spikey

Table 59.1 Principal effects of (complete) tooth loss	
Facial changes	Alteration to vertical nasiolabial angle also affects vermillion border Alteration to lip support affects philtrum May, in time, induce a pseudoprognathic appearance
Intraoral changes	Maxilla resorbs inwards, therefore arch becomes more narrow Incisive papilla appears to move anteriorly Mandible appears to widen Residual ridge resorption – this is irrevocable
Physiological changes	Loss of proprioception from periodontal membrane Reduction of masticatory efficiency Decreased ability to adapt to the edentulous state in older patients, including phonetic problems Need to select appropriate freeway space
Psychological changes	Varies with person to person – may be severe antagonism to loss of teeth May affect confidence
Social changes	Current change in social (non) acceptance of edentulousness Greater emphasis on facial aesthetics

ridges or retained roots; Figure 59.1). This will also include prescribing an appropriate freeway space (FWS) in older patients with atrophic mandibular ridges – here clinical wisdom would suggest providing a larger FWS to avoid discomfort in mastication. This is the one factor that the clinician should be able to assess accurately and diminish the potential for failure, as retention and stability problems cannot always be overcome.

Dentistry at a Glance. First Edition. Edited by Elizabeth Kay. © 2016 John Wiley & Sons, Ltd. Published 2016 by John Wiley & Sons, Ltd.
Companion website: www.ataglanceseries.com/dentistryseries/dentistry

Table 59.2 Basic aspects to consider in planning complete dentures (C/Cs)

Factor to consider	Definition	What to watch out for
Support	A feature of the denture-bearing tissues (DBTs) resisting movement of the denture towards these tissues	Assess ability of DBTs to withstand digital pressure Assess nature of DBA (i.e. bony, fibrous) Is DBA inflamed or is there any mucosal pathology present?
Retention	A feature of the denture periphery resisting movement away from the denture-bearing tissues	Need to provide a peripheral seal Need to determine form and displacability of post dam tissues/ presence of a palatal fissure Assess quality and quantity of saliva
Stability	A feature of the denture resisting anterior–posterior and lateral movements of the denture	All C/Cs require occlusal balance in RCP Check if your patient should have balanced articulation Always ensure that the C/Cs are in harmony with the periodenture musculature (muscle balance) Patient's ability to control denture(s)
Other patient-related factors	Appearance Form Denture-wearing experience	Establish what the patient wants and (also if this is appropriate!) Inform the patient of the design of the denture – if you plan to leave off some teeth (e.g. 7s) tell the patient why Good denture-wearing history might indicate that replica dentures should be prescribed where indicated and where practicable
Dentist-related factors	Experience Laboratory quality Staff experience	Know your limitations! Ensure you have and maintain good communication with your technician Good teamwork is essential for a successful outcome

Retention: Retention requirements mean that the denture need to create a peripheral seal – essentially a triangle incorporating the post dam as the base and the right and left flanges of the upper denture. The presence of a cleft palate or a palatal cleft (Figure 59.2) can jeopardise a peripheral seal, as can muscle attachments that obliterate the sulcus. Also, absence of saliva will mean that the small but beneficial role of surface tension in the retention of a denture will be impaired.

Stability: This is the most complex and uncertain aspect of complete denture prescription. It is dependent on a combination of occlusal balance (OB), muscle balance (MB) and patient skills; the latter are, in the main, beyond the clinician's ability to control and many dentures have been prescribed which satisfy prosthodontic norms yet fail to gain patient acceptance. The converse is also true. Muscle balance requires care in recording the definitive impressions, while occlusal balance needs assessment at the initial consultation. Clinicians ought to prescribe OB in retruded contact positions (RCPs) for all dentures by ensuring that the registration stage is recorded properly, using specialised techniques if necessary. However, it will not be possible to ensure that balanced articulation can be prescribed. As this is required for stability in for ruminatory movements in eating, and stability problems must be anticipated in most patients.

Other patient-related factors

These will include perceptions of how the dentures should look, the number and form of teeth on the denture and denture-wearing experience. A balance must be struck between what is desired and what is feasible. For example, patient preferences for tooth selection may very well have to hold sway against that of the

clinician, but in cases where stability indicates that second molars should be left off the denture, then the patient should be made aware of the fact that stability matters have to take precedence. Contentment with a particular form of the denture periphery may well mean that the clinician should opt to prescribe a replica or template denture. In this case the clinician must ensure that the peripheral form is faithfully reproduced and that the occlusal form of the replacement denture does not induce instability as, in most cases, a worn-down occlusal surface will be being replaced by teeth with cusps.

Dentist-related factors

The art of complete denture prosthodontics is a problem area to younger graduates, who now treat fewer complete denture patients than undergraduates of 20 years ago. As the number of adults who are edentulous falls, undergraduates who are edentulous will become more problematic to treat – yet their expectations of success may very well be raised by virtue of the power of advertising in the media. One consequence of this is that a combination of lack of training allied to fear of failure may mean that many clinicians may fail to inspire patient confidence. In a clinician who is treating a complete denture patient with any lack of this quality, the chances of realistic success are much diminished.

Finally, the provision of complete dentures does require the harmonious integration of the dental team including the clinician, the dental technician/ clinical dental technician, the dental surgery assistance and the receptionist. The incorporation of available leaflets with the practice booklet will, in addition, keep the patient informed of what is required, for after care and maintenance.

60 Pulp therapy (deciduous teeth)

Figure 60.1 A healthy deciduous (a) upper arch, (b) lower arch and (c) dentition

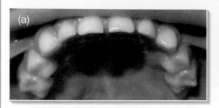

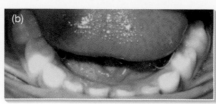

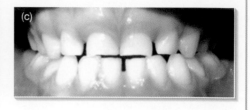

Figure 60.2 Indication for indirect pulp cap – pulp not involved

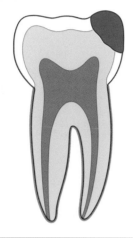

Figure 60.3 Indication for pulpotomy – pulp inflamed or partially necrotic

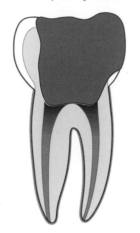

Figure 60.4 Indication for pulpectomy – pulp completely necrotic

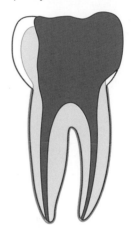

Introduction

The aim of pulp therapy in deciduous teeth is to remove inflamed pulp tissue, conserve the damaged tooth and restore function until the permanent successor erupts (Table 60.1). The main reason for the pulp of a tooth to become inflamed or infected is dental caries. It is important to take an accurate pain history in order to determine the level of pulp involvement and preoperative radiographs are useful to assess the extent of the carious lesion and its proximity to the pulp. Once caries has been removed from the tooth, it is easier to assess the level of pulpal exposure. Blood will be present at the exposure site if the pulp tissue is still vital.

Signs that may indicate pulp treatment is necessary are:
- Occlusal caries extending into the pulpal tissue (usually 4 mm or more in depth)
- Proximal caries extending into the marginal ridge
- Tooth mobility
- Sinus formation
- Furcation radiolucency on radiograph.

Symptoms that may indicate pulp treatment is necessary are:
- Reversible pulpitis pain – pain on stimulus
- Irreversible pulpitis pain – pain is spontaneous and lasts
- Swelling.

There are various treatment options for deciduous teeth with pulpal involvement:
- Indirect pulp capping
- Vital pulpotomy
- Non-vital pulpotomy (desensitising)
- Pulpectomy.

Indirect pulp capping

The purpose of this technique is to maintain pulp vitality by placing a lining onto deep dentine in order to eliminate bacteria and to stimulate secondary dentine.

- **Indications:**
  - An otherwise healthy mouth, similar to that shown in Figure 60.1a–c
  - Minor reversible pulpitis symptoms, e.g. pain on a stimulus only
  - Deep caries but no abscess or swelling
  - Caries not extending into pulp, so no pulpal exposure (Figure 60.2).
- **Contraindications:**
  - Extensive caries into the pulp
  - Irreversible pulpitis symptoms, e.g. pain waking child at night or pain that lingers without a stimulus.

Vital pulpotomy

This procedure involves removing the coronal pulp that is inflamed and infected (Figure 60.3), leaving healthy radicular pulp. The coronal pulp will bleed as it is still vital.

- **Indications:**
  - Co-operative child
  - Compliant child and parent with regard to diet and oral hygiene
  - Caries extending into the pulp in anaesthetised tooth
  - No furcation involvement

- No abscess
- When extraction is not possible due to a bleeding disorder.
- **Contraindications:**
  - Tooth close to exfoliation
  - Children who are immunosuppressed
  - Children with congenital heart disease
  - Poor general condition of the mouth, e.g. more than one or two teeth with likely pulpal involvement
  - Insufficient coronal tooth tissue to ensure an effective coronal seal.

Devitalising pulpotomy

This is a two-visit procedure used when adequate anaesthesia cannot be gained. At visit one Ledermix paste on cotton wool is sealed into the cavity with a temporary cement for 7–14 days. At the second visit the necrotic pulp can be removed and restored as per a pulpectomy.

Pulpectomy

This is used when there is non-vital tissue in the root canals (Figure 60.4). The canals are instrumented with files and then filled with zinc oxide cement or calcium hydroxide.

- **Indications:**
  - Co-operative child
  - Compliant child and parent with regard to diet and oral hygiene
  - Irreversible pulpitis of primary molars
  - Necrotic pulps
  - Furcation involvement
  - Acute or chronic abscess
  - When a tooth needs to be maintained in the arch or extraction is contraindicated to due health reasons
  - No permanent successor.
- **Contraindications:**
  - Medically compromised child
  - Poor general condition of the mouth, e.g. more than three teeth with likely pulpal involvement
  - Insufficient coronal tooth tissue to ensure an effective coronal seal
  - Tooth close to exfoliation.

Antibiotics may be administered, initially to relieve acute symptoms if there are systemic effects present or if there is an acute abscess or cellulitis present. The pulpectomy can be performed following the subsidence of acute symptoms.

Table 60.1 Summary of deciduous pulp treatments, techniques and medicaments

Procedure	Indications	Technique	Medicament
Indirect pulp cap	Symptoms of reversible pulpitis Caries not extending into the pulp	Remove all caries from periphery of cavity walls Deep soft dentine may be left at the floor of the cavity following gentle excavation Do not expose the pulp Place calcium hydroxide as a lining over the dentine floor Place a well-sealed permanent restoration, e.g. composite or stainless steel crown Review regularly	Calcium hydroxide
Vital pulpotomy	Deep carious lesion extending into the pulp Vital pulp No abscess or sinus Extraction is contraindicated, e.g. bleeding disorder	Remove caries Remove roof of pulp chamber Remove coronal pulp Apply ferric sulphate soaked on cotton wool for up to 60 seconds to the radicular pulp – this will help to arrest bleeding Place zinc oxide eugenol cement (Kalzinol) or MTA over the pulp Restore the tooth ensuring a good coronal seal is obtained, e.g. composite, amalgam or a stainless steel crown Review regularly	Ferric sulphate 15.5% MTA or zinc oxide eugenol
Devitalising pulp therapy leading to a pulpectomy (2 stages)	When anaesthesia cannot be gained (hyperalgesic)	Ledermix (polyantibiotic and steroid paste) is placed on cotton wool and sealed into the cavity with temporary cement for 7–14 days At the second visit the pulp can be removed and restored as per a pulpectomy	Visit 1: Ledermix Visit 2: zinc oxide eugenol or calcium hydroxide
Pulpectomy	Irreversible pulpitis Necrotic pulp Furcation radiolucency Abscess No permanent successor or as space maintenance	Remove caries, roof of pulp chamber, coronal pulp and identify the root canals Use endodontic instruments to remove necrotic tissue Irrigate canals (chlorhexidine, sodium hypochlorite, saline or EDTA) Dry the root canal with paper points Fill the root canal with zinc oxide eugenol using spiral root fillers Definitively restore the tooth ensuring a good coronal seal is obtained – this can be achieved with composite, amalgam or a stainless steel crown	Zinc oxide eugenol or calcium hydroxide

Administration of local anaesthesia (LA) and placement of rubber dam is deemed best practice for all procedures except desensitising pulpotomy, when LA cannot be gained due to behavioural reasons or LA has not worked.
EDTA, ethylene diaminetetra acetic acid; MTA, mineral trioxide aggregate.

61 Pulp protection procedures for traumatised teeth

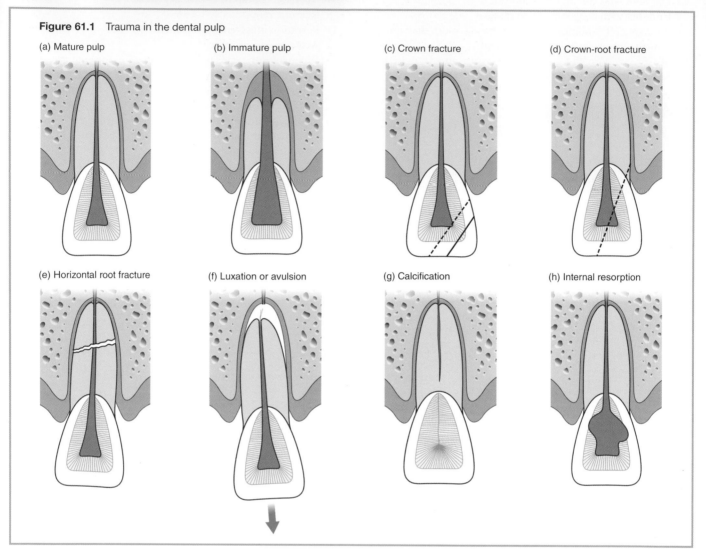

Figure 61.1 Trauma in the dental pulp

(a) Mature pulp

(b) Immature pulp

(c) Crown fracture

(d) Crown-root fracture

(e) Horizontal root fracture

(f) Luxation or avulsion

(g) Calcification

(h) Internal resorption

Types of tooth injury

• When the crown is fractured dentine and pulp may be exposed (complicated crown fracture in the Andreasen classification).

• An oblique fracture may involve both root and crown with pulpal exposure (complicated crown root fracture).

• In horizontal root fractures, the pulp may be torn or may remain intact (horizontal root fracture).

• In teeth that are avulsed or displaced, the pulp is separated from its vascular supply (luxations or avulsion).

• In teeth that are traumatised but neither fractured nor displaced the pulp may 'bruise', and/or there may be calcification or internal resorption (concussion or subluxation).

Diagnosis and prognosis are based on the following factors:

• Time since the tooth was traumatised
• Age of the patient
• Stage of root development
• Size of the pulpal exposure
• Extent of contamination
• Feasibility of restoration
• Vitality.

A traumatised tooth may not respond to vitality tests shortly after the trauma but a response may return later (up to 3 months).

Treatment (Table 61.1)

Crown fractures (Figure 61.1c)

• Small clean exposures seen immediately:
  • Cap directly using white mineral trioxide aggregate or calcium hydroxide
  • Restore
• Larger exposures in immature teeth:
  • Pulpotomy and apexogenesis
• Large exposure in mature teeth:
  • Pulpectomy
  • Root canal treatment
• Pulp is not exposed:
  • Treat fractured dentine as an indirect pulp exposure.

Oblique fractures (Figure 61.1d)

• Both crown and root fractured:
  • A complex problem with both periodontal and restorative challenges

- Cap the exposed pulp with mineral trioxide aggregate (MTA) or calcium hydroxide
- Place a temporary and sealing restoration
- If tooth remains vital:
  - Final restoration
- If tooth remains non-vital:
  - Root canal treatment
  - Restoration
- If root apex open:
  - Apexogenesis/apexification.

Horizontal root fractures (Figure 61.1e)
- Flexible splint
- Check vitality at 3 months
- If apical root fragment pulp necroses:
  - Remove surgically
- If coronal fragment necroses:
  - Root canal treatment
- If crown fragment separated:
  - Post and core
  - Crown lengthening
  - Extrusion

Avulsion and luxations (Figure 61.1f)
- Mature tooth:
  - Reimplant
  - Stabilise
  - Monitor
  - Root canal therapy if vitality does not return (luxations)
  - Most often vitality does not return and root canal treatment is indicated (avulsion)
- Immature tooth:
  - Reimplant
  - Stabilise
  - Monitor

Pulpal bruising
- Discoloured but vital:
  - No pulpal treatment
  - Monitor for loss of vitality or possible internal calcification (Figure 61.1g) or resorption (Figure 61.1h)
    - Root canal therapy if vitality lost
  - If no pulpal treatment indicated, consider improving aesthetics.

Procedures for treatment of traumatised teeth

Indirect pulp capping
1 Anaesthesia
2 Isolation
3 Cleaning
4 Placement of liner (calcium hydroxide base liner)
5 Restoration

Direct pulp capping
1 Anaesthesia
2 Isolation
3 Cleaning
4 Placement of capping material (MTA or calcium hydroxide)
5 Restoration.

Pulpotomy
1 Anaesthesia
2 Isolation
3 Debride the pulp chamber with a spoon excavator or high-speed drill
4 Copiously irrigate with sodium hypochlorite
5 Apply appropriate medication (MTA or calcium hydroxide) to the canal orifices
6 Cover pulpal floor with cement
7 Restore.

Table 61.1 Pulpal treatment of traumatised teeth

Condition	Clinical findings	Symptoms	Concerns	Treatment
Crown fracture (Figure 61.1c)	Loss of enamel and dentine Possible pulp exposure	Sensitivity Bleeding	Stage of root development Extend of exposure Time since injury	Indirect pulp capping Direct pulp capping Pulpotomy Pulpectomy
Crown-root fracture (Figure 61.1d)	Loss of enamel, coronal and radicular dentine Possible pulp exposure Fragments possible still in place	Sensitivity Bleeding	Stage of root development Extend of exposure Level of root fracture Time since injury	Indirect pulp capping Direct pulp capping Pulpotomy Pulpectomy Consider crown lengthening or extrusion
Horizontal root fracture (Figure 61.1e)	Increased mobility Usually detected on radiographic evaluation	Increased mobility Sensitive to percussion and or chewing	Stage of root development Extend of exposure Position of fracture Time since injury	Flexible splint (4–12 weeks) Check for vitality at 3 months If apical root fragment pulp necroses remove fragment surgically If coronal fragment necroses RCT If crown fragment separated post and core perhaps with crown lengthening and or extrusion
Luxation or avulsion (Figure 61.1f)	Tooth dislodge from socket or displaced Increased mobility or tooth maybe wedged in the socket	Pain on palpation and percussion Increased mobility	Stage of root development Degree of displacement Time since injury	Reposition teeth Flexible splint (2–4 weeks) Check for vitality at 3 months RCT if not vital and root completed Apexification/apexogenesis if root not completed
Pulpal bruising (Figure 61.1g,h)	Crown colour change: pink if internal resorption darker if calcification	Asymptomatic	Extend of resorption Aesthetic needs Possible presence of periapical lesion	RCT for internal resorption Follow-up observation for discoloration External bleaching Veneer

RCT, Root canal treatment.

62 Pulp removal (permanent teeth)

Figure 62.1 Pulp removal steps and materials: (a–c) diagnostic X-rays for tooth #36 (#19) diagnosed with necrosis and symptomatic apical periodontitis; (d) access opening on anterior tooth; (e) access opening on upper molar, buccal canal straight-line access; (f) palatal canal straight-line access; (g) access opening under rubber dam isolation, four canals found, distolingual canal access shown; (h,i) apex locator used to determine initial working length (WL); (j) four files placed, one for each canal; (k) distal angle X-ray taken to confirm WL; (l) working length X-ray, distal canals join and short; (m) Gates glidden drills for coronal flare; (n) hand file NiTi files (profile system); (o) protaper rotary NiTi system used for crown down technique, #15 file used to recapitulate; (p) copious irrigation with sodium hypochlorite used between files; (q) rotary file handpiece and control motor unit; (r) rotary instrumentation in progress

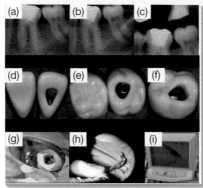
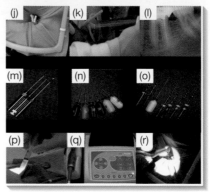

Figure 62.2 Pulpal removal/instrumentation techniques: (a) Working length determination to apical constriction. Crown-down technique; (b) Coronal flare; (c) Middle third preparation; (d) Apical third preparation; (e) Root canal prepared to #40 file. Step-Back technique: (f) Coronal flare; (g) Apical instrumentation to size #25 file; (h) Step-back increasing file size and reducing length; (i) Root canal prepared to size #25 file

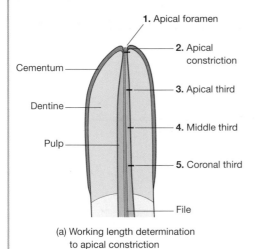
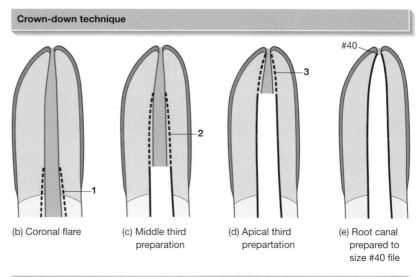

1. Apical foramen
2. Apical constriction
Cementum
3. Apical third
Dentine
4. Middle third
Pulp
5. Coronal third
File

(a) Working length determination to apical constriction

Crown-down technique

(b) Coronal flare
(c) Middle third preparation
(d) Apical third prepartation
(e) Root canal prepared to size #40 file — #40

Step-back technique

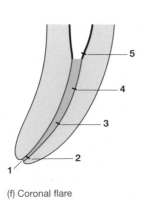
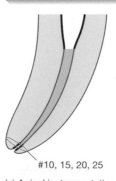
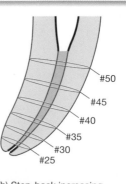
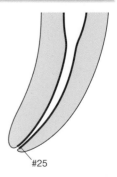

(f) Coronal flare

(g) Apical instrumentation to size #25 file — #10, 15, 20, 25

(h) Step-back increasing file size and reducing length — #50, #45, #40, #35, #30, #25

(i) Root canal prepared to size #25 file — #25

Dentistry at a Glance. First Edition. Edited by Elizabeth Kay. © 2016 John Wiley & Sons, Ltd. Published 2016 by John Wiley & Sons, Ltd.
Companion website: www.ataglanceseries.com/dentistryseries/dentistry

Partial pulp removal (pulpotomy)

Indications for partial pulp removal are:

• Symptomatic irreversible pulpitis: partial pulp removal is as effective in relieving pain as pulpectomies. This is usually a temporary procedure, executed quickly in an emergency.

• Incomplete root development: the aim of partial pulp removal is to amputate the coronal pulp in a tooth with incomplete root development while adding medication to encourage root growth and apical closure.

This technique has been used as a permanent procedure, applying a variety of medications to the root canal orifices followed by restoration. This is not universally approved of but deserves consideration when time, expertise and funds are available.

Complete pulp removal

Indications for complete pulp removal are:

• Symptomatic irreversible pulpitis (pulpectomy)
• Pulp necrosis (pulpal debridement).

Procedure for pulp removal

The availability of a pretreatment bitewing and at least one good periapical radiograph is essential before initiating pulp removal (Figure 62.1a–c). The stages of pulp removal are:

• Local anaesthesia
• Rubber dam isolation – this is mandatory
• Prepare occlusal access cavity for posterior teeth and lingual cavity for anterior teeth following the shape of the chamber and effectively removing its roof to allow straight-line access to the canal orifices (Figure 62.1d–f)
• Debride pulp chamber and canals.

The length to which each canal should be cleaned and shaped (the working length) is determined either by taking radiographs with files in the canals and/or using electronic apex locators. Sufficient radiographs should be taken at different angles to determine the local anatomy in detail. The length should be measured from a reproducible reference point on the crown to the apical constriction (the cementodentinal junction). This point is not always discernible by tactile exploration but can be safely estimated as lying 0.5–1.5 mm from the radiographic root end (Figure 62.1g–l).

Shape and clean the canals as follows:

• Widen the canal orifices and the coronal third of the canal (coronal flaring) by using hand or rotary instruments (Figure 62.2), allowing for minimal difficulty negotiating any curvature in the apical third.

• There are many types of instruments available, both hand and rotary (Gates–Glidden drills, nickel–titanium files) (Figure 62.1m–o).

• Confirm the working length as removing the curvature reduces the length of the canal.

• Prepare the apical third of the canal to a size determined individually for each canal (Figure 62.2).

• Prepare an apical 'stop' at or close to the cement–dentinal junction.

• Shape the apical segment of the canal by either the 'crown down' or the 'step back' technique (Figure 62.2).

• The apical constriction is likely to be absent in teeth with chronic periapical lesions as both bone and root resorption will have occurred. In such cases, an apical stop must be created artificially and is best placed further from the apex than it would be in a resorption-free root.

• Recapitulate the filing to full working length between each step, including copious irrigation with sodium hypochlorite, using a file of the same size as the apical preparation (Figure 62.1p–r).

• Rinse the canal with ethylene diamine tetracetic acid (17% EDTA) to remove dentinal debris.

• If a second appointment is needed prior to obturation, the canals can be medicated with calcium hydroxide or antibiotic paste.

• Place a cotton pellet in the pulp chamber and apply a sealing temporary restoration.

63 Pulp canal obturation (permanent teeth)

Figure 63.1 Obturating techniques: (a–d) lateral condensation; (e–i) vertical condensation. Red, shaped canal walls; yellow, sealer; pink, gutta percha; s, spreader; c, condenser

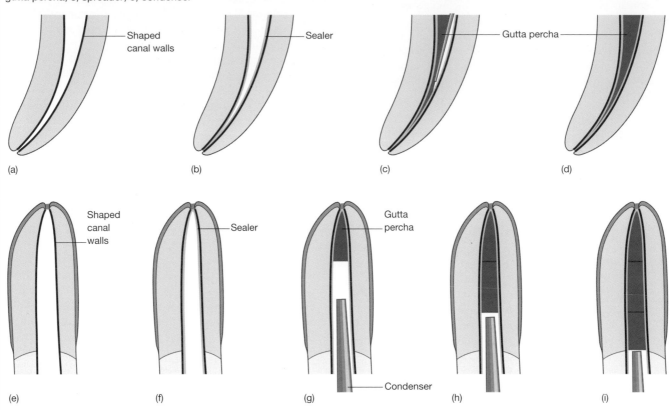

Figure 63.2 Instruments and materials for root canal obturation: (a) finger spreaders for lateral condensation; (b) standardised gutta percha cones and cement; (c) heat spreader for vertical condensation; (d) condensers; (e) gutta percha master cones in place; (f) gutta percha master cones X-ray; (g) system B and heat spreader; (h) heat spreader inside the canal to remove part of the master cone; (i) thermoplastised gutta percha to back-fill the canal; (j) injection of themoplastised gutta percha in the canal; (k–l) final obturation X-rays

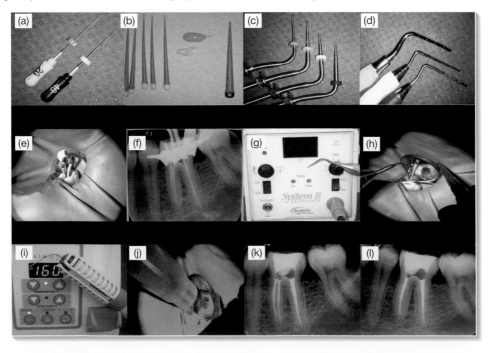

Dentistry at a Glance. First Edition. Edited by Elizabeth Kay. © 2016 John Wiley & Sons, Ltd. Published 2016 by John Wiley & Sons, Ltd.
Companion website: www.ataglanceseries.com/dentistryseries/dentistry

Aims of pulp obturation

Once the diseased pulp has been removed from a tooth and the pulp chamber and canal space cleaned and shaped these spaces should be obturated. The root canal obturation will impede the bacterial growth and favour the periapical healing.

Obturating materials

Obturating materials are available in several forms including solid, semisolid and hybrid. Properties of an ideal root canal filling material are listed in Box 63.1. All are used in combination with a sealing cement to improve adhesion and sealing ability (Table 63.1).

Box 63.1 Properties of an ideal root canal filling material

- Easy to place in canal
- Hermetic seal at coronal end and root apex
- Should not shrink
- Bactericidal or bacteriostatic
- Radiopaque
- Non-staining
- Biocompatible
- Easy to remove

Sealers: All sealers are flowable and are applied to the clean walls of the prepared canal using a file and can also be added as a coating to solid obturating materials (Table 63.2).

Obturating techniques

Some materials are available as cones. The initial cone (master cone) should be placed into the sealer-coated canal to full working length and condensed using spreaders to conform the cone to the canal shape and to provide space for further material. This condensation can be carried out cold or warm.

Two techniques are commonly used to fill the remaining space with cones. In **lateral condensation** (Figures 63.1a–d and 63.2a,b), small cones are placed sequentially with condensation between each cone until the canal is filled. Excess cone is cut off at the canal orifices. In **vertical condensation** (Figure 63.1e–i and 63.2c–l), after the master cone has been placed, it is cut down to a short length and vertically condensed with warm instruments. The rest of the canal will be backfilled with thermoplasticised obturating material.

The final restoration should now be placed. If this is not possible or not desirable, a strong-sealing temporary restoration should be used.

Table 63.1 Obturating materials

Material	Composition	Properties	Technique
Gutta percha cones	Zinc oxide 70% Gutta percha (isoprene) 20% Colouring/ fillers 10%	Semirigid low melting point Non-toxic	Lateral condensation Vertical condensation
Rigid core in gutta percha (hybrid)	Gutta percha with solid plastic or metal core	Rigid centre Easy insertion	Thermoplasticised – warm and insert
Thermoplasticised gutta percha	Special formulation of gutta percha	High melting point	Injection and condensation
Synthetic polymers (hybrid)	Coated gutta percha cones	Possibly good sealing Difficult to re-treat	Cones condensed with methacrylate resin sealer
Pastes	Zinc oxide and eugenol with added medication	Variable consistency Medicaments sometimes toxic	Injection – best placed after apical plug Widely regarded as ineffective due to difficulty in placement, leakage and toxicity
Mineral trioxide aggregate	Tricalcium silicate Dicalcium silicate Tricalcium aluminate Tetracalcium aluminoferrite Calcium sulphate Bismuth oxide	Highly biocompatible Slow setting	Difficult to place in current formulations Best placed after firming apical plug (collagen)
Silver points	Silver alloy	Very rigid Easily placed Non-adaptable	Insert with cement Prone to leakage and corrosion Commonly re-treated

Table 63.2 Sealers

Material	Composition	Properties
Zinc oxide and eugenol	Zinc oxide 42% Isoprene resin 27% Bismuth and barium salts	Eugenol toxic but resorbable Easily removed for re-treatment Stains Antimicrobial
Resin	Epoxy resin	Toxic Non-resorbable
Glass ionomer	Polyalkenoate cement	Good adhesion
Silicone	Polydimethylsiloxane Silicone oil	Shrinks Biocompatible
Calcium hydroxide	Calcium oxide Toluene salicylate	Stimulates hard tissue deposition Antimicrobial
Bioceramics	Alumina, zirconia, bioactive glass, glass ceramics, calcium silicates, hydroxyapatite calcium phosphates	Injectable Radiopaque Biocompatible Hydrophilic Difficult to re-treat

64 Patient management

Figure 64.1 (a, b) Reinforcement of toothbrushing instructions at recall visits

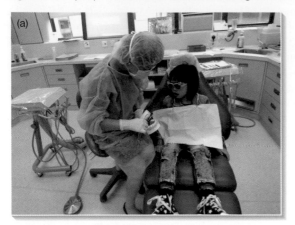

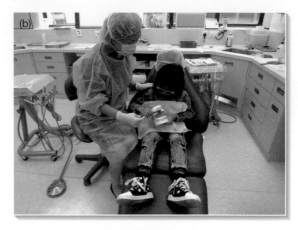

Figure 64.2 Demonstration of prophylaxis on the child's finger nail

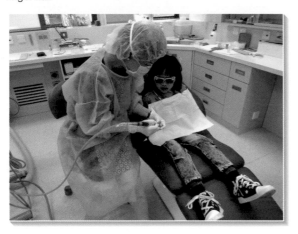

Figure 64.3 Child raises her hand up when she feels discomfort during treatment

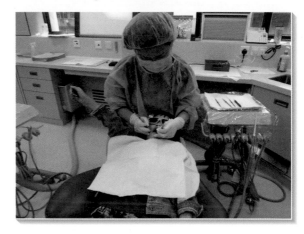

Dentistry for children is very different from dentistry for adult. Effective management of children is a team effort involving the parent, the dentist and the dental team. It is important that parents are involved in the decision-making process regarding treatment of their children. Gaining rapport from parents is essential for providing good dental care to children. Parent's active participation is likely to enhance the successful management of dental diseases as children rely entirely on the parent for compliance to dental appointments and preventive regimes.

Each member of the dental team (receptionist, dental surgery assistants and dental hygienist) should be supportive of each other in making the dental visit a smooth and pleasant experience for the child. Successful management of the child patient requires proper office procedures and positive dentist-and-patient relationship.

Office procedures

A preappointment letter, which informs the parent and the child's expectations for the first visit, often helps to reduce the child's dental anxiety and increases the likelihood of a successful first appointment. When the child arrives, the receptionist, being the first member of the dental team to meet the child, should show a positive and caring attitude and greet the child using his or her name. A child-friendly waiting area with colourful walls, children's books and toys will help to allay children's anxiety while waiting for dental treatment. The dental surgery assistant plays a major role in assisting the dentist and at the same time calming and supporting the child throughout treatment.

The objective of the first appointment is to introduce dentistry to children in a favourable manner. The appointment will usually involve history taking, clinical and radiographic examinations. Simple preventive treatments like prophylaxis and topical fluoride application can also be performed in the first appointment if the patient is co-operative. A well-organised treatment plan, developed based on the child's caries risk assessment, will enhance efficiency in provision of dental treatment. Following the first appointment, the receptionist assists the dentist by arranging a sequence of appointments in accordance with the dentist's treatment plan.

Usually, the child will need to be seen on a weekly basis, initially to familiarise with the dental environment and the procedures.

Dentistry at a Glance. First Edition. Edited by Elizabeth Kay. © 2016 John Wiley & Sons, Ltd. Published 2016 by John Wiley & Sons, Ltd.
Companion website: www.ataglanceseries.com/dentistryseries/dentistry

The restorative care should be completed by quadrants and as rapidly as possible in subsequent appointments, starting with simple restorative work to more complicated pulp treatments and extractions. The dental team should also be flexible and be prepared to make changes in treatment at times according to the child's behaviour at each visit.

Parental presence is essential for young and very unco-operative children. Older children, after the first consultation, may prefer not to have their parent in the surgery, so that the dentist will be the sole communicator with the child. This does reduce communication confusion and establishs appropriate dentist–patient roles. The choice of parental presence or absence should be discussed and agreed upon by the parent and child.

Once the planned course of treatment has been completed for the child, a recall interval should be decided. The recall interval depends on the caries risk and oral health needs of the child. The recall dental appointments for children give the dentist an opportunity to reinforce proper oral hygiene habits (Figure 64.1) and establish a trusting dentist–child patient relationship.

The dentist–child relationship

Establishing good communication with both the child and the parent is the key to develop positive dentist–child relationship. The dentist's communication is a major factor in patient satisfaction. Both verbal and non-verbal communications are equally important. Generally, verbal communication with children is best initiated with compliments, such as on their outfits and belongings. The words used have to be age-specific and at a level that the child understands. The tone of the voice should be caring, soft and kind, while expressing empathy. Truthfulness is important in communicating with children to build trust in the relationship. Non-verbal communication, including positive facial expressions, appropriate contact, posture and body language are all critical elements of child management. A smile or a gentle pat on the child shoulder often decreases the child's anxiety level and improves behaviour in the dental chair.

Behaviour management techniques

Good behavioural management is essential to obtain cooperation in child patients and allows successful delivery of dental treatment. The goals of behavioural management are to enable the dental team to provide treatment safely and efficiently and to develop positive dental attitudes in the child. These goals are achieved via communication and trust. Behavioural management can also be enhanced with pharmacological and non-pharmacological means. The non-pharmacological techniques described are mainly for co-operative and potentially co-operative children. Although the techniques are described individually, they are usually used in combination.

Behaviour shaping and positive reinforcement: This involves careful planning and introduction of the treatment procedures in small steps, from simple to complex, so that the child gradually accepts treatment in a relaxed and co-operative manner. Verbal phrases should be specific in encouraging helpful behaviour such as 'thank you for keeping your mouth open so that I can see clearly' or 'thank you for raising your hand when you need a rest', so that the desired behaviour will continue at the next appointment. At the end of the appointment, the child can be given tangible rewards such as stickers, balloons or toys as positive reinforcement and approval for positive behaviour. Any unhelpful behaviour during treatment should be ignored.

Tell–show–do: This is a classic technique for communicating with children and introducing them to a new procedure. The 'tell' phase includes an age-appropriate explanation of the procedure to be carried out. The 'show' phase involves demonstration of the procedure (Figure 64.2) and this is followed by the 'do' phase, in which the procedure is being conducted without delay.

Voice control: This is a controlled alteration of voice volume, tone or pace to influence or direct a patient's behaviour. The technique aims to gain the patient's attention and compliance, and negative behaviour. The technique is effective for inattentive but communicative children. However, it may not be appropriate for very young children or for those with intellectual or for those with emotional impairment.

Systematic desensitisation: This is usually used in children with existing dental fear. It is important to understand the causes of dental fear so that the child can be desensitised through exposure to the fear-producing stimuli. Three common stimuli for children in the surgery are injection, rubber dam application and cavity preparation using a high-speed handpiece. The patient is trained to relax in the first few appointments by showing them that they are in safe hands. Then, a hierarchy of fear-producing stimuli related to the patient's principal fear will then be constructed and applied on the child in the subsequent appointments, starting with the stimulus that causes the least fear and progressing to the next when the patient no longer fears that stimuli.

Distraction: This is often used to shift the patient's attention from the dental setting to some other situation or from a potentially unpleasant procedure to something else. Forms of distraction include cartoon films and music. Placement of a salivary ejector inside the patient's mouth may help to distract the patient's attention and discomfort associated with giving an injection. Similarly, asking the child to move their arms and legs during impression taking may divert the child's attention.

Modelling: This will help to decrease anxiety by showing a positive outcome in others to a procedure the children require themselves. For best results, the model should be of similar age as the target child. It is hoped that the relaxed, co-operative behaviour of the model will be imitated by the anxious child. This technique is best used on young children between 3 and 5 years of age. It is particularly useful for their first visit to a dentist. Tell–show–do and positive reinforcement should be used to supplement the modelling procedure.

Enhancing control: A feeling of loss of control can enhance anxiety and helplessness. A sense of control can be given by introducing choices such as asking the patient to raise a hand as a stop signal from treatment or to pause for a rest (Figure 64.3). The dentist must respond immediately on seeing the sign.

Other methods: Most patients can be managed using these basic behavioural management techniques. However, in some children, especially the young, extremely anxious children and patients with special healthcare needs, pharmacological approaches under sedation or general anaesthesia may have to be used.

65 Local anaesthesia

Table 65.1 Local anaesthetic agents – amide type

Local anaesthetic agent	Duration of anaesthesia		Properties
	pulpal (min)	soft tissues (hour)	
Lidocaine 2% plain	5–0	1–2	less effective anaesthesia witnout a vasoconstrictor
Lidocaine 2% 1:100 000 epinephrine	60	3–5	profound anaesthesia
Lidocaine 2% 1:50 000 epinephrine	60	3–5	for procedures requiring increased bleeding control no additional pain control achieved as compared to 1:100 000 concentration increases risk of cardiovascular reactions
Mepivacaine 3% plain	20 (infiltration) 40 (block)	2–3	short procedures where profound anaesthesia is unnecessary can be used when a vasoconstrictor is contraindicated
Mepivacaine 2% 1:20 000 levonordefrin	60–90	3–5	equivalent depth and duration of anaesthesia as compared to lidocaine with epinephrine levonordefrine does not produce the same intensity of haemostasis as epinephrine
Prilocaine 4% plain	5–10 (infiltration) 40–60 (block)	1.5–2 (infiltration) 2–4 (block)	can be used when a vasoconstrictor is contraindicated
Prilocaine 4% 1:200 000 epinephrine	60–90	3–8	slightly longer duration of anaesthesia than lidocaine with 1:100 00 epinephrine used when longer duration of anaesthesia is required used in ASA category 111 (severe systemic disease) patients who are epinephrine sensitive
Articaine 4% 1:100 000 epinephrine	60–75	3–6	better diffusion through bone than lidocaine or mepivacaine
Articaine 4% 1:200 000 epinephrine	45–60	3–6	used in patients with significant cardiovascular system diseases in patients onmedications that enhance the systemic effects of epinephrine
Bupivacaine 0.5%	90–180	4–9	most potent and toxic of all amide anaesthetics increased risk of systemic toxicity

Table 65.2 Local anaesthetic dosage

Local anaesthetic agent	Maximum dose		Dosage per dental cartridge	Maximum total dosage	
	mg/kg	mg/lb	mg/1.8ml cartridge	mg	no. of 1.8ml
Lidocaine	4.4	2.0		300	
2% plain			36		8.3
2% + 1:50 000 epinephrine			36		8.3
2% + 1:100 000 epinephrine			36		8.3
Articaine	7.0	3.2		500	
4% + 1:100 000 epinephrine			72		6.9
Prilocaine	6.0	2.7		400	
4% plain			72		5.5
4% + 1:200 000 epinephrine			72		5.5
Mepivacaine	4.4	2.0		300	
3% plain			54		5.5
2% + 1:100 000 epinephrine			36		8.3
2% + 1:20 000 levonordefrin			36		8.3
Bupivacaine	1.3	0.6		90	
0.5% + 1:200 000 epinephrine			9		10

Dentistry at a Glance. First Edition. Edited by Elizabeth Kay. © 2016 John Wiley & Sons, Ltd. Published 2016 by John Wiley & Sons, Ltd.
Companion website: www.ataglanceseries.com/dentistryseries/dentistry

Local anaesthesia

Pain control is an important aspect of dentistry and achieving profound local anaesthesia is essential to allow the operator to perform operative dental procedures with minimal stress to the patient.

The term local anaesthesia refers to loss of sensation resulting from a reversible blockade of nerve conduction in a circumscribed area. The chemical agents used to produce local anaesthesia are amphiphile (both hydrophilic and lipophilic) molecules of tertiary amines that stabilise neuronal membranes by inhibiting the ionic fluxes required for the propagation of neural impulses.

Most of the local anaesthetic agents used in dentistry are considered to be safe and effective with negligible soft-tissue irritation and minimal concerns for allergic reactions. The most important clinical properties of local anaesthetics are potency, onset and duration of action, as well as relative blockade of sensory and motor fibres (Table 65.1). Nonetheless, an ideal local anaesthetic agent should:
- Produce profound anaesthesia
- Be reversible
- Have a rapid onset and satisfactory duration of action
- Be non-irritating to the tissues
- Have minimal adverse local and systemic effects
- Be stable in solution and undergo biotransformation readily within the body
- Be sterile or capable of being sterilised by heat without deterioration.

Local anaesthetic agents

Articaine is a thiopene derivative, which contains an extra ester linkage and exhibits better diffusion properties through bone than lidocaine or mepivacaine. It is hydrolysed by plasma esterase in the blood and by enzymes in the liver. Approximately, 90–95% of articaine is metabolised in the blood; hence, it has a shorter half-life, thus decreasing the risk of systemic toxicity.

Lidocaine is a xylidine derivative and a potent vasodilator; hence, a vasoconstrictor (epinephrine) is used to achieve profound anaesthesia. Lidocaine exhibits a low risk of systemic toxicity and allergic reactions. It is metabolised in the liver through a complex metabolic pathway utilising several hepatic enzymes. It is contraindicated in patients with liver dysfunction and those who are on medications that utilise hepatic enzymes for metabolism.

Prilocaine is a toludine derivative, which produces less vasodilatation than lidocaine, and exhibits a similar potency as lidocaine and mepivacaine. Prilocaine is the least toxic local anaesthetic with minimal effects on the central nervous system and the cardiovascular system compared to lidocaine. A significant amount of prilocaine is metabolised in the lungs and kidney before reaching the liver. One of the by-products of metabolism, orthotoludine, can induce the formation of methaemoglobin leading to methaemoglobinaemia; therefore, it is contraindicated in patients at risk of methaemoglobinaemia and in those with oxygenation difficulties.

Mepivacaine is a xylidine derivative, produces less vasodilatation than lidocaine and is metabolised in the liver through a complex metabolic pathway utilising several hepatic enzymes. Its contraindications are similar to lidocaine.

Bupivacaine is the most potent and toxic of all amide anaesthetics with increased risk of systemic toxicity. Bupivacaine is pharmacologically similar to mepivacaine and is also metabolised in the liver; hence, it is contraindicated in patients with liver dysfunction. In addition, its use is contraindicated in young children.

Vasoconstrictors

Epinephrine (adrenaline) is a sympathomimetic amine added to local anaesthetic to cause vasoconstriction, which helps in achieving haemostasis, increases the duration of action of the local anaesthetic agent, decreases the systemic absorption and lowers systemic toxicity. Adverse effects to epinephrine include tachycardia, tremors, palpitations, arrhythmia and hypertension.

Techniques

Local anaesthesia can be achieved by:
- Field anaesthesia (infiltration)
- Conduction anaesthesia (nerve block).

In paediatric dentistry 1.8-mL cartridges are most commonly used but 1.7-mL and 2.2-mL cartridges are available on the market. Most often, for maxillary procedures, infiltration anaesthesia is sufficient as the cortical plate of the alveolus is thin and porous so making infiltration anaesthesia effective. Very rarely are posterior superior alveolar and infraorbital nerve block administered in children. Conversely, for mandibular procedures most often nerve block anaesthesia of the inferior alveolar, lingual and buccal nerves would be required when the operator decides that infiltration anaesthesia would be insufficient to obtain profound anaesthesia. The techniques used to obtain inferior alveolar nerve block are:
- Halstead method (nerve is blocked as it enters the mandibular foramen)
- Akinosi technique (higher level of injection, anaesthetises the inferior alveolar, lingual and buccal nerves in a single injection)
- Gow–Gates technique (uses external landmarks to direct the needle to a higher puncture point to deposit the solution above the lingula)

Complications
- Lip biting due to paraesthesia
- Toxicity
- Allergic reactions are rare – minor such as skin reactions (itching, redness, swelling); major such as bronchospasm and anaphylaxis
- Postinjection pain and paresis
- Facial nerve paresis
- Lingual nerve injury
- Broken needle.

An allergic reaction usually occurs due to a non-anaesthetic compound, such as sodium bisulphite which is used as a preservative for epinephrine in local anaesthetic solutions.

Reversing the effects of local anaesthetics

Phentolamine mesylate (OraVerse) is an alpha-adrenergic receptor antagonist that reverses the effects of local anaesthetics that contain vasoconstrictors. It acts as a vasodilator, resulting in faster diffusion of the local anaesthetic into the vascular system and away from the site, thereby reducing the unwanted side effects of lingering lip and tongue numbness.
- It must be injected in the same volume and at the same site as the local anaesthetic with vasoconstrictor was administered, e.g. 1 carpule of lidocaine = 1 carpule of OraVerse.
- It is not recommended for use in children younger than 6 years of age or weighing less than 15 kg (33 lbs).

66 Sedation and general anaesthesia

Figure 66.1 Pulse oximeter for measurement of oxygen saturation

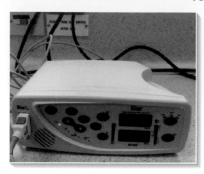

Figure 66.2 Nitrous oxide inhalation sedation delivery system

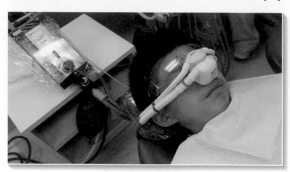

Figure 66.3 The use of local anaesthesia with nitrous oxide sedation

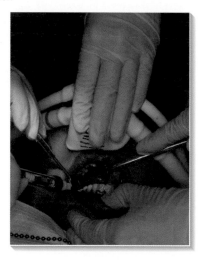

Figure 66.4 Nasotrachael intubation

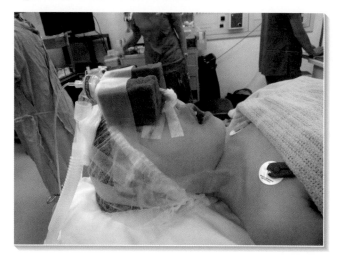

Figure 66.5 (a, b) Provision of dental treatment under mouth prop placement and rubber dam isolation

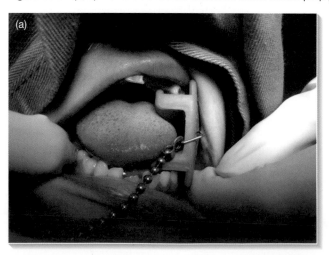

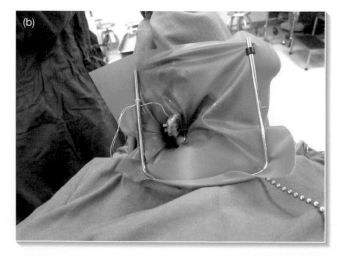

Conscious sedation

Conscious sedation is a technique in which the use of a drug or drugs produces a state of depression of the central nervous system enabling treatment to be carried out, but during which verbal contact with the patient is maintained throughout the period of sedation. The drugs and techniques used to provide conscious sedation for dental treatment should carry a margin of safety wide enough to render unintended loss of consciousness unlikely. The level of sedation must be such that the patient remains conscious, retains protective reflexes and is able to understand and to respond to verbal command

Indications for conscious sedation are:
- Fearful, anxious patients
- Prolonged or traumatic procedures.

Patient assessment: A full medical and dental history should be taken, followed by oral, radiographic examination and treatment planning. Patients with American Society of Anaesthesiologists (ASA) I and ASA II can be considered as outpatients. People who are chronically ill (ASA111 or above) should be treated in a hospital setting.

Patient information and consent: The patient or their parent or guardian must be given clear pre- and postsedation instructions verbally and in writing. Informed consent must be obtained prior to the conscious sedation appointment.

Fasting instructions: Fasting is not required for patients undergoing inhalation sedation. Patients who undergo all other forms of sedation should be fasted prior to the procedure as follows:
- No solid food within 6 hours
- No milk within 4 hours
- No clear fluid within 2 hours.

Documentation:
- Before treatment – consent, a clear treatment plan and presedation assessment
- During treatment – details of sedation used, dental treatment provided and monitoring performed
- After treatment – postsedation assessment and instructions.

Monitors: Alert clinical monitoring is essential throughout treatment. The other monitors for sedation are pulse oximeter (Figure 66.1), precordial stethoscope, capnograph and automated blood pressure cuff. Electronic monitoring is indicated in all types of conscious sedation, except nitrous oxide inhalation sedation.

Discharge: Patients should be alert and oriented before discharge. Parents or an adult must accompany a child and be given verbal and written postoperative instructions.

Routes of administration of conscious sedation: The commonly used sedation routes are inhalation, oral and intravenous.

1 Inhalation: This is the most common form of conscious sedation for paediatric dental patients. Dedicated dental nitrous oxide inhalation sedation delivery systems must be used (Figure 66.2). Nitrous oxide is a very weak analgesic and the use of local anaesthetic agent is required for painful procedures (Figure 66.3).
- Advantages associated with the use of nitrous oxide sedation are:
  - Rapid onset and recovery time
  - Ease of dose control
  - Lack of serious adverse effect.
- Disadvantages associated with the use of nitrous oxide sedation are:
  - Weak agent
  - Lack of acceptance in some patients
  - Potential chronic toxicity.

2 Oral: Benzodiazepines, in particular midazolam, are commonly used for oral sedation. The advantages of this route are universal acceptance by patients, ease of administration and decreased incidence of allergic reaction. However, the effects are unpredictable in children due to unreliable absorption.
3 Intravenous: This is the most effective method of ensuring rapid onset and predictable sedation. Intravenous sedation is not recommended for preco-operative children because of the difficulty in placing and maintaining an intravenous catheter. As the drugs are injected directly into the blood stream, the complication risk is higher than other routes.

General anaesthesia

A controlled state of unconsciousness accompanied by a loss of protective reflexes, including the ability to maintain an airway independently and respond purposefully to physical stimulation or verbal command.

Indications for general anaesthesia are:
- Severe dental disease in very young child, extremely uncooperative patient or children with special healthcare needs
- Patients requiring minor surgical procedures
- Patients who have sustained extensive orofacial and/or dental trauma.

Patient assessment: Full medical and dental histories must be taken. Clinical and radiographic examinations are performed for development of a comprehensive treatment plan.

Preanaesthetic assessment: The anaesthetist is responsible for the preanaesthetic assessment. Information on general anaesthesia (GA), its associated risk and benefits will be given to the parent and the consent form should be completed and signed.

Fasting instructions:
- No solid food for 6 hours preoperation
- No milk for 4 hours preoperation
- No clear fluids for 2 hours preoperation.

Operating theatre environment: The choice of premedication and general anaesthetic technique to be used is determined by the anaesthetist. Nasotracheal tube is preferred to orotracheal because it does not interfere with the working space in the mouth and reduces the chance of laryngeal oedema (Figure 66.4). The patient has his/her throat packed with gauze prior to provision of dental treatment.

Clinical procedures: Operative procedures are performed under rubber dam isolation and placement of a mouth prop (Figure 66.5). For restorative care, stainless steel crown is the preferred restoration for posterior primary molars. Pulp therapies should be performed cautiously, taking into consideration the long-term prognosis of the tooth. Grossly broken down teeth are routinely extracted. Local anaesthetic solution is given prior to extraction to reduce postoperative bleeding and discomfort. After completion of treatment, the throat pack is removed and the nasotracheal tube by the anaesthetist.

Documentation:
- Before treatment – informed consent, a comprehensive treatment plan and pre-GA assessment
- During treatment – name of the drug, dosage, route and duration of GA, dental treatment performed and monitoring performed
- After treatment – post-GA assessment and instructions.

Discharge: The patient is discharged on the day following the operation if no complication arises. Parents should be given verbal and written postoperative instructions.

67 Caries in deciduous teeth

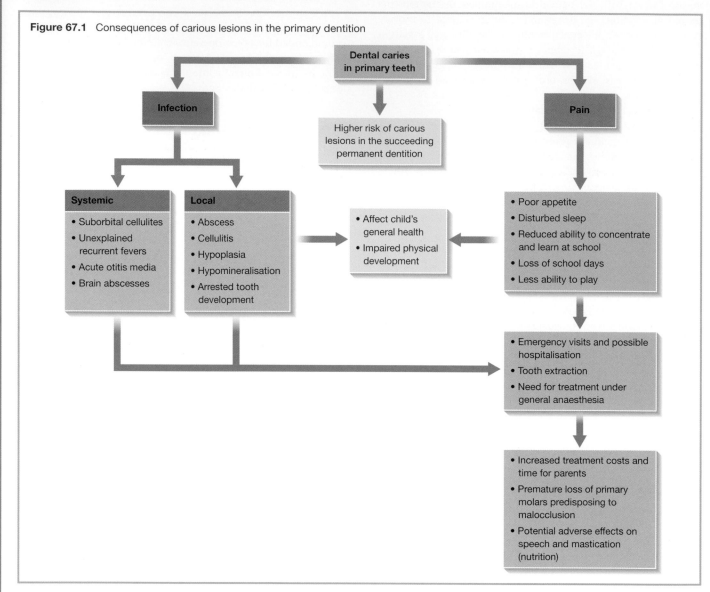

Figure 67.1 Consequences of carious lesions in the primary dentition

Dental caries

Dental caries is the localised destruction of susceptible dental hard tissue by acidic by-products from bacterial fermentation of dietary carbohydrates. Therefore, it is a bacterial driven, site-specific, multifactorial dynamic disease process that is general, chronic and results from an imbalance in the physiological equilibrium between tooth mineral and plaque fluid.

The caries process is the dynamic sequence of biofilm–tooth interactions that can occur over time on and within a tooth surface. This process involves a shift in the balance between destructive factors (favouring demineralisation) and protective factors (favouring remineralisation). This disease process can be moderated, or even arrested, at any time by therapies that enhance the remineralisation process.

Primary teeth play a critical role in the growth and development of a child. In addition to their roles in aesthetics, mastication, speech, normal oral function and expected growth, another major function of the primary teeth is to provide space for their permanent successors until the permanent teeth erupt.

The condition of the primary dentition and the occlusal relationship of the maxillary teeth to the mandibular teeth directly influence both the functional and morphological development of the permanent dentition. The primary teeth maintain the natural length of the dental arch and so permit the permanent teeth to erupt in an orderly fashion with adequate space. Some of the permanent teeth (premolars) are smaller than their primary predecessors while others are larger (permanent incisors and canines). Furthermore, the eruption pattern is not a uniform sequence. Therefore, without the primary teeth, the permanent successors cannot assume their correct position in the dental arch.

Consequences of leaving untreated carious primary teeth

The consequences of leaving dental caries in primary teeth untreated, which are illustrated in Figure 67.1, may include short- or long-term consequences or even rare sequelae.

- Short term:
  - Pain
  - Infection, e.g. abscess, cellulitis
  - Emergency visits and possible hospitalisation
  - Poor appetite
  - Disturbed sleep
  - Loss of days at school, kindergarten and playgroups with restricted activity and ability to play
  - Reduced ability to learn and concentrate at school
  - Need for tooth extraction
  - Need for treatment under general anaesthesia
  - Premature loss of primary molars predisposing to malocclusion in the permanent dentition
- Long term:
  - Higher risk of new carious lesions in other primary teeth and the succeeding permanent dentition
  - Poor oral health and dental disease often continues into adulthood
  - Affects child's general health, resulting in insufficient physical development especially in height and weight
  - Increased treatment costs and time for parents
  - Potential adverse effects on speech, nutrition and quality of life

- Rare sequelae:
  - Suborbital cellulitis
  - Unexplained recurrent fevers
  - Acute otitis media
  - Brain abscess.

Management of carious primary teeth

Preventive measures

Expectant mothers should be educated about:
- The importance of nutrition throughout pregnancy
- Good oral health and hygiene for themselves
- Infant dietary habits
- Early dental visits
- Tooth brushing and fluoride preparations
- The value of early dental check-ups for the child.

Fissure sealants

These are recommended for primary and permanent molars in children with a history of dental caries and those who are in high-risk groups. Fissure sealants have been proven to be effective; however, they need regular maintenance and repair.

Restorative management

Prior to any definitive treatment plan the following factors must be considered:
- Extent of the disease
- Child's age and level of co-operation
- Parents' attitude and motivation towards dental treatment.

Primary anterior teeth

The reason for restoring carious primary incisors and canines is to allow the child to retain these teeth, so as to allow natural exfoliation without any pulpal complications. The treatment options available are:
- Restorations with composite resin strip crowns, compomer, glass ionomer cements or stainless steel crowns
- Pulp therapy (pulpotomy or pulpectomy)
- Extraction.

Primary molars

Depending on the extent of a carious lesion, one of the following materials can be used for the restoration of primary molars.
- Composite resin
- Compomer
- Stainless steel crowns
- Glass ionomer cement
- Amalgam
- Pulp therapy (pulpotomy or pulpectomy)
- Extraction.

Space maintainers

Premature loss of primary teeth by extraction can have an influence on the occlusion and space for the teeth of the permanent dentition. Very rarely it is thought necessary to use space maintaining appliances in an attempt to retain the space for the succeeding permanent teeth. Numerous factors, such as the age of the patient, teeth present, caries status, level of oral hygiene, the willingness of the parents to bring the child for treatment and the patient to accept the treatment, need to be considered prior to deciding to insert a space maintainer.

68 Paediatric dental materials

Figure 68.1 Stainless steel crowns placed on lower primary molars

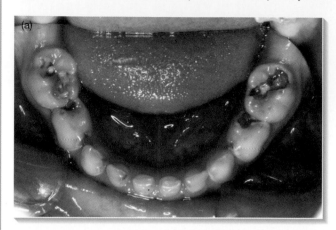
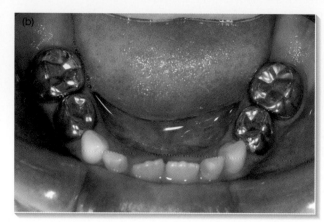

Figure 68.2 Composite strip crowns placed on the upper primary incisors

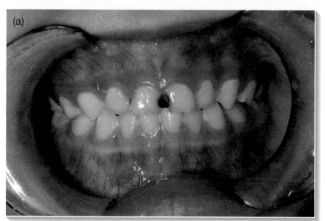
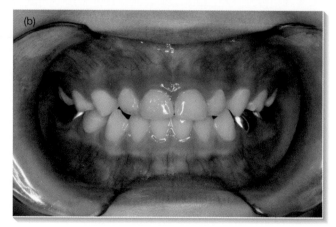

A diversity of restorative materials is now available for restoration of carious lesions in the primary and permanent teeth of children. It is imperative that clinicians understand the advantages and disadvantages associated with each type of restorative material and select the most appropriate material for use in their patients. The choice of material in a given clinical situation depends on the age, caries risk and cooperation level of the child, the compliance of the parents and the type of cavities to be restored.

Stainless steel crowns

Stainless steel crowns (SSCs) are widely recognised as the most effective and durable restoration for primary molars. They are mainly used to restore large multisurface carious lesions (Figure 68.1), following pulp therapy in primary molars as well as hypoplastic or hypomineralised primary or permanent molars.

Recently, the Hall technique, which involves sealing caries beneath SSCs, provides a simple method of managing early to moderately active dentinal lesion in primary molars. The crown is cemented over the tooth without caries removal, tooth preparation or the use of local anaesthesia. The technique is gaining popularity with good evidence of effectiveness and acceptability to children and parents.

Some parents or patients may find the appearance of metal SSCs unacceptable. Alternatives to this technique are prefabricated tooth-coloured crowns. However, these crowns are more expensive and require significantly more preparation due to their greater bulk, resulting in a lack of natural appearance and poorer gingival health. The aesthetic facings of the crowns are also prone to fracture.

Resin-based composites

Current composites are available as microfilled, hybrid and packable composites, depending on the size and percentage of the fillers. The microfilled composites are mainly used as class V restorations, non-stress-bearing class III restorations and small class I restorations. Flowable composites are a subclass of microfilled composites with a lower volumetric filler percentage than traditional hybrid resins. They are less rigid with a favourable modulus of elasticity and less polymerisation stress. However, they have inferior mechanical properties and are mainly used for very small class I occlusal restorations in low-stress areas as well as liner under posterior composite restorations.

Hybrid resins are indicated for class III and IV restorations, as well as class I and II restorations in load-bearing surfaces. Packable composites generally have a chemically modified resin matrix with a higher filler content of 65–70%. They are denser with a stiffer consistency than conventional resin composites. However, there is no clinical evidence that their properties are better than conventional composites.

The advantages associated with resin-based composite restorations include: excellent aesthetics qualities, ease of use, reparability and preservation of tooth structure in cavity preparation (Figure 68.2). The disadvantages of composite are: polymerisation shrinkage, postoperative sensitivity, marginal discoloration and secondary caries.

Resin infiltration

Recently, caries infiltration was introduced as a microinvasive treatment to arrest non-cavitated, small proximal caries lesions. The method is based on the penetration of low-viscosity light-cured resins into the non-cavitated pores of an incipient lesion. Consequently, a barrier is created that blocks further bacterial diffusion and halts lesion development. The technique involves removal of the covering surface layer by 15% hydrochloric acid gel to enable the penetration of the infiltrant into the lesion body. Subsequently, the lesion is properly desiccated with ethanol to allow capillary action to soak the resin into the lesion body. Finally, the infiltrant is applied for sufficient time to infiltrate the lesion deeply and be light cured. A major advantage of caries infiltration is that treated lesions change their optical properties and appear similar to sound enamel. Hence, resin infiltration can also be used to camouflage aesthetically disfiguring white spot lesions on buccal surfaces.

Glass ionomer cement

Conventional glass ionomer cements (GIC) are based on fluoroaluminosilicate glass powder mixed with polyalkenoic acid, which set by acid–base reaction. The moisture susceptibility and inferior mechanical properties of conventional GIC have led to the development of metal-modified GIC and resin-modified GIC. Although metal-reinforced GIC were formulated to improve the mechanical properties of the cement, their use in high-stress-bearing areas is not recommended.

Resin-modified glass ionomer cements have been developed with improved aesthetics, wear resistance and command set. They are used as class I, II, III and V restorations in primary teeth as well as class III and V restorations in permanent teeth in high-risk patient or teeth that cannot be isolated. Recent improvements in conventional GICs have led to the development of high-viscosity GIC for use in atraumatic restorative treatment.

Glass ionomers are also been used as luting cements for stainless steel crowns and orthodontic bands, as cavity liner and base. More recently, it is used as interim therapeutic restorations (ITR). The indications for ITR are very young patients, unco-operative patients or patients with special healthcare needs, for whom traditional cavity preparation and/or placement of traditional dental restorations are not feasible or need to be delayed. ITR may also be used for caries control in children with multiple open carious lesions before definitive restoration of the teeth.

Compomer

Compomers are polyacid-modified composite resins. The primary setting reaction of compomers occurs by photoinitiation, followed by a secondary acid–base reaction. A limited release of fluoride ions occurs following water sorption. The increased water sorption of compomer compared to conventional composite, results in marginal staining affecting the aesthetics of the tooth-coloured restorations. Adhesion to tooth structure is the same as composite resin and the use of an adhesive system is recommended. The main clinical applications of compomer are class I and II restorations in primary molars and class V restorations in primary and permanent teeth.

69 Fissure sealants

Figure 69.1 Fissure sealant

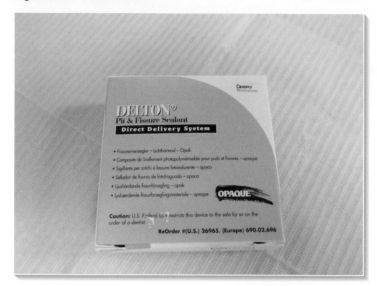

Figure 69.2 Light cure

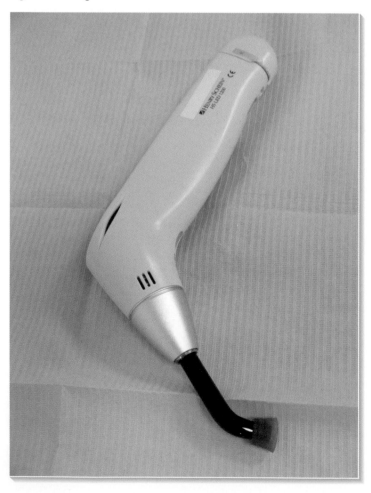

Dentistry at a Glance. First Edition. Edited by Elizabeth Kay. © 2016 John Wiley & Sons, Ltd. Published 2016 by John Wiley & Sons, Ltd.
Companion website: www.ataglanceseries.com/dentistryseries/dentistry

The fissures of the teeth retain plaque more readily than the smooth surfaces and are therefore more susceptible to caries. Not all fissures will decay, however, and therefore only susceptible teeth in children with moderate to high caries risk should be sealed. The following factors should be taken into account when the decision to seal a fissure is being considered:

• **Tooth morphology** – deep fissures are more susceptible
• **Caries history** – decayed deciduous molars are an indicator that the first permanent molars should be sealed
• **Caries risk factors** – diet, medication and oral hygiene.

Types of sealant

Both filled and unfilled resins and glass ionomer cements have been used as sealants (Figure 69.1). Resins have better retention rates and flow more easily into deep and complex fissures. However, the effectiveness of glass ionomers and resins at preventing caries are similar. Glass ionomers are less affected by moisture contamination and therefore may become the material of choice in, for example, very small children for whom rubber dam and total moisture control are overly challenging.

Steps in fissure sealing

1 Clean the pit and fissure surfaces: First, clean all plaque and debris from the surface to be sealed (Box 69.1). A prophy cup or brush with pumice is most commonly used for this purpose although probes, toothbrush or air polishing with sodium hydrogen carbonate is also effective.

2 Isolate the tooth: Any contamination of the fissure by saliva will reduce the likelihood of a sealant being retained. Therefore the tooth in question must be completely isolated using either cotton wool rolls or rubber dam, the latter being preferable.

3 Etch the enamel: To ensure that the sealant adheres to the enamel it must be etched with 37% orthophosphoric acid. Etchants may be in liquid or gel form but both offer equal surface penetration and there is no difference in sealant retention rates with one or the other. Coloured gels are helpful as it is easier to see where the etchant has been applied. Gel can be applied with a brush or syringe. The etching should continue for 15 seconds and thoroughly rinsed off, then dried. The etched area should have the appearance of frosted glass. If the surface is contaminated at any point by saliva the etching must be repeated.

Sealant application

The fissure sealant is then applied to the etched area using a small applicator or brush. If a light-cured sealant is being used the curing light should be brought adjacent to the sealant for 20 seconds (Figure 69.2). Once cured, it is best to wipe the surface of the sealant with a cotton pledget as oxygen inhibits the surface layer from polymerising, and unpolymerised sealant has a most unpleasant taste.

Evaluation

Coverage of all parts of the fissure should be checked and a periodontal probe should be used to ensure that the sealant has bonded to the enamel. The dentist should also confirm with the patient, and with the use of articulating paper, that the occlusion has not been affected. If it has, a finishing bur can be used to correct this.

Box 69.1 Steps in fissure sealing

1 Clean the pit and fissure surfaces
2 Isolate the tooth
3 Etch the enamel
4 Rinse and dry the tooth
5 Apply the sealant
6 Polymerise
7 Evaluate

70 Dietary control

Figure 70.1 (a) Biscuits are high in NMES. (b) Confectionery is designed to be attractive to children. (c) High NMES foodstuffs are widely available and (d) made to appeal. (e) The majority of sugars consumed are found in fizzy drinks, (f) with wide ranges available.

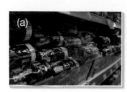
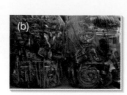
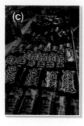
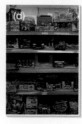
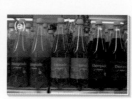
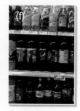

Figure 70.2 Some of the five a day (a). Vegetables are good value for money (b), and healthy options can be attractive alternatives

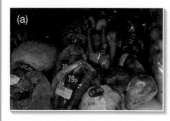

Figure 70.3 Diet diaries require careful explanation

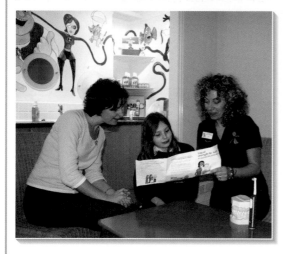

Figure 70.4 Three-day diet and 24-hour diet assessment sheet

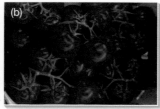

3 day diet assessment

- Please write down all the food and drink you have consumed for **three days**. Please include a Saturday or Sunday.

- Please write down the **time of day** and try and **describe how much** has been eaten or drunk. For example, one cup, one tablespoon, one portion. Please leave the comments column blank.

- Please then **bring this sheet back** to your next dental appointment so you and your dentist can look together at the effect your diet may be having on your teeth.

DAY 1

TIME	FOOD OR DRINKS	AMOUNTS	COMMENTS

DAY 2

TIME	FOOD OR DRINKS	AMOUNTS	COMMENTS

DAY 3

TIME	FOOD OR DRINKS	AMOUNTS	COMMENTS

There are two types of extrinsic sugar: milk extrinsic sugars and non-milk extrinsic sugars (NMES). NMES are found in sweet foods and drinks such as confectionary, soft drinks, biscuits, honey and, of course, table sugar (Figures 70.1). In order to avoid caries, evidence suggests that:

• People should limit both the amount of NMES they consume and the number of times they are consumed in a day. If at all possible NMES should only be consumed at meal-times.

• Restricting NMES consumption to less than four times a day is advised.

• NMES should provide less than 5% of total energy in the diet and should not exceed 60 g per day per person.

• Consumption of five portions of fruits or vegetables per day is health promoting (Figures 70.2). These contain intrinsic sugars.

If dentists are to offer advice to patients with respect to their diet, it is important that the information that they give patients does not conflict with general nutritional requirements for good health.

Sugar consumption in the UK

Sugar consumption in the UK peaked in the 1950s. During the war years, rationing had greatly limited consumption of NMES, but as rationing faded, sugar consumption rose dramatically. Subsequently, it reduced year on year but there has also been an increased consumption of manufactured and processed foods and drinks, many of which contain considerable amounts of sugar – often this is referred to as 'hidden sugar'.

Sugar and caries

Epidemiological studies have shown that there is a clear association between caries experience and mean sugar consumption. When sugar consumption declined during the war, because of rationing, caries prevalence also fell. Isolated communities with restricted diets containing little sugar have very low caries experience and countries consuming the greatest amounts of sugar have the highest. It has also been noted that long-term use of sugary medicines increases caries risk. Other studies have shown that increasing or decreasing the sugar in a person's diet affects the increment in caries they experience.

If electrodes are placed into plaque, when sugar solution is applied, the pH falls and remains low (acidic) for a considerable time (20 minutes–2 hours).

Changing people's eating habits

It is recommended that people who are at higher risk of caries should receive dietary advice. It is insufficient and completely ineffective to add a 'don't eat so many sweets' to the end of a dental visit. Dietary advice needs to be 'SMART' (see Figure 70.4).

Identifying patients requiring dietary counselling

All patients should be given appropriate information about diet and its effect on oral health. However, if patients have active caries, a high caries rate, or erosion, they should be given more specific counselling and help to reduce their caries risk. In general, caries rates tend to be highest in preschool children, teenagers, the elderly and those taking sugary medicines. Caries is also more prevalent in people from lower socioeconomic groups. If a patient belongs to any of these groups and has active caries, the dentist should take a careful diet history.

Box 70.1 'SMART' dietary advice

- **Specific** – tailor the advice to the person you are speaking to, making it particular to that individual and their current habits and lifestyle.
- **Measurable** – make sure you know what their sugar consumption is currently so that you (and they) can measure the difference when they change their behaviour.
- **Appropriate** – the advice must be appropriate to the problem. Recommending complete abolition of sugar to someone with low caries rates is clearly inappropriate.
- **Realistic** – try not to ask for the impossible. Set goals which the patient has a real chance of achieving.
- **Time related** – make it clear that the behaviour needs to change within a given period, not just sometime in the future.

Taking a dietary history

Obtaining an accurate picture of the entirety of a person's food and drink intake is difficult and requires skill and sufficient time if it is to be done successfully. Fortunately, for the purpose of caries prevention only key aspects of the diet require in-depth exploration. You need, firstly, to establish:

- The frequency of food intake
- The frequency of NMES-containing food intake
- NMES food intakes prior to sleeping.

The way in which this information should be sought is by the use of a 3-day diet diary (Figure 70.3). The patient should be asked to record each food and drink intake, a description of exactly what was eaten, the time and place it was eaten and the amount of each food and drink, and also an indication of what time the person retired to bed.. The diary should include at least one weekend day (as dietary patterns alter when routine is changed).

This is clearly quite an onerous request to make of a patient and, unless they clearly understand why it is needed and are motivated, they are very unlikely to complete the diary accurately or give you a complete picture of their dietary habits. In addition, do not simply ask the patient to 'fill in a diet diary'. You need to give them very careful and precise instructions about what you wish them to do and why. Ideally, these instructions should be given both verbally and in a written format. You also need to allow the patient to ask you anything they wish about the process.

Once the diet diary is returned, time should be set aside to analyse its content and discuss it in detail with the patient. The diary should give the dentist an idea of any dietary habits that may relate to the patient's oral health problems.

Setting goals

The ultimate goal of dietary advice is to reduce both the amount and frequency of NME consumption. The dentist must set very clearly delineated goals such as 'missing out the biscuits at coffee and tea time' or 'replace your sugar with sweeteners in your tea'. Vague goals will not be effective.

Usually the bulk of NMES are consumed in soft drinks, confectionary, biscuits and cakes. Therefore setting goals that specifically focus on reduction of these items should reduce the patient's caries risk. The goals should be agreed by the patient. Simply telling them what you wish them to do will not work.

Action points

Help the patient by suggesting ways of altering their routines so that the situations when they are most likely to consume NMES are avoided. Also, suggesting alternative foods, such as drinks and snacks that are not cariogenic, is extremely useful.

Monitoring

It is essential that a regular and serious review of progress takes place. To ask a patient to do something as difficult as changing their diet and then not even ask about their achievements is dispiriting and demotivating for the patient. Continued support, encouragement and feedback is needed in order that positive changes are maintained. This should occur every time the patient is seen.

Summary

Altering the way and what a person eats is a very difficult thing to do. Always bear the following in mind:
- The aim is to reduce the frequency and amount of sugar whilst maintaining a healthy eating pattern.
- Taking a diary is essential.
- No change will take place unless the patient wants to achieve caries risk reduction.
- Monitoring, reviewing and supporting the patient's efforts is crucial.

71 Fluoride supplements

Figure 71.1 Toothpaste should be at least 1000 ppm fluoride

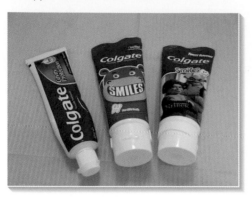

Figure 71.2 Patients should be encouraged to select an appropriate toothbrush

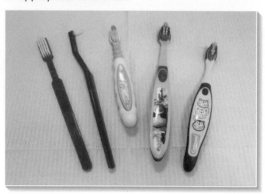

Figure 71.3 Chlorhexidine rinse

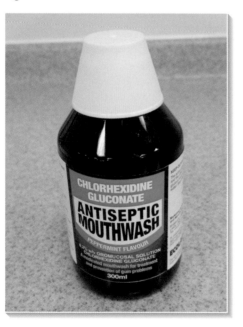

Figure 71.4 Fluoride varnish

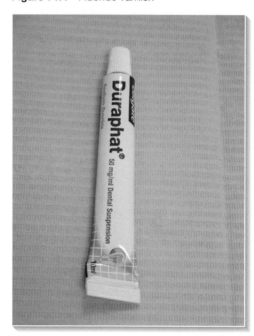

Fluoride produces an anticaries affect in a number of ways, and these act simultaneously to bring about observed improvements in oral health (Box 71.1).

Box 71.1 When to apply fluoride in the surgery

- High smooth surface caries rate
- Evidence of susceptibility to root caries
- Patients at increased caries risk
- Orthodontic
- Patients undergoing head and neck irradiation
- Decreased salivary flow

Remineralisation: Even small amounts of fluoride in plaque and saliva change the chemical balance so that enamel is more prone to remineralise than demineralise. Furthermore, not only is the carious process reversed but the new crystals that are deposited are more acid resistant.

Reduced acid production: Plaque concentrates fluoride and its presence prevents plaque bacteria from so easily converting dietary sugars into acid.

Fluoride substitution: Fluoride ingested in the diet is incorporated into developing teeth. The fluohydroxyapatite is more resistant to acid attack than unfluoridated hydroxyapatite.

Dentistry at a Glance. First Edition. Edited by Elizabeth Kay. © 2016 John Wiley & Sons, Ltd. Published 2016 by John Wiley & Sons, Ltd.
Companion website: www.ataglanceseries.com/dentistryseries/dentistry

Reduced fissure depth: The fissures of the teeth are the most susceptible to caries. It seems that when fluoride is in the bloodstream during teeth formation they have less pronounced (shallower) fissures. This is thought to reduce their susceptibility to caries.

Forms of fluoride delivery

Six methods of utilising fluoride's caries-preventive effect for the benefit of the population and patients are available. They are:

- Fluoride toothpaste
- Fluoridated water
- Fluoride tablets and drops
- Fluoridated milk
- Fluoride varnishes
- Fluoride gel and foam.

Fluoride toothpaste

Fluoride toothpaste, which has been widely available in the UK since the early 1970s, has been responsible for the rapid improvements in dental health seen over the last 30 plus years. Toothpastes containing 1000–1500 ppm fluoride are highly effective in reducing caries risk (Figure 71.1).

All patients should be advised to brush twice daily with a fluoride toothpaste (Figure 71.2). Patients at particularly high risk of caries should be prescribed toothpastes with higher concentrations. Children should be encouraged to use a pea-size amount of 1000-ppm toothpaste. Fluorosis is dependent on the fluoride dose ingested whilst the anticaries properties are correlated with fluoride concentration.

Brushing is best carried out prior to sleeping as acids in the mouth are less well buffered due to the reduction of salivary flow during sleep. Most people like to brush their teeth in the morning as part of their hygiene routine and this is appropriate. Further brushing after mealtimes will give additional benefit. It is best if patients use a minimal amount of water to remove toothpaste from their mouths after brushing as the anticaries effect of the toothpaste is reduced by vigorous rinsing.

So, advice to patients should be:
- Use a standard fluoride toothpaste
- Brush at least twice a day, including once before bed
- Spit after brushing rather than rinsing.

Fluoridated water

There is unassailable evidence that fluoride in public water supplies substantially reduces caries rates (by approximately 50%). At a concentration of 1 ppm there are no adverse health effects other than a possibility of increased fluorosis. Where water is fluoridated less children undergo general anaesthetics and extractions.

Fluoride tablets

Fluoride supplementation is no longer considered effective as a public health measure and at present may be inappropriate even on an individual basis, although they may have a place for those in whom dental decay might have life-threatening consequences. This is because compliance problems often produce poor effectiveness whilst the risk of fluorosis or even poisoning is present.

Fluoride rinses

Unlike fluoride tablets, fluoride mouth rinses have a good risk to benefit ratio (Figure 71.3). They present little risk of fluorosis whilst having a measurable effect on caries reduction. Rinses are not usually recommended for children below the age of 7 years because of the possibility that the rinse may be accidently swallowed by the child. Rinses may be for daily use (0.05% sodium fluoride; 227 ppm fluoride) or weekly (0.2% sodium fluoride; 909 ppm fluoride), with daily rinsing being marginally more effective.

Fluoridated milk

School-based fluoridated milk programmes are now operating in 15 countries around the world. The fluoride in the milk has an anticaries effect and the milk may act as an alternative to caries-promoting soft drinks. Fluoridated milk programmes appear to be almost as effective in reducing caries as water fluoridation.

Fluoride varnishes

Fluoride varnishes deliver fluoride at sites in the mouth that are at risk of caries (Figure 71.4). The varnish hardens on the tooth and contains high levels of fluoride. The most widely used is Duraphat, which contains 5% sodium fluoride (22600 ppm) suspended in alcohol. The resin in which the suspension is held sets on contact with saliva (Box 71.2). They are highly effective, giving caries reductions of 38%. Their mechanism of action is possibly the formation of calcium fluoride, which then releases fluoride over a longer time period.

Box 71.2 Applying fluoride varnish

- Dry teeth
- Apply varnish to teeth using brush or cotton wool pledget
- Avoid varnish contacting gingival tissues
- Advise patient to avoid hard foods for 4 hours
- Advise patients not to brush until bedtime

Fluoride gels and foam

Fluoride gels are more commonly used in the US and Canada compared to the UK. The acidulated phosphate fluoride (APF) gel is applied to the teeth via a Styrofoam mouth tray (Box 71.3). In the permanent dentition regular annual or 6-monthly fluoride gel application prevents 20–30% of caries.

Fluoride foams are relatively new products, which have not yet been thoroughly evaluated in clinical trials. They are applied in the same way and the concentration of fluoride is the same as gels. They claim to give better fluoride enamel uptake than gels.

Box 71.3 Applying fluoride gel

- Try mouth trays in patient's mouth; trim if necessary
- Ensure suction functional and comfortable in patient's mouth
- Air dry teeth
- Place 2 gram of gel in the tray and place in mouth to completely cover teeth
- Insert upper and lower trays separately
- Apply gel for 4 minutes
- Allow patient to spit out but they should avoid rinsing, eating or drinking for 30 minutes

---

72 Classification of trauma

Figure 72.1 Concussion

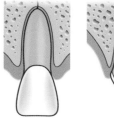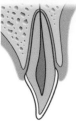

Figure 72.2 (a) Subluxation; (b) subluxation of teeth 51 and 52

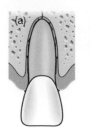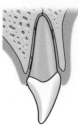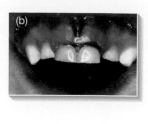

Figure 72.3 (a) Extrusion; (b) extrusion of teeth 11 and 21

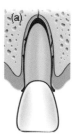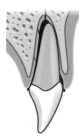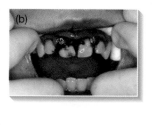

Figure 72.4 (a) Luxation; (b) luxation of tooth 52

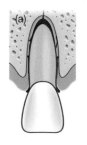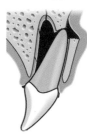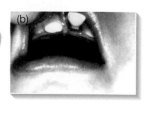

Figure 72.5 (a) Intrusion; (b) intrusion of tooth 21

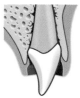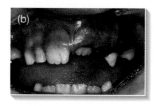

Figure 72.6 (a) Avulsion; (b) avulsion of tooth 22

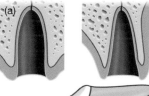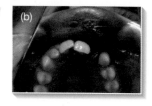

Figure 72.7 Transillumination to observe cracks and infractions in enamel

Source: Duggal M, Cameron A, Toumba J (2013). *Paediatric Dentistry at a Glance*. Reproduced with permission of John Wiley and Sons, Ltd.

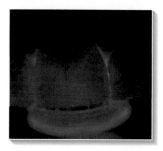

Figure 72.8 (a) Enamel fracture; (b) enamel fracture of tooth 21

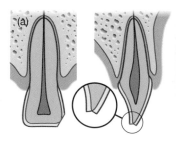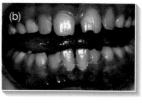

Figure 72.9 (a) Enamel–dentine fracture; (b) enamel–dentine fracture of teeth 11 and 21

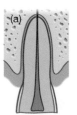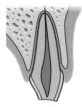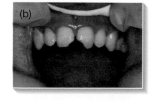

Figure 72.10 (a) Enamel–dentine–pulp fracture; (b) enamel–dentine–pulp fracture of teeth 11 and 21

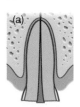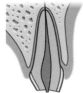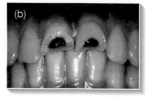

Source: Figures 72.1–72.6, 72.8–72.13 and 72.16 Andreasen JO, et al. (2011). *Traumatic Dental Injuries: A Manual*, 3rd edn. Reproduced with permission of John Wiley and Sons, Ltd.

Figure 72.11 Uncomplicated crown root fracture

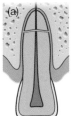
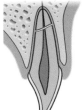

Figure 72.12 (a) Crown–root fracture; (b) Crown–root fracture of tooth 21

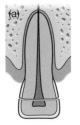
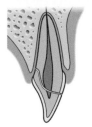
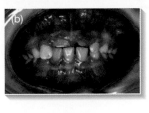

Figure 72.13 (a) Root fracture; (b) anterior maxillary occlusal radiograph showing coronal third root fracture of tooth 21

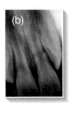
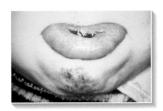

Figure 72.14 Laceration of tongue and abrasion of chin

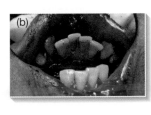

Figure 72.15 Contusion of the upper labial mucosa and fraenum

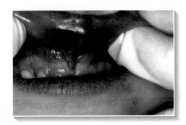

Figure 72.16 Dentoalveolar fracture encompassing all four permanent lower incisors

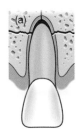
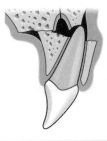

Periodontal injuries

Concussion: No mobility or displacement of the tooth but marked tenderness to percussion is present. No gingival bleeding (Figure 72.1).

Subluxation: Increased mobility without displacement of the tooth. Gingival bleeding is present in the acute injury (Figure 72.2a,b).

Extrusion: Partial displacement of the tooth out of its socket in an axial direction (Figure 72.3a,b).

Lateral luxation: Displacement of the tooth in any direction other than axially, with comminution or fracture of the alveolar socket (Figure 72.4a,b).

Intrusion: Displacement of the tooth into the alveolar bone with comminution or fracture of the alveolar socket (Figure 72.5a,b).

Avulsion: Complete displacement of the tooth from its socket (Figure 72.6a,b).

Tooth injuries (enamel, dentine or pulp fractures)

Enamel infraction: Incomplete fracture (crack) of enamel without loss of tooth substance (Figure 72.7).

Enamel fracture: Loss of tooth substance confined to enamel (Figure 72.8a,b).

Uncomplicated crown fracture (enamel–dentin fracture): Loss of tooth substance confined to enamel and dentine with no exposure of the pulp (Figure 72.9a,b).

Complicated crown fracture (enamel–dentin–pulp fracture): Fracture of enamel and dentine with exposure of the pulp (Figure 72.10a,b).

Uncomplicated crown–root fracture: Fracture of enamel, dentine and cementum but no exposure of the pulp (Figure 72.11).

Complicated crown–root fracture: Fracture of enamel, dentine and cementum with exposure of the pulp (Figure 72.12a,b).

Root fracture: Fracture involving radicular dentine, cementum and pulp. Can be subclassified into apical, middle and coronal (gingival) thirds (Figure 72.13a,b).

Injuries to gingiva or oral mucosa

Laceration: Wound resulting from a tear (Figure 72.14).

Contusion: Bruise not accompanied by a break in the mucosa, usually causing submucosal haemorrhage (Figure 72.15).

Abrasion of gingiva or oral mucosa: Superficial wound produced by rubbing or scraping the mucosal surface (Figure 72.14).

Injuries to bone

Comminution of alveolar plate: Crushing and compression of socket walls as found in intrusive and lateral luxation injuries.

Fracture of alveolar plate: Fracture of alveolus confined to socket walls.

Fracture of alveolar process: Fracture of the alveolar process that may or may not involve the tooth sockets (Figure 72.16a,b).

Fracture of supporting bone: May or may not involve the alveolar socket.

73 Accidental injury to primary teeth

Figure 73.1 Maxillary occlusal radiograph demonstrating the relationship between the primary and permanent incisors

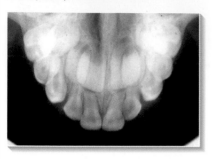

Figure 73.2 Avulsion of tooth 61 and mild extrusion of tooth 51

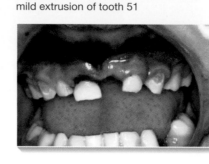

Figure 73.3 Lateral luxation of teeth 51 and 52 with the crowns displaced palatally

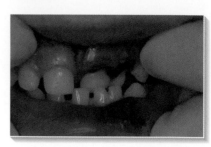

Figure 73.4 Intrusion of tooth 51 with a small enamel fracture at the distal-incisal corner

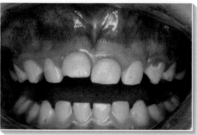

Figure 73.5 An avulsed primary upper central incisor tooth

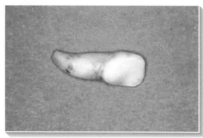

Figure 73.6 Enamel–dentine fracture of tooth 61

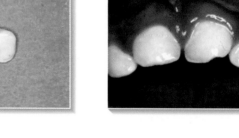

Figure 73.7 Internal discoloration of tooth 51 displaying a mild pink hue

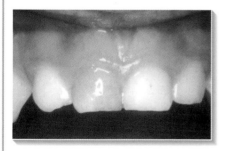

Figure 73.8 Hypoplasia of enamel of tooth 21 as a result of primary tooth trauma

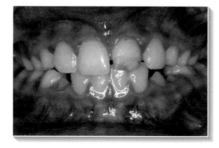

Figure 73.9 Severe dilaceration of a permanent central incisor at the crown–root junction from trauma to the primary precursor

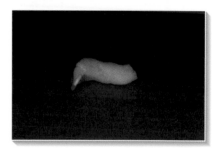

General information

Approximately 1 in 4 children will suffer trauma to their primary teeth, most commonly between 2 and 4 years of age as a result of falling. This is at a time when children are becoming increasingly adventurous whilst having little understanding of danger and consequence. Due to the relative position of the primary tooth and the developing permanent tooth germ (Figure 73.1), trauma in this age range can result in damage to both. In general, due to the age of the child and the risk of damage to the permanent successor, treatment options are usually limited to either simple observation or extraction of the offending tooth. A compliant child, however, can be a candidate for more advanced restorative procedures where the operator's skills allow. In all injuries, it is most important to ensure parents/carers maintain high oral hygiene standards with tooth brushing to optimise prognosis. This is combined with a soft diet and regular review of the dentition until the permanent successors erupt.

Periodontal injuries

In general, injuries involving the periodontal ligament (PDL) of a primary tooth are either managed conservatively with soft diet, appropriate analgesia and observation. Or the other alternative is to extract the tooth.

Dentistry at a Glance. First Edition. Edited by Elizabeth Kay. © 2016 John Wiley & Sons, Ltd. Published 2016 by John Wiley & Sons, Ltd.
Companion website: www.ataglanceseries.com/dentistryseries/dentistry

Concussion

There is generally no damage to the neurovascular bundle but there may be some bleeding and oedema in the PDL, hence the tooth being tender to percussion (TTP), but the majority of the PDL remains intact and the tooth will require no active treatment.

Subluxation

The neurovascular bundle may be damaged, and there will be bleeding and oedema in the PDL with evidence of bleeding in the gingival sulcus in fresh trauma. The tooth will be mobile but as it is in the correct position and placing a splint in a young child can be difficult, it is often left to simple observation.

Extrusion

A minimally extruded tooth that remains relatively firm can be observed without active treatment; however, anything greater than 1–2 mm of extrusion will result in severance of the neurovascular bundle and notable mobility, necessitating extraction (Figure 73.2).

Lateral luxation

The permanent successor of a traumatised primary tooth is at risk of damage as the result of displacement of the primary tooth. Repositioning such a displaced tooth risks further damage and, in general, a luxated tooth is best extracted. The exception is a firm and minimally palatally displaced tooth, which is not interfering with the occlusion. The apex of such a tooth will have been displaced buccally away from the developing successor (Figure 73.3).

Intrusion

Intrusive luxation is the commonest displacement injury in the primary dentition and is commonly the result of a downward fall onto an object, causing axial displacement into the developing tooth germ. Often, it is combined with a degree of lateral luxation. If the apex is intruded with a degree of buccal displacement, then the tooth can be left to re-erupt; however, if it is intruded palatally towards the tooth germ, it should be extracted. If not re-erupted within 6 months, the tooth should be extracted as it will have ankylosed and will prevent the permanent successor from erupting (Figure 73.4).

Avulsion

To prevent damage to the permanent successor, avulsed primary teeth should not be replanted. Either a periapical or a maxillary anterior occlusal radiograph will rule out an intrusion where no tooth tissue can be seen due to the severity of the impaction; however, a notable clinical difference between the two, which can also help in making the diagnosis, is the relative lack of gingival disruption in an avulsion compared with marked gingival trauma in an intrusion (Figures 73.2 and 73.5).

Tooth injuries (enamel, dentine or pulp fractures)

Infraction and enamel fracture

Infraction of the enamel requires no intervention whilst a fracture can either be left untreated or smoothed if rough. A child unable to cope with the use of a handpiece may yet be able to manage to have a tooth smoothed with an abrasive disc or strip held in the fingers (with gauze suitably placed for airway protection)

Enamel–dentine fractures

Exposed dentine should be sealed to avoid sensitivity, pulpitis and potential loss of vitality. For the compliant child, this can involve restoring the tooth to full anatomical form whilst for the preco-operative or less co-operative child, this can be effectively managed with a one-stage etch/prime/bond followed by just enough flowable composite resin to simply seal the exposed dentine (Figure 73.6).

Pulpally involved fractures

Fractures of the crown and/or root involving the pulp almost invariably result in the need for extraction. The exception is the root fractured tooth that is not notably mobile, which can be observed. Where there is a root fracture with a mobile coronal portion, extraction of the coronal portion should be carried out whilst leaving the apical fragment in situ, due to the potential for further damage to the permanent successor, and attempting to remove an apical portion, which will most often resorb uneventfully in any case.

Alveolar fracture

If the teeth involved in the fracture are to be kept, the teeth may be utilised to splint the associated fractured bone. The alveolar fracture should be reduced under appropriate anaesthetic (local or general) and the teeth involved in the segment of fractured alveolus splinted to the adjacent teeth for a period of 4 weeks to allow bony healing.

Sequelae

Following trauma to the primary dentition, the primary and/or secondary teeth may suffer the following outcomes.

- **Primary tooth:**
  - **Primary/pulp death:** In the absence of any other signs or symptoms the vast majority of such teeth will exfoliate naturally in normal sequence without concern and therefore should simply be left *in situ* (Figure 73.7). Where there is pain, sepsis or increasing mobility, such teeth should be extracted to prevent increased risk of damage to the permanent successor.
  - **Pulp canal obliteration:** Previously considered a poor outcome, the pulp's defensive process of rapidly laying down dentine to obliterate the pulpal space is now considered a favourable response, which demonstrates the continued vitality of the pulp. Pulpal necrosis subsequent to obliteration is rare.
  - **Resorption/early loss:** A traumatic injury to the PDL of a primary tooth may hasten the otherwise physiological process of root resorption. As a result, a traumatised primary tooth may exfoliate earlier than a non-injured contemporary, but this is rarely associated with negative outcome.
- **Permanent successor:**
  - Due to the physical impact from the traumatic injury, either directly or vicariously via the primary tooth, the permanent successor may, dependent upon the patient's age, stage of permanent tooth development and type and severity of injury, undergo pathological changes such as discoloration, hypoplasia (Figure 73.8), dilaceration (Figure 73.9), odontome formation, failure of eruption or arrest of formation.

74 Non-accidental injury

Figure 74.1 Palatal petechial contusion as a result of oral sexual abuse

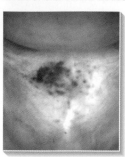

Figure 74.2 Pinch contusion of the pinna as a result of abusive tugging of the ear

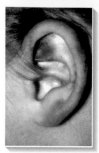

Figure 74.4 Diagram to show areas of the body that are uncommon for accidental injuries to occur and raise suspicion of non-accidental injury

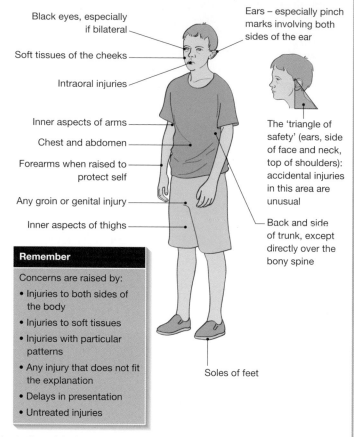

Black eyes, especially if bilateral

Soft tissues of the cheeks

Intraoral injuries

Inner aspects of arms

Chest and abdomen

Forearms when raised to protect self

Any groin or genital injury

Inner aspects of thighs

Ears – especially pinch marks involving both sides of the ear

The 'triangle of safety' (ears, side of face and neck, top of shoulders): accidental injuries in this area are unusual

Back and side of trunk, except directly over the bony spine

Soles of feet

Figure 74.3 Diagram to show areas of common sites for accidental injuries to occur

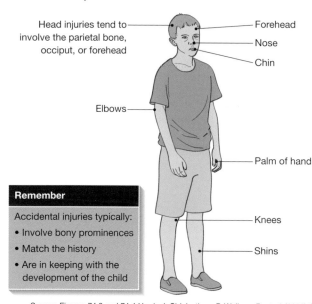

Head injuries tend to involve the parietal bone, occiput, or forehead

Forehead

Nose

Chin

Elbows

Palm of hand

Knees

Shins

Remember

Accidental injuries typically:
- Involve bony prominences
- Match the history
- Are in keeping with the development of the child

Remember

Concerns are raised by:
- Injuries to both sides of the body
- Injuries to soft tissues
- Injuries with particular patterns
- Any injury that does not fit the explanation
- Delays in presentation
- Untreated injuries

Source: Figures 74.3 and 74.4 Harris J, Sidebotham P, Welbury R, *et al*. (2006) *Child protection and the dental team: an introduction to safeguarding children in dental practice*. Reproduced with permission from COPDEND: Sheffield. Available at: www.cpdt.org.uk.

Figure 74.5 Responding to concerns of abuse

1. You have concern about a child's welfare

- If you have concerns you must advise a safeguarding officer
- Talk to the child about the cause of the injuries without asking leading questions
- A child who makes a disclosure of abuse should always be taken seriously
- If requested to keep a secret, you should not do so but should explain that you may have to share information

2. Where to go for help

- Local child protection guidelines (available in all dental practices)
- National child protection guidelines (available at: www.cpdt.org.uk)
- Experienced dental colleague
- Consultant paediatrician
- Child protection nurse
- Social services (informal discussion)
- Others: the child's health visitor, school nurse or general medical practitioner

A 'non-accidental injury' is a physical harm, which has occurred either as the result of an act of physical abuse or as the result of wilful failure to prevent such an injury.

Over 50% of children suffering physical abuse will display signs of such abuse in their head and neck region – exactly the area of the body where the dental team is best placed to identify these children.

Although many children are poor and infrequent dental attenders within the UK, the often periodic and episodic nature of dental pain and dental injury in those who are dentally neglected or physically abused is one which can bring an abused child to the attention of a dental team, who are then in a position of being able to intervene and prevent further abuse. This is only possible when the dental team is aware of the signs of abuse and the appropriate procedures to follow in highlighting any concerns of such abuse to the relevant child protection agencies. If you have any concerns you MUST alert the safeguarding team.

The role of the dental team

It is not the role of the dental team to diagnose abuse. It is, however, the role of all members of the dental team to be aware of, and have concern for, the signs and symptoms that may suggest abuse and to highlight such concerns to the relevant child protection agencies for them to consider, investigate and manage.

How abuse presents

When determining whether signs and symptoms are of concern, it is important to consider a number of factors related to the injury. The type, location and explanation for the injury should all be weighed up in conjunction with consideration of the child's demeanour and interaction within the dental surgery, along with any general information known about the broader social picture of the child and family. In some cases it may be that one over-riding factor alone is sufficient to raise concern, whilst for others it may be a more subtle combination of factors that provokes unease. Whatever the cause for concern, it is imperative that ALL concerns are acted upon.

Particular types of injury, occurring in certain areas of the body, can be highly suggestive of abuse, but is important to be aware that there are no injuries that are pathognomonic for abuse (meaning they occur only in or prove abuse).

Types of injuries of potential concern

Types of injury affecting the head and neck that may raise the suspicion of physical abuse are listed in Table 74.1.

Locations of injuries of potential concern

Other lesions may present that are unusual in their location, such as petechial haemorrhage at the junction of the hard and soft palate, as seen in Figure 74.1, which is the result of trauma from oral sexual abuse.

Body maps have been constructed to demonstrate locations of injuries and their potential for being non-accidental, as shown in Figures 74.3 and 74.4.

Features of presentation of potential concern

Particular aspects of the presentation may in themselves raise concern, such as a delay in presentation, conflicting explanations between the child and their parent/carer regarding the cause, timing, location or those present at the time of injury. It is important to note the general demeanour of the child, their state of hygiene, how well they appear to be growing and how they interact with their parents, carers or others.

Responding to concerns of abuse

See Figure 74.5.

Table 74.1 Injury that may raise suspicion of physical abuse

Injury	Features raising suspicion of abuse
Bruising	Occurs in babies or non-mobile children (no reason to bruise) Bizarrely shaped with uniform borders (implement outline) Bruising to 'protected' areas such as the neck and the inner folds or back of the ears (Figure 74.2)
Abrasions and lacerations	Injury and history provided are inconsistent
Burns	Circular punched-out lesions of 6–10 mm in diameter may be due to cigarette burns Well-delineated burns may be due to placement of a heated implement upon the skin Intraoral burns in a child unable to feed themselves (force feeding of hot foodstuffs)
Bite marks	Difficult to differentiate abusive bite marks from 'innocent' marks caused by other children such as young siblings Presence of bite marks requires careful questioning to determine if explanation is in keeping with injury
Eye injuries	Periorbital bruising in children, particularly bilaterally
Bone fractures	Facial fractures in children are rare and require substantial force to occur Suspicion of abuse merits a full skeletal survey in liaison with a paediatrician/child protection team
Dental injuries	Type of injury, age of child and a thorough history are imperatives for determining if injury is abusive

75 Treatment of tooth fractures

Figure 75.1 Radiograph of a foreign body in the lower lip

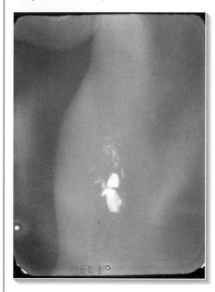

Figure 75.2 Enamel fracture of tooth 21

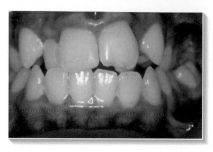

Figure 75.3 Buccal view of rebonded incisal fragment with discoloration of tooth 21

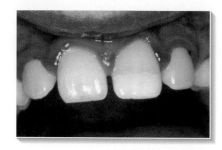

Figure 75.4 Palatal view of rebonded incisal fragment with discoloration of tooth 21

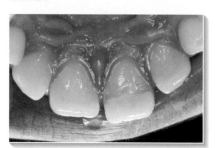

Figure 75.5 Enamel–dentine fracture of teeth 11 and 21

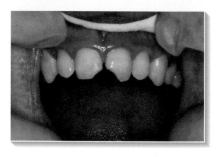

Figure 75.6 Enamel–dentine fracture of teeth 11 and 21 restored with composite resin

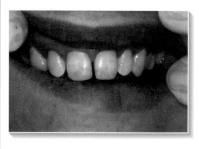

Figure 75.7 Enamel–dentine–pulp fracture of the crown

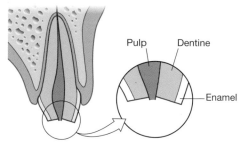

Pulp   Dentine

Enamel

Figure 75.8 2 mm of pulp tissue has been removed

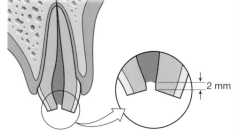

2 mm

Figure 75.9 MTA or calcium hydroxide is placed over the exposed pulp tissue

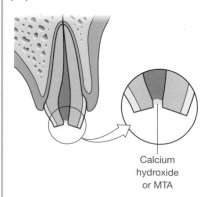

Calcium hydroxide or MTA

Figure 75.10 Glass ionomer is placed over the MTA or glass ionomer

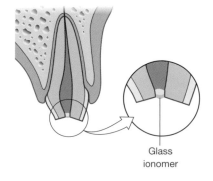

Glass ionomer

Figure 75.11 The fracture site is hermetically sealed with composite resin

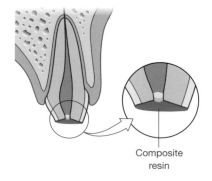

Composite resin

Dentistry at a Glance. First Edition. Edited by Elizabeth Kay. © 2016 John Wiley & Sons, Ltd. Published 2016 by John Wiley & Sons, Ltd.
Companion website: www.ataglanceseries.com/dentistryseries/dentistry

The management of dental hard tissue injuries, that is crown and/or root fractures in permanent teeth, is unrelated to the degree of root development or apical closure and therefore the following is applicable to both mature and immature permanent teeth.

It is important to exclude additional injuries beyond what can be clinically observed, such as root or alveolar fractures or displacement injuries, particularly in the early mixed dentition when subtle degrees of extrusion and intrusion can be overlooked. Clinical examination should be supplemented by periapical and anterior maxillary occlusal radiographs taken from more than one angle.

Breaches of the soft tissues where there is loss of tooth fragment, restoration or suspected foreign body requires radiographic examination of the soft tissues at a reduced exposure to exclude their embedment (Figure 75.1).

All dental injuries should be followed up to ensure timely management of any negative sequelae that may arise.

Enamel and enamel–dentine fracture

Small fractures of enamel may be left untreated unless rough, when they may benefit from being smoothed with an abrasive stone or disc. Larger fractures, although not extending into dentine, would aesthetically benefit from composite repair (Figure 75.2).

Exposed dentinal tubules require prompt coverage, ideally with a bonded resin restoration or with a temporary 'composite bandage'. Whilst glass ionomer can be quick to place and potentially helpful for the uncooperative or pre-cooperative child, it will not achieve the preferred robust seal of a bonded restoration, which will improve the prognosis.

A fractured distal fragment of a tooth can be rebonded; however, it can be subject to desiccation and delayed colour mismatch with the remaining tooth (Figures 75.3 and 75.4). If it is rebonded with resin, it should have a gutter cut around the fracture line after rebonding and this should be in-filled with composite to improve fragment bond strength and mask the fracture line.

Restoration of anatomical form is often best achieved by composite resin build up of the crown, either free hand or with cellulose crown forms. Layered restorations utilising modern composite systems with dentine and enamel subshades can provide very pleasing aesthetic outcomes. The amount of enamel available for bonding can be increased by incorporating a subtle bevel in the fractured enamel edge prior to build up (Figures 75.5 and 75.6). Clinical and radiographic follow-up should be arranged for 2 and 12 months postinjury.

Enamel–dentine–pulp fracture

Where there is exposure of pulpal tissue in a crown fracture (Figure 75.7), a minimal (Cvek) pulpotomy is now the preferred procedure to maximise a favourable prognosis for pulp vitality, root growth and continued deposition of radicular dentine.

Until recently, trauma guidelines would typically determine pulp treatment based on size of pulpal exposure and time elapsed between exposure and restoration; however, pulp capping is now considered to have a slightly poorer prognosis than pulpotomy for all exposures.

Where there has been complete loss of vitality, pulpectomy will be required. Where there is incomplete root growth, the options for management are apical closure (apexification) with calcium hydroxide, mineral trioxide aggregate (MTA) or the more novel technique of encouraging continued root formation (apexigenesis) via the regenerative endodontic technique (RET).

Procedure for pulpotomy

- Local anaesthesia
- Isolate with a rubber dam if possible
- Clean the area with saline or chlorhexidine
- Perform pulpotomy to a depth of 2 mm using a round diamond bur with water or saline coolant (Figure 75.8)
- Place a moistened cotton pledget until the pulp wound stops bleeding
- Apply calcium hydroxide or MTA (Figure 75.9)
- Seal with calcium hydroxide or MTA as well as sealing the dentine with glass ionomer (Figure 75.10)
- Then restore with composite resin (Figure 75.11).
  Clinical and radiographic follow-up should be arranged for 2 and 12 months postinjury.

Crown–root fracture and crown–root–pulp fracture

Dependent upon the extent of the fracture and its relationship to the gingival and alveolar margin, the options for management include:

- Removal of minimal enamel sliver only
- Repair with composite resin
- Gingivectomy with repair
- Surgical/orthodontic extrusion
- Decoronation for bone preservation for implant in adulthood
- Extraction.
  Clinical and radiographic follow up should be arranged for 2 and 12 months postinjury.

Root fracture

The site of the fracture within the root determines the classification, splinting regimen and prognosis (Table 75.1).

The more apical portion of any fracture is likely to remain vital whilst the greater the displacement and mobility of the coronal fragment, the greater the likelihood of loss of vitality of the coronal portion.

If the coronal portion becomes non-vital, the pulp need only be extirpated and the tooth obturated up to the fracture line. Obturation can only be completed following barrier formation at the fracture line by one-stage MTA or multiple-visit calcium hydroxide changes. The apical portion is likely to retain vitality.

Clinical and radiographic follow-up should be arranged for 2, 4, 6 and 12 months postinjury.

Table 75.1 Classification and prognosis of root fracture

Root third classification	Duration of splinting	Survival at 10 years
Apical	4 weeks	10%
Middle	4 weeks	10%
Coronal	4 months	50%

76 Tooth displacement injuries

Figure 76.1 Flexible composite and wire splint stabilising traumatised permanent upper incisors

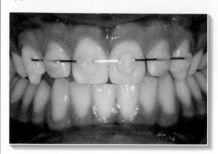

Figure 76.2 Mild intrusion of tooth 11

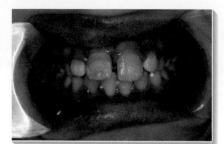

Figure 76.3 Severe intrusion of permanent upper incisors

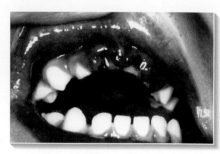

Figure 76.4 Mandibular oblique occlusal radiograph demonstrating dentoalveolar fracture of lower permanent incisors

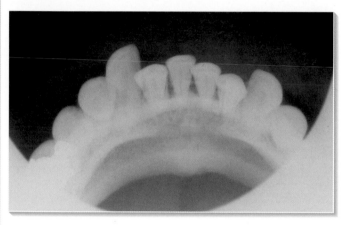

Figure 76.5 Dentoalveolar fracture of permanent lower incisors reduced and splinted

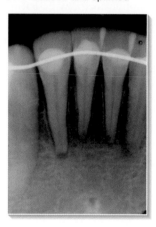

Due to the varied nature of trauma presentation, the potential for concomitant injuries and the varying age and stage of patient/tooth development, there are myriad permutations for managing dental trauma and determining outcomes. An invaluable resource when working clinically is the free to access to the online Dental Trauma Guide provided by the International Association for Dental Traumatology, available at: www.dentaltraumaguide.org, which gives invaluable step by step advice on the diagnosis, treatment, follow-up and prognostication of dental trauma.

General information

Approximately 35% of boys and 20% of girls will suffer trauma to their permanent teeth by the time they enter secondary school, most commonly around 8 years of age, resulting in enamel/dentine fractures of the maxillary incisors as a result of falls or collisions whilst playing. The incidence of sports and cycling-related injuries increase as children grow into adolescence and for males, the later teens and early twenties is a time where they may become involved with dental trauma as a result of interpersonal violence.

A very important cause of dental injury that must always be borne in mind when dealing with trauma is that of non-accidental injury, that is physical abuse. This is discussed more fully in Chapter 76.

The aims of managing injuries to the periodontal ligament (PDL) are:
• To reduce the risks of infection (wound cleansing, tetanus prophylaxis for prone wounds, antibiotics for significant tissue breaches and good oral hygiene measures)
• To reduce displaced teeth and/or bone/soft tissues to return the tissues to appropriate anatomical form
• To fixate any mobile teeth or associated tissues to maximise optimal healing (splinting and/or suturing)
• To protect the teeth and associated tissues from further damage (dietary/ lifestyle modification and splinting)

In all injuries, it is most important to ensure patients/parents/carers maintain high oral hygiene standards with tooth brushing to optimise prognosis. This is combined with a soft diet and regular review of the dentition as per follow-up protocols described.

Dentistry at a Glance. First Edition. Edited by Elizabeth Kay. © 2016 John Wiley & Sons, Ltd. Published 2016 by John Wiley & Sons, Ltd.
Companion website: www.ataglanceseries.com/dentistryseries/dentistry

Concussion

There is generally no damage to the neurovascular (NV) bundle but there may be some bleeding and oedema in the PDL, hence the tooth being tender to percussion (TTP), but the majority of the PDL remains intact and the tooth will require no active treatment.

Subluxation

The NV bundle may be damaged, there will be bleeding and oedema in the PDL with evidence of bleeding in the gingival sulcus in fresh trauma. The tooth will be mobile and to minimise further damage to the NV bundle, the tooth should be splinted for 2 weeks to stabilise the tooth (Figure 76.1).

Extrusion

The tooth should be repositioned with finger pressure and splinted for 2 weeks. The pulp of a tooth with an open apex has a 95% chance of retaining vitality whilst the pulp in a tooth with a closed apex is likely to remain vital in less than 50% of cases and therefore it is important to be vigilant for the signs and symptoms of loss of vitality:

- Crown discoloration
- Radiographic periapical radiolucency
- Repeated negative sensibility testing
- If untreated, eventually mobility will manifest.

Prompt extirpation followed by endodontic obturation is required when loss of vitality is diagnosed to prevent both the occurrence and progression of external inflammatory resorption.

Lateral luxation

Local anaesthesia will be required to reposition the tooth. As the apex of the tooth can be displaced out with its bony cradle, the tooth may firstly require an extrusive force applied to slightly withdraw the tooth outwards in an axial direction prior to relocating the tooth to overcome what is termed the 'bony lock'. The tooth should be splinted for 4 weeks and any gingival lacerations sutured.

Intrusion

The degree of intrusion, the stage of root end closure and the time elapsed between injury and reduction of the intrusion will dictate the options available as per Table 76.1.

There is no difference on the outcomes between surgical and orthodontic repositioning and therefore in those situations described in the Table 76.1 where both are possible, surgical repositioning is preferred when the injury is relatively fresh,

that is within 24–48 hours, before extensive healing has occurred. Orthodontic repositioning is often favoured with late presentation due to it avoiding further trauma to the healing/ healed tissues (Figures 76.2 and 76.3).

Avulsion

Good telephone first aid is essential as the tooth is best replanted as soon as possible by the patient, parent, carer, friend or colleague. Advice should be as listed in Box 76.1.

Box 76.1 Telephone dental first-aid advice for the immediate management of an avulsed permanent tooth by a non-dentally qualified person

- Find the tooth and pick it up by the crown (the white part). Avoid touching the root.
- If the tooth is dirty, wash it briefly (10 seconds) under cold running water before repositioning it.
- Try to encourage the patient/ parent to replant the tooth. Bite on a handkerchief to hold it in position.
- If this is not possible, place the tooth in a glass of milk. The tooth can also be transported in the mouth, keeping it between the molars and the inside of the cheek. Avoid storage in water and seek emergency dental treatment immediately.

The further treatment you will need to provide will depend on:

- The extra alveolar dry time (EADT), i.e. how long the tooth has been out of the mouth and dry
  - EADT >60 minutes will result in PDL cell death and the need to remove the PDL before replantation, which will result in ankylosis.
- Whether the apex is open or closed
  - If the tooth has an open apex and the EADT is less than 60 minutes, the pulp may survive and vitality should be monitored (although there is a significant drop in the probability of pulp survival after more than 5 minutes EADT).
  - If the apex is closed and the EADT is greater than 60 minutes, both the pulp and PDL will not survive and therefore endodontics can be completed out with the mouth prior to replantation and splinting for 4 weeks.

Alveolar fracture

Unlike fractures of the long bones where fractures are fixated with casts, the teeth are utilised to splint fractured alveolar bone. The fracture should be reduced under local anaesthetic and the teeth involved in the segment of fractured alveolus splinted to

---

Table 76.1 Treatment guidelines for intruded permanent teeth dependent upon degree of root development and intrusion level

		Repositioning type		
	Degree of intrusion	Spontaneous	Orthodontic	Surgical
Open apex	<7 mm	√		
	>7 mm		√	√
Closed apex	<3 mm	√		
	3–7 mm		√	√
	>7 mm			√

the adjacent teeth for a period of 4 weeks to allow bony healing. The teeth themselves often maintain vitality but close follow-up is mandated (Figures 76.4 and 76.5).

Splinting

Splinting of teeth utilises a flexible splint, which is commonly an acid-etch-wire composite splint attached to the traumatised tooth/teeth and one uncompromised tooth either side (Figure 76.1).

Other methods include acid-etch flexible resin splint, acid-etch composite nylon line splint, acid-etch orthodontic wire splint and titanium trauma splint (TTS).

Rigid splinting aims to avoid any functional movement of the PDL and is limited to the stabilisation of alveolar fractures only. This utilises a thicker diameter of wire with less 'free' wire unattached to composite between the teeth to reduce the flexibility of the wire (Figure 76.5).

Longer splinting time is indicated for avulsions where the extra-alveolar dry time (EADT) is more than 60 minutes as these teeth will always ankylose and the intention is to stabilise the tooth in the correct position until union has been established directly between bone and cementum/dentine (Table 76.2).

Prognosis

The prognosis for tooth displacement injuries is most often considered in terms of pulp and tooth survival. The likelihood of survival is largely dependent upon the type of injury sustained and whether the tooth apex is open or closed, as seen in Table 76.3.

Follow up

Follow-up of traumatic injuries aims to detect pathological changes in the tooth, particularly loss of vitality, resorption and failure of healing. The recommended intervals for clinical and radiographic re-evaluation are dependent upon the type of injury sustained and in the case of avulsion on the duration of EADT (Table 76.4).

Table 76.2 Splinting duration guidelines for displaced permanent teeth dependent upon injury type

Displacement type	Splinting duration
Concussion	Not required as no mobility
Subluxation	2 weeks
Extrusion	2 weeks
Intrusion	2 weeks
Avulsion	2 weeks if <60 min EADT 4 weeks if > 60 min EADT
Lateral luxation	4 weeks
Alveolar fracture	4 weeks (rigid)

Table 76.3 Pulp and tooth survival percentages for 1, 3 and 10 years postinjury in relation to injury type

Displacement Type	1-year survival (%)		3-year survival (%)		10-year survival (%)	
	Pulp	Tooth	Pulp	Tooth	Pulp	Tooth
Concussion	100 (100)	100 (100)	100 (100)	100 (100)	100 (100)	100 (100)
Subluxation	100 (87.5)	100 (100)	100 (87.5)	100 (100)	100 (87.5)	100 (100)
Extrusion	94.1 (43.5)	100 (100)	94.1 (43.5)	100 (100)	94.1 (43.5)	100 (100)
Lateral luxation	95.3 (34.9)	100 (100)	95.3 (27.2)	100 (100)	95.3 (24.7)§	100 (100)
Intrusion	94.4 (0)	50 (100)	38.9 (0)	94.4 (94.7)	32.4 (0)	88.5 (71.1)
Alveolar fracture	30 (0)	97.3 (99)	29.1 (0)	77 (88.1)	29.1 (0)	52.7 (54.9)

Figures without parentheses, teeth with an open apex at time of injury; figures in parentheses, teeth with a closed apex.

Table 76.4 Postinjury follow-up guidelines for timing of clinical and radiographic review and splint removal dependent upon injury type

Displacement type	Follow up periods					
	2 weeks	1 months	2 months	3 months	6 months	12 months
Concussion		R	R			R
Subluxation	S	R	R			R
Extrusion	S	R	R		R	R
Intrusion	S	R	R		R	R
Avulsion	S*	S**/R		R	R	R
Lateral luxation	R	S/R	R		R	R
Alveolar fracture		S/R	R	R	R	R

R, radiographs and clinical review; S, splint removal.
*, if EADT <60 min; **, if EADT >60 min.

77 **Instruments**

Figure 77.1 Disposable No. 15 blade with reusable handle

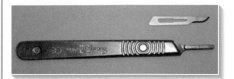

Figure 77.2 Disposable scalpel with No.15 blade attached

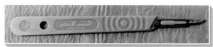

Figure 77.3 Bowdler Henry Rake retractor

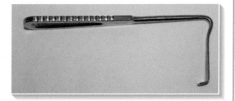

Figure 77.4 Lack's tongue depressor

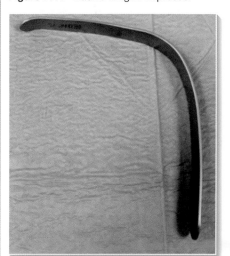

Figure 77.5 Rongeurs forceps

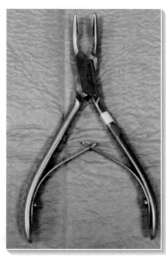

Figure 77.6 Bone file

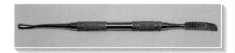

Figure 77.7 Surgical handpiece with round and fissure burs

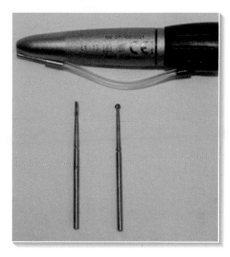

Figure 77.8 Suture cutting scissors, needle holder and Gillie's tissue forceps

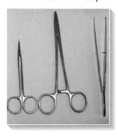

Figure 77.9 Kilner cheek retractor

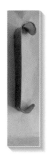

Figure 77.12 Set of Coupland elevators 1, 2 and 3

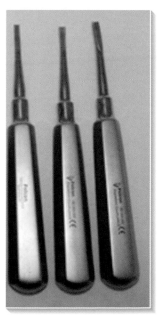

Figure 77.10 Maxillary forceps for anteriors, premolars and molars (right and left)

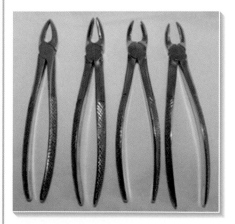

Figure 77.11 Mandibular forceps for anteriors, premolars and molars

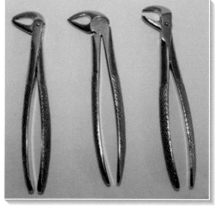

Dentistry at a Glance. First Edition. Edited by Elizabeth Kay. © 2016 John Wiley & Sons, Ltd. Published 2016 by John Wiley & Sons, Ltd.
Companion website: www.ataglanceseries.com/dentistryseries/dentistry

Figure 77.13 Set of Cryer elevators with triangular blades (R and L)

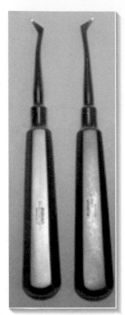

Figure 77.14 Set of Warwick James elevators right, straight and left

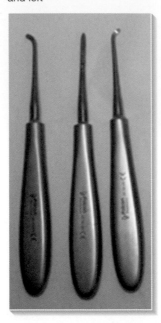

Figure 77.15 Set of luxators

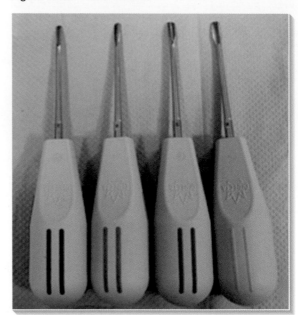

Figure 77.16 A layout of standard instruments for minor oral surgery

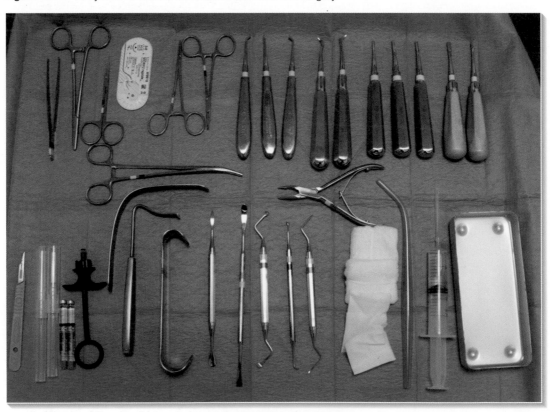

Introduction

Selection of appropriate instruments is fundamental to the practice of oral surgery. While a wide range of instruments are available, it is wise to select a small range of instruments initially. A clinician must understand the function of each instrument and use the correct instrument at each stage of a procedure. It is also important to choose high-quality instruments and maintain them with care. This section describes the basic instruments used for minor oral surgery, including exodontia.

Instruments for surgical flaps (incision, reflection and retraction)

- **Scalpel:** Primary instrument for surgical incisions. It is available as a re-usable handle with a disposable sterile blade (Figure 77.1) or as a single-use plastic handle with a fixed blade (Figure 77.2). The most commonly used handle is No. 3 and the most commonly used scalpel blade is No. 15.
- **Periosteal elevator:** Following incision, a surgical flap is reflected from the bone using a periosteal elevator. A variety of designs are available. No. 9 Molt and Howarth's are used commonly.
- **Bowdler Henry rake retractor:** This is a rake-shaped instrument with a serrated end which helps retraction of a mucoperiosteal flap (Figure 77.3).
- **Lack's tongue depressor:** This may be used to depress or retract the tongue, e.g. during suturing (Figure 77.4). It is also helpful for protection of the airway to prevent accidental displacement of tooth and bone fragments into the aerodigestive tract, especially during removal of teeth with elevators.
- Alternate instruments for tongue retraction include Austin and Weider retractors

Instruments for bone removal

- **Rongeurs forceps:** May have side-cutting or end-cutting blades and incorporate a spring mechanism between the blades (Figure 77.5). These may be used to carry out gross trimming of bone, e.g. removal of inter-radicular bone or sharp edges of bone around an extraction socket.
- **Bone file:** May be used to carry out fine smoothing of bone in a pull stroke (Figure 77.6).
- **Surgical handpiece and burs:** A surgical handpiece on a micromotor with a tungsten carbide bur is the most efficient method of bone removal as well as tooth sectioning, e.g. during a surgical extraction (Figure 77.7). Generally, a round bur is used for bone removal and a fissure bur is used for tooth sectioning. Bone removal must be carried out under copious saline irrigation to prevent heat damage to the tissues. It is important not to used air turbines during surgical extractions due to the risk of surgical emphysema.
- **Mallet and chisel:** May be used for bone removal, e.g. during removal of teeth and reduction of tori, but are not suitable for inexperienced operators.

Instruments for suturing

- **Needle holder:** Intraoral suturing is carried out using a needle holder, usually 15 cm in length (Figure 77.8). It has a pair of short, cross-hatched, thick beaks that, along with a locking handle, permit a secure grasp of the suture needle. The Mayo design is quite popular.
- **Gillie's tissue holding forceps:** These are used to hold and stabilise soft tissues during dissection and suturing.
- **Suture scissors:** These have short cutting edges and come in a variety of designs and sizes.

Miscellaneous instruments

- **Dissecting scissors:** McIndoe's scissors are used for dissection and undermining of soft tissues.
- **Mitchell's trimmer:** This instrument has one pointed end, which is helpful in raising a flap. The other end is spoon-shaped and can be used to curette granulation tissue.
- **Bone curettes:** A range of spoon-shaped curettes is available and may be used to separate soft tissue (e.g. granulation tissue or cyst lining) from the bone.
- **Haemostat:** A haemostat has a pair of long delicate beaks and handles with a locking mechanism. The beaks may be curved or straight. It is used to clamp a blood vessel before ligation or cauterisation. It may also be used to remove granulation tissue or residual follicular tissue after tooth extraction.
- **Kilner cheek retractor:** This is a C-shaped instrument, and is available in a range of sizes (Figure 77.9). It is used for retraction of cheeks to improve visibility and protect soft tissues.

Instruments for tooth extraction
Extraction forceps

Forceps are the most recognised instruments for tooth extraction. All forceps consist of two blades and handles joined at a hinge. Forceps blades are wedge shaped and used to dilate the socket. The blades are concave on the inner surface to fit the root accurately, with sharp edges to cut the periodontal ligament. The blades of forceps are applied labiolingually parallel to the long axis of a tooth.

Maxillary forceps (Figure 77.10) have a straight design with the blades and handles in line while the mandibular forceps (Figure 77.11) have beaks at a right-angle bend to allow positioning along the long axis of the tooth. There are numerous designs and variations in forceps and a clinician needs to select a design that works best for them.

Elevators

Elevators are single-bladed instruments used as levers or wedges. They are placed between tooth and bone and turned on their long axis to dislodge the tooth/root. Elevators can only move the tooth/root in one direction, that is away from the point of application.

- **Coupland elevators:** Straight elevators with a blade width of 3, 3.5 and 4 mm (numbered as 1, 2 and 3, respectively) and often used in succession (Figure 77.12).
- **Cryer elevators:** Paired elevators (right and left) with triangular blades (Figure 77.13). They are used to remove fractured roots and upper third molars.
- **Warwick James elevators:** Consist of two curved (right and left) and one straight elevator (Figure 77.14).
  - The curved design is used for removal of upper third molars and separation of gingival tissue at the neck of a tooth.
  - The straight design is used similar to Coupland's elevator.

Luxators

Luxators have a shape similar to straight elevators but the blade is finer, sharper and flexible to some degree (Figure 77.15). They are used to incise the periodontal ligament with minimal force.

Layout of instruments

A layout of instruments for minor oral surgery is depicted in Figure 77.16.

78 The patient in pain

Introduction

Pain is one of the commonest reasons for attendance at a dental clinic. Although in a vast majority of cases pain is related to dental disease, it is not unusual for patients to present with pain not related to teeth (Table 78.1). This section provides an overview of a range of disorders that may present with pain in the oral and perioral region (based on the source of pain).

Teeth

Odontogenic causes are the most common source of orofacial pain and must be ruled out before considering other disorders. Routine dental examination accompanied by appropriate investigations (vitality tests, radiographs) is usually sufficient to exclude dental causes.

Temporomandibular joint

Myofascial pain and internal derangement of the temporomandibular joint (TMJ) are common and can be identified by careful examination of the masticatory muscles and TMJ (tenderness, clicking, reduced mouth opening etc.). A majority of patients are managed conservatively (patient education, analgesics, night guard, relaxation therapy, etc.). Other options include arthrocentesis, arthroscopy and meniscoplasty.

Jaw disease

Infected cysts and tumours in the jaw bone may present with localised swelling, tenderness, tooth mobility and local nerve paraesthesia. Appropriate radiographs (e.g. orthopatntomogram) usually help identify the size of the lesion and relationship to teeth, nerves etc. Alveolar osteitis, osteoradionecrosis and bisphosphonate-related osteonecrosis of jaws (BRONJ) are discussed in Chapter 84.

Sinus disease

Maxillary sinusitis is common and may simulate a maxillary toothache. It is often caused by viral or bacterial infection and may be unilateral or bilateral. It can present as a constant ache, typically localised to the involved sinus, and may worsen with change of posture (bending over or when lying down).

Salivary glands

Acute sialadenitis may be viral (e.g. mumps) and presents with parotid involvement. It is managed conservatively with non-aspirin analgesics and bed rest. Bacterial sialadenitis may be secondary to sialolithiasis and often involves the submandibular gland. Management includes removal of a stone if present. Chronic cases may warrant removal of the affected gland. Mucoceles and ranula are not painful! Pain related to malignant tumours (e.g. adenoid cystic carcinoma) is accompanied by swelling, with possible facial nerve paresis and regional lymphadenopathy.

Table 78.1 Disorders that may present with pain in the oral and perioral region

Origin	Common disorders

Teeth	Dentin sensitivity
	Pulpitis
	Infected periapical lesions
	    Periapical granuloma
	    Periapical abscess
	    Radicular cyst

Periodontium	Periodontal abscess Pericoronitis Necrotising periodontal disease HIV-associated periodontal disease
Temporomandibular joint	Arthritis Facial arthromyalgia
Jaws	Alveolar osteitis (dry socket) Fractures Osteomyelitis Osteoradionecrosis Bisphosphonate-related osteonecrosis of jaws (BRONJ) Infected cysts and malignant neoplasms
Maxillary antrum	Acute sinusitis Malignant neoplasms
Salivary glands	Acute sialadenitis Ductal obstruction Malignant neoplasms Advanced Sjögren syndrome HIV-associated salivary gland disease

Nerves	*Primary neuralgias*
	    Trigeminal neuralgia
	    Vagoglossopharyngeal neuralgia
	Secondary neuralgias
	    Postherpetic neuralgia
	    Multiple sclerosis neuralgia
	    Causalgia
	    Neuralgia inducing cavitational osteonecrosis
	    Intracranial mass lesions
	    Extracranial mass lesions
	    Nasopharyngeal carcinoma (Trotter's syndrome)
	    HIV-associated neurological disease

Blood vessels	Migraine Cluster headaches Temporal arteritis
Psychogenic	Facial arthromyalgia Atypical facial pain Atypical odontalgia Oral dysaesthesia Factitious ulceration
Referred pain	Ischemic heart disease (angina pectoris and myocardial infarction) Nasopharyngeal, ocular and aural disease

Dentistry at a Glance. First Edition. Edited by Elizabeth Kay. © 2016 John Wiley & Sons, Ltd. Published 2016 by John Wiley & Sons, Ltd.
Companion website: www.ataglanceseries.com/dentistryseries/dentistry

Nerves
Trigeminal neuralgia

The first accurate account of trigeminal neuralgia is credited to John Fothergill who presented his *On a Painful Affliction of the Face* before the medical society of London in 1773. Although considered idiopathic, the condition may be related to central vascular compression. It is usually seen in the fifth decade or later with a female predilection. It is characterised by intense paroxysmal electric or shooting pain unilaterally. Each bout of pain may last few seconds to 2 minutes. Pain is often initiated by touching an area on the face often referred as a **trigger zone**. Any branch of the nerve may be involved. The pain may be so severe that patients may avoid washing the face or shaving.

Diagnosis is based on history, clinical examination, local radiographs and more sophisticated investigations like computed tomography (CT) scan (to rule out central mass lesions) and magnetic resonance imaging (MRI) (to rule out central vascular compression).

Medical management is usually the first-line treatment. Carbamazepine (Tegretol) is one of the most commonly used medication. Other drugs include: gabapentin, phenytoin, oxcarbazepine and clonazepam.

Operative options include microvascular decompression (MVD), gamma knife radio surgery (GKR) and percutaneous stereotactic radiofrequency thermal rhizotomy (PSRTR) are currently popular options. Historically, partial sensory rhizotomy (PSR), glycerol injections, alcohol injections and cryotherapy have also been tried with variable success.

Vagoglossopharyngeal neuralgia

Vagoglossopharyngeal neuralgia is probably 100 times less common than trigeminal neuralgia. Presentation is similar to trigeminal neuralgia except for the location (base of tongue, pharynx and tonsillar areas and ear and infra-auricular areas). Management principles are also similar to those for trigeminal neuralgia.

Postherpetic neuralgia

Pain lasting for more than 1 month after herpes zoster infection is termed postherpetic neuralgia. It may represent destruction of large myelinated fibres. It may resolve spontaneously in 6–24 months. Management options includes tricyclic antidepressants, ibuprofen, topical lignocaine and entonox for acute attacks.

Blood vessels
Cluster headaches (migrainous neuralgia)

This is a unique condition characterised by pain occurring in clusters of weeks. Generally regarded as idiopathic, it may have a vascular basis possibly mediated by abnormal hypothalamic function. It is common in the third and fourth decades with a strong male predilection. It is characterised by intense, paroxysmal pain (15 minutes–3 hours) with most attacks occurring in the middle of night (**alarm clock headache**). The pain is unilateral and involves the midface, especially the circumorbital region, often accompanied by nasal stuffiness, facial flushing and lacrimation. It may mimic a maxillary toothache. A variety of medications have been used to treat this condition including sumatriptan, prednisone, lithium and calcium channel blockers.

Temporal arteritis

Autoimmune vasculitis of temporal artery may present with unilateral throbbing headache followed by intense aching, burning temporal and facial pain. It is more commonly seen in women aged 50–85 years. It may be accompanied by prodromal gastrointestinal tract symptoms and involvement of retinal arteries (retro-orbital pain), which carries a risk of blindness. Elevated erythrocyte sedimentation rate (ESR) and biopsy of temporal artery (vasculitis) help in the diagnosis. Management is based on systemic corticosteroids.

Psychogenic pain

Patients with psychogenic pains are often seen in practice and their pain may be related to depression or hypochondria. Patients may present with bizarre descriptions of relentless pain which does not seem to respond to any treatment. Often there is a history of repetitive visits to multiple clinicians, to no avail! The site, distribution and duration of pain are often inconsistent and do not conform to any specific diagnosis. Antidepressant medications are the main stay of treatment.

Key points in orofacial pain management

- Local causes of pain are by far the most common.
- Never extract teeth without justification, an accurate diagnosis of the pain is always required.
- Always exclude organic causes before labelling the pain as psychogenic.
- Remember that patients with psychogenic disease are not exempt from organic disease.
- Refer patients in pain if you cannot diagnose a reason for their pain.

79 Extraction of teeth

Figure 79.1 Extensive root resorption of a root treated lower right second molar precludes restorative treatment; extraction may be the most appropriate option.

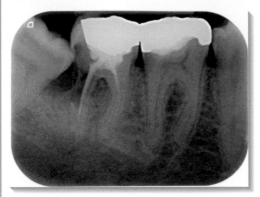

Figure 79.2 A large radicular cyst involving the left mandible molar region; the lesion extends to the lower border of the mandible and failed to resolve following endodontic treatment of the lower left first and second molars

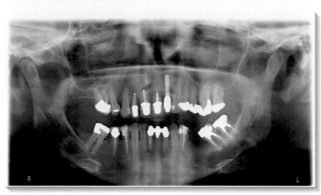

Figure 79.3 A supernumerary tooth (mesiodens) in the anterior maxilla; this was removed due to persistent discomfort

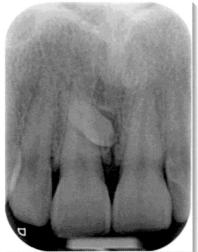

Figure 79.4 (a) Correct way to hold extraction forceps in a palm grip and using little finger to open and close forceps blades; (b) application of forceps on an upper right central incisor with appropriate support of the alveolus using the non-dominant hand

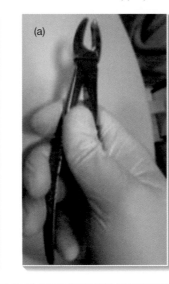

(a)

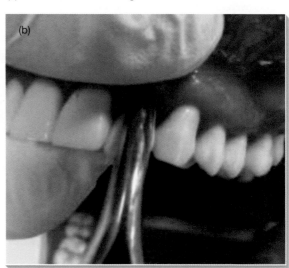

(b)

Introduction

Tooth extraction is a minor surgical procedure and may present with a wide range of difficulty level. Good preoperative assessment and sound extraction technique are essential to achieve a successful outcome with minimal trauma. Straight-forward extractions may be carried out using a closed extraction technique, while more difficult ones may require a surgical approach.

Indications

The most common reasons for tooth extraction are unrestorable caries and advanced periodontal disease. Other indications include extensive root resorption (Figure 79.1), involvement of teeth by pathological lesions (Figure 79.2), symptomatic impacted and supernumerary teeth (Figure 79.3), and orthodontic prescriptions. Trauma to teeth and jaw bone may warrant extraction(s). Prophylactic extractions may be required prior to

Dentistry at a Glance. First Edition. Edited by Elizabeth Kay. © 2016 John Wiley & Sons, Ltd. Published 2016 by John Wiley & Sons, Ltd.
Companion website: www.ataglanceseries.com/dentistryseries/dentistry

radiotherapy or chemotherapy. Finally, financial constraints may preclude extensive restorative treatment making extraction(s) the more feasible option.

Contraindications

Local contraindications include a spreading cellulitis and limited mouth opening. However, a localised abscess is not a contraindication as removal of the diseased tooth may offer the most rapid resolution of infection. Nevertheless, obtaining effective local anesthesia may be difficult and this must be considered. Lastly, teeth involved by a malignancy or suspected vascular lesions should not be removed but should be referred for appropriate management.

Preoperative assessment

History: Presenting complaints, medical history and patient factors including race, age, and gender.
Clinical assessment: Crown form, caries, periodontal health, status and alignment of adjacent teeth, mouth opening.
Radiographic assessment: Radiographic assessment may be carried out using a periapical view or an orthpantomogram, or both if appropriate:
- Relationship to vital structures (maxillary antrum, inferior alveolar nerve canal, mental foramen)
- Root morphology (number, shape, size, curvature)
- Evidence of root caries, root resorption, hypercementosis, ankylosis or previous endodontics
- Periradicular pathology (granuoloma, cyst, etc.)
- Sclerosis of alveolar bone.

Technique

Closed tooth extraction may be carried out using forceps alone but more commonly the tooth is loosened first using an elevator. It is essential that the operator gains adequate access and visualisation of the operative field with correct positioning, use of supporting hand and suction (role of the assistant). An unobstructed path of withdrawal of the tooth must be established and controlled force should be used throughout the extraction. A step-wise approach is as follows:
1 Detach gingival tissues around the cervical margin of the tooth atraumatically using a periosteal elevator to facilitate application of forceps beaks more apically. This is primarily indicated when extracting a grossly decayed tooth with minimal residual crown.
2 Loosen the tooth using a luxator and/or a straight elevator (see Chapter 80).
3 Adapt the forceps to the tooth and carry out appropriate movements to deliver the tooth (see section Forceps extractions).

Chair and operator position

Correct position of the patient, chair and operator is vital during extractions. Ensure that it is comfortable for the operator to approach the tooth, allows adequate visualisation of the field and permits maximal control over force application. Many operators perform extractions in the standing position. For maxillary extractions, the chair is reclined so that the maxillary occlusal plane is 60° to the floor and level with the operator's elbow. For mandibular extractions, the chair is more upright so that the occlusal plane is parallel to the floor and usually 15 cm below the operator's elbow. For all teeth, except mandibular lower right posteriors, the right-handed operator stands in front of the patient on the right side. For mandibular right posteriors, the operator stands behind the patient. These positions are reversed for left-handed operators.

Role of non-dominant hand

- Reflect the soft tissues (lips, cheeks and tongue) to improve visualisation and minimise trauma.
- Support the alveolus buccopalatally; this helps to stabilise the patient and gain tactile information to discern tooth movements during extraction.
- Support the mandible to avoid undue forces being transmitted to the basal bone and temporomandibular joint.

Forceps extractions

Extraction forceps are used on the wedge principle and facilitate extraction by expanding the socket. After adapting the forceps blades parallel to the long axis of the tooth (Figure 79.4), apical pressure is applied to force the beaks into the gingival sulcus, partially severing the periodontal ligament. Subsequent movements are specific to individual teeth and are summarised below. Slight traction force (pull) is necessary to complete the extraction:
- **Maxillary central incisor** (single root): rotation, delivered in a labio-occlusal direction
- **Maxillary lateral incisor** (single root): labial displacement, delivered in a labio-occlusal direction
- **Maxillary canine** (single root): labial force followed by rotation, delivered in a labio-occlusal direction
- **Maxillary first premolar** (two roots): progressive buccopalatal displacement, delivered in an bucco-occlusal direction
- **Maxillary second premolar** (single root): buccal displacement, delivery in bucco-occlusal direction with a rotational traction
- **Maxillary molars** (three roots): progressive buccopalatal displacement, delivery in bucco-occlusal direction
- **Mandibular incisors and canine** (single root): labiolingual displacement followed by rotation, delivery in a labio-occlusal direction
- **Mandibular premolars** (single root): rotation, delivery in bucco-occlusal direction
- **Mandibular molars** (two roots): initially squeeze the beaks into the bifurcation followed by controlled buccal or figure-of-eight movements, delivery in bucco-occlusal direction.

Postextraction management

Remove any obvious debris such as amalgam, calculus or residual tooth fragments using suction; any residual periapical pathology may be gently curetted. Firmly compress the socket walls using finger pressure buccolingually, taking care not to over-compress if an implant is contemplated. Ensure there are no residual sharp bony projections, which may require smoothening with a bone file. Place a moist gauze pack over the extraction socket for 10 minutes to achieve haemostasis prior to discharging the patient. Written and verbal postextraction instructions should be provided. A review appointment may be arranged for difficult extractions or when complications are likely.

80 Surgical extractions

Figure 80.1 A three-corned flap design to remove a fractured UR6

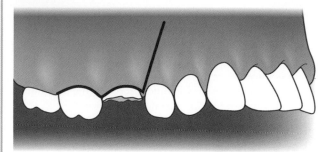

Figure 80.2 An envelop flap design for removal of a fractured UR4

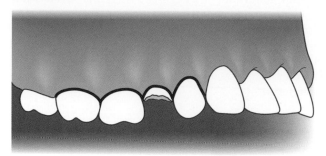

Figure 80.3 Surgical flap design for removal of a fractured LR6; the releasing incision is extended to the mesial aspect of the LR4 to avoid damage to the mental nerve

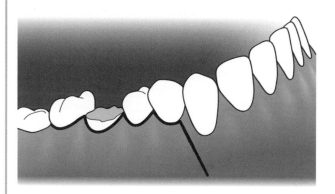

Figure 80.4 Surgical exposure of a 'mesiodens' using a palatal envelope flap

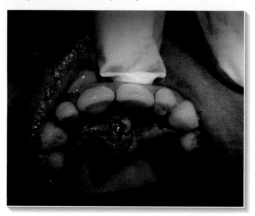

Introduction

Removal of most teeth may be accomplished by closed extraction technique (see Chapter 79). However, it may be necessary to carry out surgical extraction if a tooth fractures during routine extraction, for complicated extractions (marked dilacerations of roots, supernumerary roots, ankylosis, etc.) or if removal of retained roots is required.

Preoperative assessment

Preoperative assessment is carried out using the same principles as outlined in Chapter 79. If a surgical extraction is planned following fracture of the tooth during routine extraction, it is important to obtain an appropriate radiographic view following the event to clearly evaluate the residual tooth and identify any possible displacement.

Preoperative preparation

It is important to prepare and lay out all the instruments and equipment necessary to accomplish a surgical extraction. It is not advisable to start with a few instruments and repeatedly ask for more instruments during the procedure. It not only adds to the operating time but may also add to the patient's stress during a surgical procedure.

Surgical technique

Anaesthesia: Local anaesthesia (preferably with a vasoconstrictor) is usually adequate in most cases. Intravenous sedation or general anaesthesia may be considered where appropriate (multiple extractions, difficult extractions, unco-operative patients).

Surgical flap: A buccal approach is recommended for most surgical extractions. A variety of flap designs are in use for surgical access and the design for a given case may depend on a number of factors (Figures 80.1–80.4). Irrespective of the flap design, the incision must extend down through the periosteum to the crestal bone to allow reflection of a full-thickness mucoperiosteal flap. Some key principles that must be observed when planning surgical flaps are as follows:

- The base of the flap should be broader than the free margin to ensure adequate vascular supply.
- Must provide adequate access.
- Flap margins must rest on sound bone.
- Avoid injury to vital structures (mental and lingual nerves, see below)
- Vertical releasing incisions must involve the full width of interdental papilla.
- Avoid tension during reflection of the flap.
- Adequate flap reflection is needed to allow placement of a retractor on sound bone.
- Flap design must be amenable to tension-free closure to avoid wound dehiscence.

The following flap designs may be used:

- A three-cornered flap: An incision in the gingival sulcus of the tooth to be extracted and involving one tooth on either on either side with a vertical releasing incision, usually anteriorly.
- A four-cornered flap: Same as above with two vertical releasing incisions.
- If the involved tooth is completely covered by soft tissues, or located in an edentulous jaw, an incision is placed on the crest of the alveolar ridge overlying the buried tooth, with or without releasing incisions.
- Isolated apical root fragments may be exposed using a semilunar flap design.

Releasing incisions should not be placed in the lower premolar region (to avoid mental nerve damage). Also, distal crestal incisions in the lower third molar region must be placed on the bone and flare bucally to avoid damage to the lingual nerve.

Flap elevation: Use a periosteal elevator to lift a full-thickness mucoperiosteal flap and retract it bucally with minimal tension using an appropriate instrument (e.g. Bowdler Henry rake retractor).

Bone removal: This is accomplished using a round tungsten carbide bur on a surgical handpiece under saline irrigation. Adequate buccal cortical bone is removed, exposing the cement enamel junction along the diameter of the root. It helps to establish a point of application for an elevator and a path of withdrawal. Multirooted teeth may be sectioned vertically with a fissure bur to divide the roots. This makes their removal a lot easier and also helps minimise the extent of bone removal. The latter is particularly important if tooth replacement with an implant is contemplated.

Extraction of tooth: The tooth or roots can now be removed using appropriate elevators. Dental elevators are used primarily as levers. Adequate training and use of controlled force is mandatory to avoid unnecessary trauma when using elevators and the following principles must be strictly observed:

- The elevator must be held in a palm grip with the index figure placed along the shank.
- The elevator must only rest on the tooth to be removed and not the adjacent teeth.
- They should be used only by rotation around their long axis.
- Ensure adequate protection of buccal and lingual soft tissues with adequate retraction and guarding with a finger rest and use of appropriate retractors.
- Ensure adequate jaw support, particularly when removing lower molars as considerable force may be generated.
- Avoid damage to restorations on adjacent teeth.

Most commonly, a straight elevator (e.g. Coupland's) is applied perpendicular to the tooth in the interdental space with the inferior portion of the blade resting on alveolar bone and the superior portion against the tooth. The elevator is then rotated toward the tooth being extracted. When removing multirooted teeth, if one of the roots is fractured an elevator with a triangular blade (e.g. Cryer) made be inserted in the empty root socket and turned to elevate the root. This manoeuvre works on the wheel and axle principle with the handle of the elevator serving as an axle and the tip of the blade as a wheel.

Once sufficiently loose, delivery of the tooth is accomplished using an appropriate instrument (e.g. Fickling's forceps).

Wound debridement: Irrigate the socket with saline and remove any debris or residual granulation tissue. Also, ensure bone at the margins of the socket is smooth.

Wound closure: This is achieved with a combination of simple interrupted and mattress sutures, preferably using monfilament sutures (e.g. Vicryl Rapide).

Postoperative phase

Written and verbal postoperative instructions must be provided. Postoperative discomfort may be controlled with non-steroidal anti-inflammatory drugs.

81 Impacted third molars

Figure 81.1 OPG showing an apparently vertical lower left third molar. However, a perpendicular line drawn through the furcation of LL7 and LL8 shows a divergence, indicating that the LL8 is distoangular. Also, note the difference in the width of interdental septum on the mesial and distal aspect of LL7; the narrower interdental septum on the distal aspect of LL7 also indicates that the LL8 is distoangular

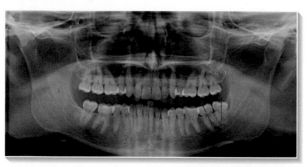

Figure 81.2 OPG showing a lower right third molar with a high risk to the inferior alveolar neve. Note the mesial root overrlapping the IAN canal; the distal root has a marked dilceration with a juxtapical radiolucency. Root outline of a recently extracted lower right second molar is also seen

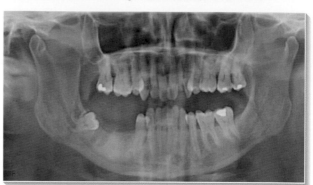

Figure 81.3 (a) OPG showing bilaterally impacted upper third molars with a distoangular inclination and no obvious dilacerations; (b, c) both third molars show marked dilacerations of roots after extraction. Also note the overlapping of IAN canal shadow by the roots of the lower third molars

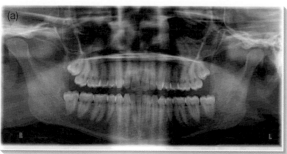

Figure 81.4 A three-cornered flap design for removal of LR8 with the releasing incision mesial to the lower second molar; note the distal incision needs to flare laterally to avoid damage to the lingual nerve

Figure 81.5 Envelope flap with crevicular incision on the buccal aspect of lower molars and a distal relieving incision; this flap design is used more commonly by experienced surgeons

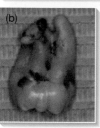
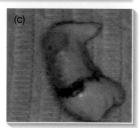
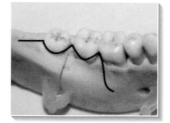
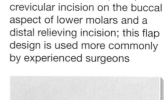

Introduction

Third molars (wisdom teeth) are the last teeth to erupt in the mouth and may become impacted due to insufficient space for eruption. Removal of third molars is one of the most common minor oral surgical procedures worldwide. In England and Wales, the National Institute for Health and Care Excellence (NICE) has produced guidelines on removal of wisdom teeth. The NICE guidelines indicate that there is no reliable research evidence to support a health benefit from prophylactic removal of pathology-free impacted third molar teeth.

Indications for removal:

- Single episode of severe pericoronitis or recurrent pericoronitis
- Unrestorable caries
- Untreatable pulpal and/or periapical pathology
- Cellulitis
- Abscess/ osteomyelitis

Dentistry at a Glance. First Edition. Edited by Elizabeth Kay. © 2016 John Wiley & Sons, Ltd. Published 2016 by John Wiley & Sons, Ltd.
Companion website: www.ataglanceseries.com/dentistryseries/dentistry

- Root resorption of the tooth or adjacent teeth
- Fracture of tooth
- Disease of follicle, including cyst or tumour
- Presence of wisdom teeth is judged to impede surgery or reconstructive jaw surgery
- Wisdom tooth involved in or within the field of tumour resection.

Removal not advisable:
- Deeply impacted third molars with no history or evidence of pertinent local or systemic pathology
- Third molars likely to erupt successfully and have a functional role
- Patients whose medical history renders removal an unacceptable risk to their overall health
- Risk of surgical complications is judged to be unacceptably high, e.g. fracture of an atrophic mandible.

Assessment

History: Presenting complaints, medical history and patient factors, including race, age, and gender.

Clinical assessment: Eruption status, soft tissue inflammation, caries, periodontal health, mouth opening.

Radio graphic assessment: The most commonly used image is an orthopatntomogram (OPG). However, there is an increasing trend to use cone beam computed tomography. The following need to be examined:
- Crown/ root morphology
- Angulation of the tooth (vertical, mesiogangular, distoangular, horizontal, transverse or inverted; Figure 81.1).
- Depth of tooth in the bone and its relationship to the anterior border of ramus
- Evidence of any associated pathology (cyst, tumour, root resporption, etc.)
- Relationship to the inferior alveolar nerve.

Risk of inferior alveolar nerve (IAN) damage is directly related to proximity of the wisdom tooth roots to nerve the IAN canal. Increased risk of nerve damage may be evident from the following observations on the OPG: narrowing or diversion of canal, darkening of root outline, overlapping of IAN canal outline by root apices, marked dilaceration of roots and a juxta-apical area radiolucency (Figure 81.2). In such cases consideration should be given to performing a coronectomy (see Section Coronectomy) as opposed to a conventional extraction.

It must be reiterated that assessment based on conventional radiographs and OPG has limitations because they provide a two-dimensional view of a three-dimensional structure (Figure 81.3).

Preoperative phase

Removal of impacted teeth is usually carried out in specialist oral surgery settings. Following a thorough assessment, informed consent must be obtained from the patient with an explanation of benefits and risks (especially damage to inferior alveolar and lingual nerves). The explanation should include details of alternative treatment options.

Surgical technique

Anaesthesia: Local anaesthesia (preferably with a vasoconstrictor) is usually adequate in most cases. Intravenous sedation or general anaesthesia may be considered where appropriate (multiple impacted wisdom teeth, difficult extractions, unco-operative or anxious patients).

Incision: A buccal approach is commonly recommended for surgical removal of wisdom teeth. A variety of flap designs are in use for surgical access and the design for a given case may depend on a number of factors (Figures 81.4 and 81.5). Nevertheless, the flap design must allow adequate access with margins (relieving incisions) resting on sound bone.

Flap elevation: Use a periosteal elevator to lift a full-thickness mucoperiosteal flap and retract it bucally with minimal trauma using an appropriate instrument (e.g. Bowdler Henry rake retractor). Elevation of a lingual flap may unnecessarily bruise the lingual nerve and is not required in most cases.

Bone removal: This is accomplished using a round tungsten carbide bur on a surgical handpiece under copious sterile saline irrigation. The aim is to remove bone on the buccal and distal aspects of the tooth creating a crater to expose the cementoenamel junction (CEJ). It allows establishment of a point of application for an elevator and a path of withdrawal. The latter may also be facilitated by sectioning the tooth (vertically or horizontally) with a fissure bur.

Extraction of tooth: Once an unimpeded path of withdrawal has been established, the tooth may be lifted from its socket using appropriate elevators (e.g. Coupland's) with minimal direct force. Finally, the tooth is delivered using an appropriate instrument (e.g. Fickling's forceps).

Wound debridement: Irrigate the socket with saline and remove any debris or residual follicular tissue. Also, ensure there are no sharp bony edges at the margins of the socket.

Wound closure: Closure of the surgical site may be achieved with a combination of simple interrupted and mattress sutures, as appropriate, preferably using monfilament sutures (e.g. Vicryl Rapide). Haemostasis must be achieved prior to discharging the patient.

Postoperative phase

The patient should be provided with appropriate written and verbal postoperative instructions. The immediate concerns are pain and swelling and are best managed with non-steroidal anti-inflammatory drugs. Antibiotics may be prescribed when indicated. Perioperative administration of steroids (e.g. dexamethasone) may be considered to reduce oedema and trismus. A review may be arranged for unusually difficult extractions or when complications are anticipated.

Coronectomy

Coronectomy refers to surgical removal of the crown of the tooth by sectioning it 3–4 mm apical to the CEJ, intentionally leaving the roots in the bone. This is a recognised alternative to conventional surgical extraction of a lower third molar when there is a higher risk of nerve damage. Following smoothing of the residual root surface with a round bur, the surgical flap is closed using sutures. A secondary procedure to remove the roots is only indicated if symptoms develop or a periradicular pathology is identified. Coronectomy is not advisable if the involved tooth is non-vital, or when sectioning of the crown itself puts the IAN at risk. Moreover, if the roots become mobile during the procedure, extraction is advisable.

82 Biopsy

Figure 82.1 A nodular growth on the right lateral border of the tongue in a 23-year-old male; following an incisional biopsy the lesion was diagnosed as a squamous cell carcinoma

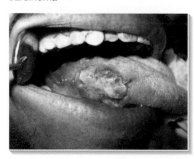

Figure 82.2 (a) A lipoma involving the right lateral border of tongue; (b) Lesion exposed during an excisional biopsy
Source: Courtesy of Professor MU Akhtar.

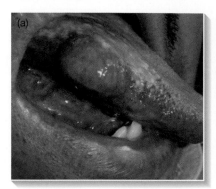

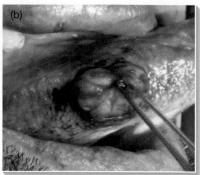

Figure 82.3 (a) A fibroma on the right buccal mucosa; (b) the lesion was excised under local anaesthesia; (c) the surgical site following excision of the lesion and suturing

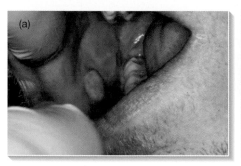

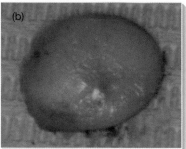

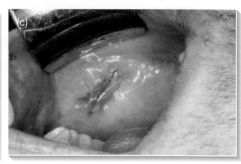

Introduction

Biopsy refers to the removal of tissue from a living body for microscopic examination. It is considered the gold standard for diagnosis of pathological lesions and the results of a biopsy dictate the future course of treatment. A systematic approach to diagnosis warrants a detailed medical history, and clinical, radiographic and other relevant investigations. A biopsy helps to establish the true nature of a lesion and may confirm or rule out a malignancy.

Biopsies are not routinely performed in general practice; if a dentist has appropriate training and experience, they may carry out biopsies of benign lesions. However, patients with suspected premalignant and malignant lesions must be referred to maxillofacial surgery colleagues. This allows the specialist colleagues to evaluate the patient and helps the formulation of a comprehensive treatment plan without delay.

Indications for a biopsy are:
- To confirm a clinical diagnosis
- To confirm or exclude malignancy
- Treatment
- May help to monitor progress of a disease.

Dentistry at a Glance. First Edition. Edited by Elizabeth Kay. © 2016 John Wiley & Sons, Ltd. Published 2016 by John Wiley & Sons, Ltd.
Companion website: www.ataglanceseries.com/dentistryseries/dentistry

Types of biopsy

Incisional biopsy

Incisional biopsy involves removal of only a small portion of a lesion. Generally, a wedge of tissue is removed at the periphery of the lesion to include some normal-appearing tissue in the specimen. It also important to ensure an adequate depth of the tissue by extending the incision margins to the base of a lesion.

Indications for an incisional biopsy are:
- Suspected premalignant and malignant lesions (Figure 82.1)
- Large lesions (usually >1 cm)
- Systemic diseases (e.g. Sjögren syndrome).

Excisional biopsy

Excisional biopsy involves complete removal of the lesion along with a margin of normal tissue (2–3 mm for benign lesions and 4–10 mm for malignant lesions) (Figures 82.2 and 82.3). Generally, a wedge of tissue is removed at the periphery of the lesion to include some normal-appearing tissue in the specimen. Ensure an adequate depth of the tissue by extending the incision margins to the base of a lesion.

Indications for an excisional biopsy are:
- Benign lesions
- Small lesions (<1 cm).

Additionally, an excisional biopsy constitutes a definitive treatment by complete removal of the lesion. Common lesions treated by this method include benign fibroepithelial polyp, mucocele and fibroma.

Methods of obtaining a specimen are:
- Scalpel
- Electrocautery
- Biopsy forceps/ punch
- Lasers.

Soft tissue biopsy

Soft tissue biopsies are mostly carried out using a No. 15 surgical blade. Generally, an excisional biopsy of small benign mucosal lesions is performed using an elliptical incisions incorporating 2–3 mm of normal tissue at the periphery. The incisions converge at the base to allow separation of the lesion from underlying connective tissue. Following the removal of a lesion, the wound margins are undermined to facilitate tension-free closure.

Incisional biopsy of large lesions or lesions with suspicion of malignancy (Figure 82.3), is most commonly carried out by outlining a wedge of tissue with a No. 15 surgical scalpel. An alternative is to use a biopsy punch. Essentially the punch comprises a circular blade attached to a plastic handle. Diameters of 2 to 10 mm are available. Multiple incisional biopsies may be required for large lesions with variable surface characteristics.

Bone biopsy

Intraosseous pathological lesions usually require exposure using a full-thickness mucoperiosteal flap. The principles of flap design described in Chapter 80 must be followed. Care must be observed to avoid damage to important neurovascular structures. Prior to biopsy, aspiration of intraosseous lesions should be done using a 16–18 gauge needle to determine the nature of the lesion (solid or cystic). The nature of aspirate (fluid, pus, blood, air, etc.) may provide valuable information.

Biopsy form

A biopsy form provides essential information to the histopathologist to help in establishing a correct diagnosis. While the format of the biopsy form may vary, generally the following must be recorded:
- Patient's demographic details
- Presenting complaint
- History of presenting complaint
- Past medical and dental history
- Social history
- Clinical description of the lesion (site, size, shape, surface, composition, relationship to nearby structures, status of local tissues, regional lymph nodes, any pertinent systemic findings)
- Any radiographic findings (bony lesions)
- Clinical photographs (soft tissue lesions)
- Findings of any other investigations.

It is also important to mention the nature of the specimen (soft tissue or bone); the type of biopsy performed (incisional or excisional); any pertinent intraoperative findings and the time-frame for biopsy report (routine or urgent).

Storage and transport of specimen

Arrangements for storage and transport of biopsy specimens must be organised before hand by liaising with the histopathology laboratory. For most biopsies, the excised specimen is placed in plastic pot containing a fixative, 10% formalin (4% formaldehyde). Ensure there is an adequate volume of fixative (usually 10 times the volume of the specimen). The specimen container must also be labelled with patient's and sender's details in case it gets separated from the biopsy form. The specimen is placed in a sealed plastic bag, which should then be placed in a rigid outer container that can be secured by adhesive tape. A further outer padded bag is recommended, which should be labelled 'Pathological specimen' and the name and address of the sender should be clearly displayed.

Adjuncts to biopsy – cytology

Cytology refers to removal of individual cells for microscopic examination. It is not as reliable as a biopsy and false-negative results are possible. Some applications of cytology for oral pathological lesions include:
- **Oral brush cytology:** This technique utilises a hand-held rotator wire brush to collect epithelial cells, which are then fixed on a glass slide for examination. It is mostly used as a tool for screening for oral cancer and monitoring oral precancerous lesions.
- **Fine-needle aspiration cytology:** This technique is primarily hospital based. It is used to collect specimens from inaccessible sites, e.g. cervical nodes or salivary glands.

83 Suturing

Figure 83.1 Common suture materials used in oral and maxillofacial surgery: Vicryl rapide 4-0; Silk 3-0 and Prolene 5-0

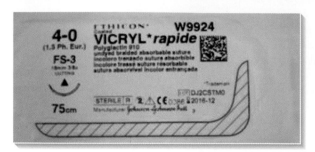

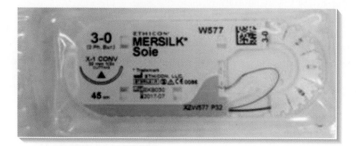

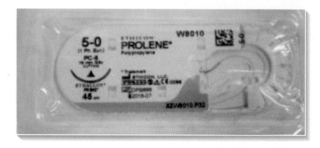

Figure 83.2 Parts of a suture needle

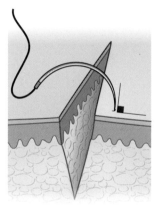

- Point
- Swaged end
- Body (shaft)

Figure 83.3 Simple interrupted suture

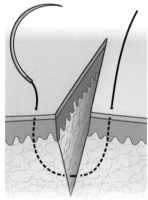
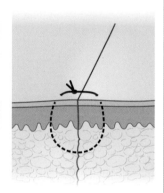

Figure 83.4 Horizontal mattress suture

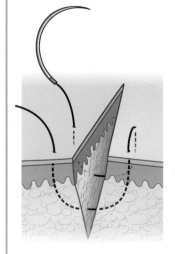
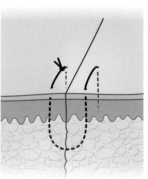

Figure 83.5 Vertical mattress suture

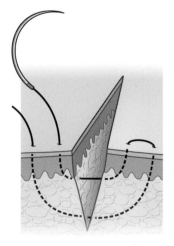
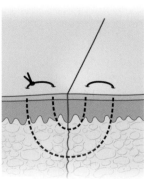

Introduction

The purpose of suturing is to hold a wound together in good apposition until such time as the natural healing process is established. Suturing of wounds promotes healing by primary intention, reduces bleeding and haematoma formation, minimises patient discomfort and lowers the risk of secondary infection. It is a fundamental skill and a dentist needs to be proficient in basic suturing skills. It may be required during a number of procedures, for example wound closure following a surgical tooth extraction. Like any operative procedure, suturing requires adequate practical training and cannot be learnt from a book alone!

Suture gauge

Suture gauge ranges from 00 (very thick, and mainly used for closure of abdominal wall) to 11-0 (very fine and typically used in microvascular surgery). For most oral surgical procedures, the recommended suture gauge is 3-0 or 4-0. A suture gauge of 5-0 or 6-0 is used on the face. Generally, finer sutures are used in children as their tissues are more delicate.

Suture needles

Suture needles may be straight (used without a needle holder) or curved (used with a needle holder). Curved needles are classified as either cutting (sharp) or tapered (round bodied). For oral and facial suturing, a curved cutting needle is recommended.

Suture materials

Suture materials may be classified in a number of ways (natural vs. synthetic, absorbable vs. non-absorbable or braided vs. monofilament) (Table 83.1). For intraoral suturing, silk, catgut and Vicryl are used most commonly (Figure 83.1). Prolene and Nylon are commonly used for facial suturing.

Correct use and handling of instruments for suturing

Safe and correct use of instruments throughout suturing is essential and also prevents needlestick injuries. The needle holder and suture scissors are held by placing the thumb and ring finger through the rings in the handles with the index finger supporting the shank. The Gillies tissue forceps are held in a pen grip to grasp soft tissues or suture needle.

- Do not handle the suture needle with your fingers.
- Hold the needle two thirds up the curvature in the jaws of a needle holder with the needle tip pointing upward (Figure 83.2).
- Ensure the needle holder is locked (audible click) before commencing suture placement.
- Use your thumb to open and close the lock on the needle holder as required.
- Never hold the suture needle at its tip as it may cause damage, making it difficult to pass the needle through the tissues.

Table 83.1 Suture materials

Suture	Absorbable	Non-absorbable
Natural	Catgut: plain chromic	Silk Cotton Linen Stainless steel wire
Synthetic	Polyglycolic acid (Dexon) Polyglactin 910 (Vicryl) Polydioxone (PDS) Polyglyconate (Maxon)	Polyamide (Nylon) Polyester (Dacron) Polypropylene (Prolene)

- Dispose of the suture needle and other sharps promptly after completion of the procedure into the sharps bin.

Guidelines for suturing

- Minimise bacterial contamination (irrigate wounds with saline to remove visible debris and foreign bodies).
- Achieve haemostasis (blood is a culture medium).
- Handle tissue gently.
- Intraoral sutures should be 3–4 mm from the wound edge and 5–6 mm apart. Facial sutures should be 2–3 mm from the skin edge and 3–5 mm apart to minimise scarring.
- Approximate wound margins without tension (do not strangulate!).
- Hold the soft tissues gently with Gillies tissue forceps to achieve better control.
- Suture from free to fixed tissue (usually facial to lingual).
- Pass the needle at right angle through the full thickness of mucosa, do not slice the needle through the tissue.
- Ensure the first knot is secure before placing the subsequent knots.
- Suture knots should rest on one side (usually buccal) clear of the wound margins.
- Cut the suture at an appropriate length (4–5 mm for Vicryl and 8–10 mm for silk).
- Ensure good postoperative care.

Common intraoral sutures

- **Simple interrupted suture** is placed and tied individually and is easiest to learn (Figure 83.3). The suture passes from one end of the wound (facial) and comes out through the other (lingual) and is then held with appropriate knots on the facial aspect.
- **Horizontal mattress suture** is particularly useful to approximate soft tissues around an extraction socket (Figure 83.4). The suture needle is passed through the mesial and distal papillae penetrating close to the base of each papilla (to avoid tearing). Involve the soft tissues across the circumference of the socket to achieve adequate compression of soft tissues against the cortical bone. The suture should be tied securely but too tightly. Do not attempt to completely cover the socket with soft tissues as this may result in haematoma formation and subsequent dehiscence.

    Another type of horizontal mattress suture is a **figure-of-eight** suture. This suture may be used to support a blood clot in the socket and retain an artificial haemostatic agent in the socket.

    Horizontal mattress sutures may also be used for closure of soft tissue incisions as they help evert wound margins and provided good contact at the connective tissue interface.

- **Continuous suture:** This is also a type of simple suture and the sutures are placed again and again without tying each individual suture. This technique is particularly suitable for closure of long span linear surgical incisions as it may be quicker and provide better hemostasis. However, if any error is made during suturing, the entire suture may need to be replaced.

    Other techniques such as **vertical mattress**, **subcuticular** sutures are more applicable in skin closure (Figure 83.5).

Suture removal

Non-resorbable sutures need to be removed in 5–7 days as they do not offer any benefit beyond this period. In fact they may harbour debris and increase wound contamination if retained for longer periods. Each suture knot is grasped firmly with a pair of Gillies forceps and pulled toward the wound margin before cutting it with the tips of sharp scissors.

84 Complications of exodontia

Figure 84.1 Displaced root of UR5 in the right maxillary antrum

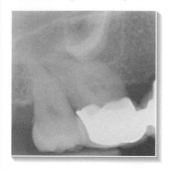

Figure 84.2 Caldwel Luc approach to remove a displaced root of the maxillary right first molar; a buccal vestibular incision is used to expose the anterior maxillary antrum followed by creation of a bony window to access the antrum and retrieve the displaced root

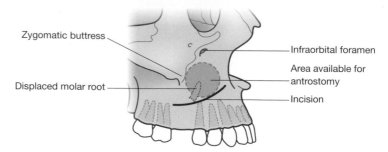

Zygomatic buttress

Displaced molar root

Infraorbital foramen

Area available for antrostomy

Incision

Figure 84.3 Partial fracture of maxillary tuberosity during extraction of a grossly carious maxillary third molar

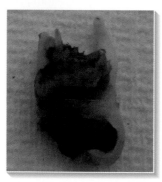

Figure 84.4 (a) Orthopantomogram showing the close relationship of the roots of the upper maxillary molars with the floor of the left maxillary antrum;(b) an oral antral communication (left maxilla) in the patient depicted in (a) following extractions of upper left molar teeth

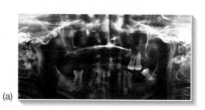

(a)

(b)

Source: Courtesy of Professor MU Akhtar.

Figure 84.5 Closure of an oroantral fistula using a buccal sliding flap: (a) Incision design of a buccal mucoperiosteal flap with two diverging releasing incisions; freshen the soft tissue across the circumference of the defect prior to outlining the flap. (b) Elevation of the flap followed by horizontal incision on the deep aspect of the flap to incise the periosteum; this helps to mobilise the flap. (c) Closure of the buccal flap to cover the defect using a combination of horizontal mattress and simple interrupted sutures.

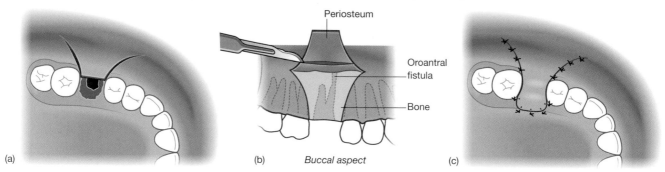

Periosteum

Oroantral fistula

Bone

(a)

(b) *Buccal aspect*

(c)

Figure 84.6 Closure of an oroantral fistula using a palatal pedicle flap: (a) Outline of palatal flap based on the greater palatine artery. (b) The palatal flap is rotated and sutured to cover the defect. The donor site is left with denuded bone. The donor site may be covered with a surgical dressing, e.g. Whitehead varnish, to reduce postoperative discomfort and facilitate healing

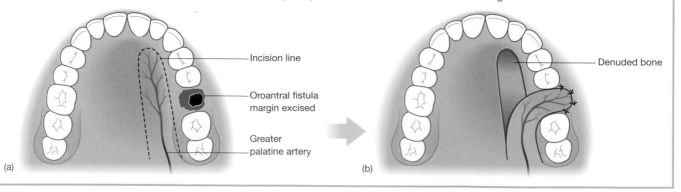

Incision line

Oroantral fistula margin excised

Greater palatine artery

Denuded bone

(a)

(b)

Introduction

A variety of complications may be associated with tooth extraction. The best approach is to prevent these complications by careful preoperative planning (medical history, clinical and radiographic evaluation) and thorough clinical technique.

Perioperative complications
Bleeding

Minor bleeding is a common occurrence during extraction. More serious bleeding may result from underlying medical disorders or medications and these should be addressed preoperatively. Damage to local vessels (e.g. inferior alveolar artery) may also cause prolonged bleeding but can be managed with local measures.

Damage to bone and adjacent soft tissues

- **Tooth fracture** is common and can be avoided with careful preoperative planning and correct technique. If removal of the retained tooth fragment is daunting, specialist referral is warranted.
- **Displacement of tooth or root fragment** into the maxillary sinus may occur during removal of upper molars or premolars (Figure 84.1); less frequently, displacement into infratemporal space (upper third molars) or sublingual pouch (lower molars) occurs. If this happens, specialist referral is recommended for possible surgical removal (Figure 84.2). If the tooth is lost in the aerodigestive tract, refer to the local hospital to rule out accidental inhalation.
- **Extraction of the wrong tooth** may occur and may have medicolegal consequences. If the wrongly extracted tooth is intact, it may be reimplanted back in the socket. In any case, the patient must be informed and meticulous clinical notes should be completed.
- **Damage to adjacent teeth or restorations** may be encountered with careless use of elevators. Correct technique to avoid any force on the adjacent teeth and protection with a finger rest is essential to avoid this complication.
- **Fracture of the alveolus** may occur if excessive force is applied using extraction forceps. It is most commonly observed in extractions of maxillary canines and molars with resultant fracture of the buccal cortex or floor of the antrum. A surgical approach may help prevent this complication.
- **Fracture of the maxillary tuberosity** (Figure 84.3) may occur when excessive force is used for extraction of the last standing tooth in the upper arch (second or third molars) and if substantial may jeopardise the construction of a maxillary denture.
- **Fracture of the mandible** may occur when excessive force is used for extraction of deeply impacted lower third molars or when removing teeth in an atrophic mandible. Immediate referral is required for appropriate management.
- **Damage to soft tissues** results from carelessness on part of the operator or from patients injuring themselves due to numbness. Small mucosal tears may heal uneventfully but more extensive damage may require surgical repair.
- **Nerve damage** is more likely with surgical extractions but is usually avoidable with a careful approach. Nerves are at risk during surgical extractionsl. These include inferior alveolar and lingual (lower third molars) and mental (lower premolars).

- **Oroantral communication** may develop following extraction of maxillary posterior teeth, especially molars (Figure 84.4). Careful examination of preoperative radiographs is essential to determine the risk of this occurring. If the roots of the tooth are in close approximation to the antral floor, a surgical approach with tooth sectioning is preferable. The presence of bone attached to the roots of the extracted tooth should alert the clinician that a communication may have developed. Even if no communication can be seen clinically, it may be wise to place a mattress suture across the socket. The patient should be advised to avoid forceful nose blowing or sneezing, use of straw and smoking. For clinically obvious communications, immediate closure with a buccal flap is advisable (Figure 84.5). Larger communication defects may require the use of buccal fat pad or a palatal pedicle flap (Figure 84.6). Persistent oroantral communication may be complicated by chronic sinusitis and establishment of an **oroantral fistula**.

Postoperative

- **Pain** and **swelling** are common after tooth extractions but are usually managed with non-steroidal anti-inflammatory drugs (NSAIDs). Excessive and persistent pain may result from traumatic extractions, infection or alveolar osteitis and may warrant further intervention. **Soft tissue bruising** may be seen after multiple extractions in the elderly and can be managed conservatively.

  Trismus may be observed, especially with lower third molar extractions. If severe and the cause thought to be infective (<20 mm), antibiotics may be prescribed.
- **Bleeding** postoperatively may result from the causes already mentioned. Additionally, poor postoperative care may encourage bleeding. Careful examination of the socket is required to determine the source of bleeding. Local measure are adequate in most cases.
- **Wound dehiscence** may occur following surgical extractions if the flap is replaced without adequate bone support or sutured under undue tension. Local infection also increases the risk of dehiscence. It may be managed conservatively or may require smoothing of exposed bone under local anaesthetic.
- **Alveolar osteitis** represents delayed healing due to failure of organisation of a blood clot in the extraction socket. However, it is not associated with infection. It is most common with lower molar extractions. It is characterised by moderate to severe pain 48–72 hours after extraction but there are no systemic features. Diagnosis is based on clinical findings and managed by irrigation of the socket with saline and placement of a medicated dressing, for example idoform gauze or Alveogyl. The procedure may be repeated on alternate days until the pain subsides.
- **Other causes of delayed healing** may include patients with a history of radiotherapy to the head and neck (**osteoradionecrosis**), chemotherapy (**osteochemonecrosis**) or bisphosphonates (bisphosphonate-related osteonecrosis of the jaw).
- **Infection**, although rare after routine extractions, may be seen more frequently with surgical extractions and in patients with immunosuppression. Infection may manifest with localised pain or swelling and suppuration. Rarely, a cellulitis or osteomyelitis may be observed and this would warrant specialist referral.

85 Surgical endodontics

Figure 85.1 Trapezoidal flap design involving an adjacent tooth on either side with a sulcular incision and two vertical releasing incisions

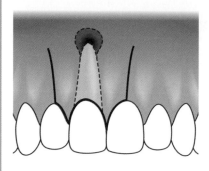

Figure 85.2 A triangular flap design involving an adjacent tooth on either side with a sulcular incision and a vertical releasing incisions on one side

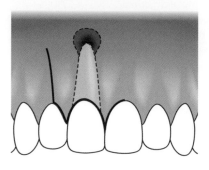

Figure 85.3 A submarginal trapezoidal flap (Ochsenbein–Luebke) design; this preserves the relationship of tooth (crown) with the marginal gingiva

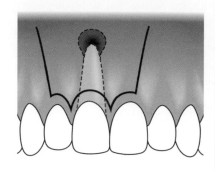

Figure 85.4 A submarginal triangular flap design with a sulcular incision and a vertical releasing incision on one side

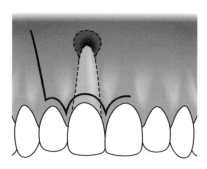

Figure 85.5 Semilunar flap design; although straightforward, this design may provide limited access to the surgical site, which may potentially compromise the result

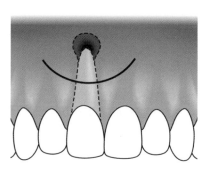

Figure 85.6 A trapezoidal muco-periosteal flap exposing a defect in the labial cortex caused by the periapical lesion; it is important to expose sound bone apical to the confines of the lesion to ensure its adequate removal

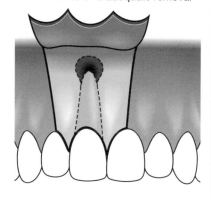

Figure 85.7 A bony window is created in the labial cortex using a round bur to allow access to the root apex of the involved tooth

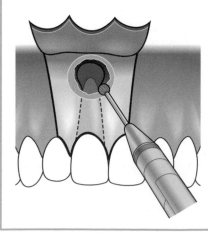

Figure 85.8 Root resection (apicectomy) with a fissure bur removing approximately 3 mm of the root apex at 90° to the long axis of the root

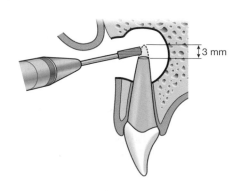

Figure 85.9 Root-end cavity preparation extending approximately 3 mm into the root end; this is best accomplished using an ultrasonic tip in line with the long axis of the root

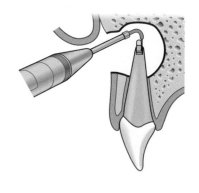

Dentistry at a Glance. First Edition. Edited by Elizabeth Kay. © 2016 John Wiley & Sons, Ltd. Published 2016 by John Wiley & Sons, Ltd.
Companion website: www.ataglanceseries.com/dentistryseries/dentistry

Introduction

Surgical endodontics offers a useful option to manage teeth with failures following conventional endodontics. However, most endodontic failures result from inadequate technique in root canal instrumentation/obturation and unsatisfactory coronal restorations. Ideally, these errors shoule be identified and rectified using re-root treatment. Conventional endodontics usually offers a better long-term prognosis.

Indications

1 Persistent periapical disease that does not resolve with conventional endodontics

2 Inability to achieve a satisfactory apical seal with conventional endodontics (obliterated root canals, perforation etc.).

Other indications include the presence of full-coverage restorations where conventional access may compromise the underlying core or when removal of a post may risk a root fracture.

Contraindications

• Uncontrolled systemic disease
• Teeth with poor prognosis (unrestorable teeth, lack of bone support)
• Risk to anatomical structures (neurovascular structures, maxillary antrum).

Assessment

Careful determination of the nature and extent of disease along with an estimate of the prognosis of the tooth is essential.

A through medical history and clinical examination should be undertaken. Note the signs of infection (lymph nodes, mouth opening, swelling, tenderness, presence of sinus tract). Long-term prognosis of the tooth should be evaluated noting the presence of caries, periodontal health, occlusion and the status of existing restorations. Radiographic assessment is based on periapical films using beam-aiming devices to ensure reproducibility. The periapical film should allow visualisation of approximately 3 mm of tissues beyond the root apex. An orthopantogram and cone beam computed tomography may be utilised in cases of larger lesions or to delineate adjacent anatomical structures, especially for posterior teeth.

Preoperative phase

It is essential that the operating dentist has appropriate skills and experience in performing surgical endodontics and the dental office has all the required facilities, that is equipment and materials. Informed consent must be obtained from the patient with an explanation of risks and benefits, including alternative treatment options.

Surgical technique

Administration of non-steroidal anti-inflammatory drugs (NSAIDs) and chlorhexidine rinse preoperatively may be beneficial. Magnification using loupes or preferably an operating microscope is also recommended. Local anaesthesia (preferably with a vasoconstrictor) is usually adequate in most cases.

Surgical flap

A variety of flap designs are in use for surgical access (Figures 85.1–85.5). The design for a given case may depend on a number of factors, including access, presence of pre-existing extracoronal restorations, surgeon's experience etc. Nevertheless, the flap design should allow adequate access with margins (relieving incisions) resting on sound bone. Atraumatic handling and protection of the flap is important.

Osteotomy

In many cases resorption of the bone due to inflammation is evident on raising a flap. Such bone defects facilitate initial visualisation and exposure of the root apex (Figure 85.6). If sound bone is encountered, an osteotomy is carried out using tungsten carbide bur on a surgical hand piece or ultrasonic tips under saline irrigation. Adequate bone removal is recommended to expose the root apex and facilitate removal of pathological tissue (Figure 85.7).

Surgical curettage

Initial debridement of inflammatory tissue should be achieved with curettes to expose the root apex. Complete removal may not be achieved until resection of the root apex. Care should be taken to avoid damage to any vital anatomical structure even if doing so necessitates leaving some residual soft tissue. The specimen should be submitted for histopathology.

Apicectomy (root-end resection)

This is achieved using a fissure bur or ultrasonic tips under saline irrigation with the aim of removing approximately 3 mm of the root apex at 90° to the long axis of the tooth (Figure 85.8). Bevelling of the root apex is no longer in vogue as it exposes a greater number of dentinal tubules. Apicectomy facilitates curettage and removes the bulk of anatomical anomalies (e.g. accessory canals).

Root-end cavity preparation

The preparation should be approximately 3 mm deep, involving the entire pulp space in the long axis of the tooth (Figure 85.9). Traditionally, root-end preparation was carried out using a miniature bur on a microhead hand piece. However, the use of ultrasonic tips offers greater ease and predictability.

Root-end filling

Currently, mineral trioxide aggregate (MTA) is the most popular material for retrograde filling. Satisfactory success rates are also reported with reinforced zinc oxide-eugenol, ethoxy benzoic acid (super EBA), and glass ionomer. However, amalgam is no longer recommended. The root-end preparation should be isolated using cotton pellets and/or haemostatic agents and the cavity dried prior to root filling. The root-end filling material should be packed with a plugger, ensuring no excess material is left in the periapical tissues. Ideally, the root end filling should be assessed radiographically before closure.

Closure is achieved with a combination of simple interrupted and mattress sutures, preferably using monfilament sutures (e.g. Vicryl).

Postoperative phase

The main considerations are pain and swelling. The use of NSAIDs may be adequate and may be supplemented by a long-acting local anaesthetics given at the end of the procedure and application of ice packs for the first 6 hours after surgery. Chlorhexidine mouthwashes may be beneficial to maintain oral hygiene. Antibiotics are not indicated routinely.

Follow-up

An initial follow-up appointment is aimed at assessing healing. Periodic follow-up with radiological monitoring is required until healing is complete. Further attempts at surgical endodontics must be approached with caution due to a lower success rate.

86 Benign swellings in the oral cavity

Figure 86.1 Ventral aspect of the tongue showing two discrete sessile papillomas
Source: Courtesy of Professor MAO Lewis.

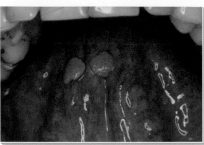
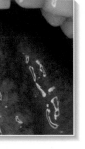

Figure 86.2 Clinical photograph of a large fibroma involving the left mandibular alveolar ridge in an edentulous subject

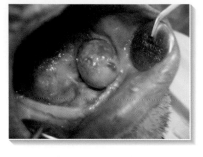

Figure 86.3 An epulis fissuratum on the lower edentulous ridge; note the groove on the surface of the lesion to accommodate the denture flange

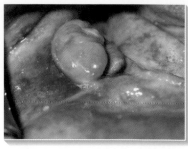

Figure 86.4 Papillary hyperplasia of the palate in a patient with a poorly fitting upper full denture

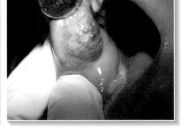

Figure 86.5 Remarkable untreated generalized gingival fibromatosis in an adult male

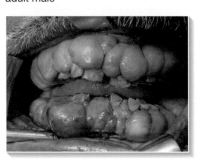

Figure 86.6 A peripheral giant cell granuloma involving the left maxilla

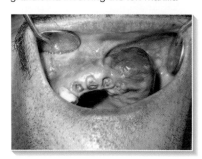

Figure 86.7 A lipoma involving the right lateral border of tongue

Figure 86.8 A large soft tissue vascular malformation involving the left buccal mucosa in a 14-year old female

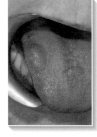

Figure 86.9 An extensive port wine stain involving the right lower face and neck

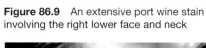
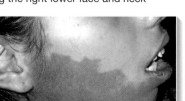

Figure 86.10 A port wine stain involving the right mid-face. The patient also had a large vascular malformation of the right maxilla

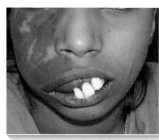

Source: Figures 86.5, 86.7 and 86.10, courtesy of Professor MU Akhtar.

Epithelial origin
Papilloma

Papilloma is a benign proliferation of stratified squamous epithelium caused by human papilloma virus (HPV). It usually presents as a soft, pedunculated, often exophytic growth. It is painless and the most common sites include the tongue (Figure 86.1), lips and soft palate. Treatment consists of conservative surgical excision. Recurrence is uncommon.

Ephelides and pigmented nevi

Ephelides and pigmented nevi are discussed in Chapter 94.

Connective tissue origin
Fibroma

Fibromas are common swellings and represent reactive proliferation of fibrous tissue secondary to local trauma or irritation.

Dentistry at a Glance. First Edition. Edited by Elizabeth Kay. © 2016 John Wiley & Sons, Ltd. Published 2016 by John Wiley & Sons, Ltd.
Companion website: www.ataglanceseries.com/dentistryseries/dentistry

They mostly occur on the buccal mucosa along the occlusal line and present as a painless, sessile, smooth-surfaced and firm lump (Figure 86.2). Treatment consists of conservative surgical excision. Recurrence is rare.

Pyogenic granuloma

Pyogenic granuloma is a common benign growth, which results from tissue response to local irritation or trauma. The term is a misnomer because neither pyogenic organisms are involved nor does it represent a true granuloma. It appears as a soft, highly vascular, pedunculated or sessile lesion. Young adults are most commonly affected with a female predilection. The lesion is painless, tends to bleed and may show rapid growth. If left untreated, most lesions tend to mature with increased collagenisation, which reduces the bleeding. Facial gingival mucosa in the anterior maxilla is the most common site. Involvement of the lips, tongue and buccal mucosa have also been reported. The lesion may develop under the influence of oestrogen and progesterone in pregnant women, hence the terms **pregnancy tumour** or **granuloma gravidarum**. The histopathological picture is marked by a lobular proliferation of numerous endothelium-lined vascular channels (**lobular capillary haemangioma**) sometimes with ulceration of the surface epithelium. Lesions mature with collagenisation and may present as fibromas. Treatment consists of conservative surgical excision. In pregnant women, treatment may be delayed until parturition to allow spontaneous regression; otherwise the recurrence rate may be high.

Denture hyperplasia

Inflammatory, reactive proliferation of fibrous connective tissue may present in several forms in association with ill-fitting dentures:
- **Epulis fissuratum:** Develops on the alveolar vestibule as multiple folds of hyperplastic tissue bordering a denture flange, usually in the anterior region (Figure 86.3).
- **Leaf-like denture fibroma or fibroepithelial polyp:** It appears as a pedunculated mass of fibrous tissue attached to the palate.
- **Papillary hyperplasia (denture papillomatosis):** Develops on the palate underneath a maxillary denture and appears as a papillary and erythematous lesion (Figure 86.4). *Candida* may possibly be involved.

Treatment consists of surgical excision and correction or replacement of ill-fitting denture. Denture papillomatosis may respond to discontinuation of denture use and antifungal therapy in early stages.

Gingival fibromatosis

Gingival fibromatosis is characterized by proliferation of fibrous connective tissue and may be localised or generalised. Although more common in children and adolescents, the condition may be observed in adults (Figure 86.5). Treatment usually requires surgical excision of the lesional tissue.

Peripheral giant cell granuloma

Peripheral giant cell granuloma is a benign reactive proliferation secondary to local irritation or trauma and may represent a soft tissue counterpart of central giant cell granuloma. It presents as a reddish blue mass on the gingivae or edentulous alveolar mucosa (Figure 86.6). It is usually seen in the fifth and sixth decades with a female predilection. The histopathological picture is characterised by the presence of multinucleated giant cells. Treatment consists of surgical excision.

Lipoma

Lipomas are benign lumps of fatty tissue and are uncommon in the oral cavity. They present as a soft, lobulated painless lump, usually involving the buccal mucosa (Figure 86.7). They are usually identified in mature adults, and there is no gender predilection. The histopathological picture is marked by proliferation of mature fat cells. Treatment consists of conservative surgical excision.

Vascular origin
Haemangioma

Haemangioma is a benign hamartomatous proliferation of endothelial cells in infants. It is most commonly observed in the first year of life, displaying rapid growth in the first few months and is more common in females. Most lesions are confined to soft tissues and are well circumscribed. Superficial lesions are usually bright red, while deeper lesions may have a bluish hue. Most lesions regress spontaneously by the fifth year and do not require any treatment.

Vascular malformations

Vascular malformations represent abnormalities of vessel morphogenesis without endothelial proliferation. They are present at birth and tend to persist throughout life (Figure 86.8). They may involve the soft tissues or bone and are classified on the basis of type of vessel involved (capillary, arterial, venous) and flow rate (low flow or high flow). A **port wine stain** represents a capillary malformation, which may appear as a pink or purple lesion in the distribution of the trigeminal nerve (Figure 86.9 and 86.10). Venous malformations are low-flow lesions while arteriovenous malformations are typically high-flow lesions with an audible bruit or thrill. Vascular malformations involving the bone may present with bony expansion and often appear as a multilocular radiolucent defect. Treatment options include sclerotherapy or therapeutic embolisation followed by surgical resection. It is wise to perform needle aspiration on an undiagnosed bony pathology in the jaws to rule out a vascular malformation prior to extractions or surgery.

Lymphangioma

Lymphangioma is a benign, hamartomatous proliferation of lymphatic vessels and presents in the first few years. The anterior part of the tongue is the most common site for oral lesions. Treatment consists of surgical excision, although complete removal may be difficult. The recurrence rate is generally high.

Neural 'lumps'
Neurofibroma

Neurofibroma is a benign lump, which develops from Schwaan cells and perineural fibroblasts. It is the most common peripheral nerve tumour and typically occurs in young adults. It presents as a slow-growing, soft, painless lump on the skin, tongue or buccal mucosa. Treatment consists of conservative surgical excision and recurrence is rare. Multiple neurofibromas may develop due to a hereditary disease, neurofibromatosis (von Recklinghausen disease).

Traumatic neuroma

Traumatic neuroma is a benign, reactive proliferation of neural tissue at the site of nerve damage due to trauma or surgery. Pain may be associated with the lesion. Most develop in the region of the mental foramen but may also be seen on the tongue and lower lip. Treatment consists of conservative surgical excision. Recurrence is rare.

87 Odontogenic tumours and tumour-like lesions

Figure 87.1 Clinical (a) and radiographic view (b) of a grotesque ameloblastoma involving the right mandible in a 40-year old female. The lesion has a classical multilocular radiographic appearance with evidence of root resorption of adjacent teeth
Source: Courtesy of Professor MU Akhtar.

Figure 87.2 OPG of a unicystic ameloblastoma involving the left mandible in a 38-year-old female; note root resorption of adjacent teeth
Source: Courtesy of Professor MU Akhtar.

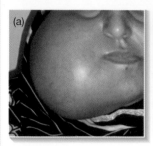
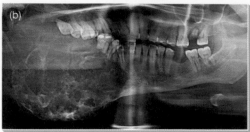

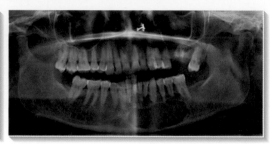

Figure 87.3 Clinical (a) and radiographic view (b) of an adenomatoid odontogenic tumour involving the right maxilla in a 13-year-old female child; the lesion has prevented the eruption of multiple teeth

Figure 87.4 A well-demarcated mixed radiopaque and radiolucent lesion associated with the mesial root of LL6; the tooth is free from caries or periodontal disease and is vital. The lesion was diagnosed as a cementoblastoma. Note the mental foramen just below the lesion.

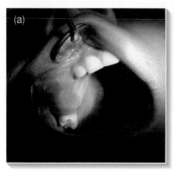
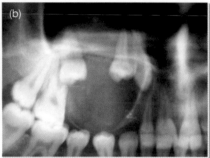

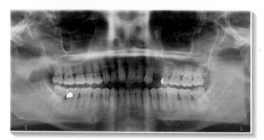

Introduction

Odontogenic tumours develop from odontogenic epithelium, odontogenic ectomesenchyme or both (mixed) and are classified accordingly. They display varied clinical and histopathological features, and treatments are different for each type of tumour.

Tumours of odontogenic epithelium
Ameloblastoma

Ameloblastoma is the most common odontogenic tumour excluding odontomas. It may originate from a variety of epithelial tissues, including the dental lamina, enamel organ, or sometimes from the lining of an odontogenic cyst. It is a slow-growing, locally aggressive neoplasm and may present with several distinct clinical radiographic appearances (Figure 87.1).

The **solid** or **multicystic** variety is the most common type and is usually seen in adult patients over a wide age range without any gender predilection. The posterior of the mandible is the most common site and the ameloblastoma usually presents as a painless expansion of the jaws. Radiographically, the multicystic type presents as a multilocular radiolucency, simulating either a 'soap bubble' or 'honey comb' appearance. Buccal cortical expansion and root resorption of adjacent teeth may be seen. The solid variety appears as a unilocular radiolucency.

The histopathological picture is varied, with the **follicular** pattern being the most common. It is characterised by islands of enamel organ-type epithelium with reversed polarity. The epithelium encloses a core of loose, stellate reticulum-type cells and is surrounded by a fibrous connective tissue. Areas of cystic degeneration are common. The **plexiform** pattern displays cords or sheets of odontogenic epithelium enclosing loosely arranged epithelium and a loose, vascular connective tissue. Other patterns include: **acanthomatous** (epithelium with squamous metaplasia and keratin formation); granular cell (epithelium displays eosinophilic granules); **desmoplastic** (a dense collagen stroma); or **basal cell** (cuboidal epithelial cells).

Multicystic or solid ameloblastoma is an aggressive tumour with a high recurrence rate. Treatment options range from enucleation to *en bloc* resection. However, marginal resection with a 1-cm border past the radiographic limits of the lesion is recommended.

Unicystic and **peripheral** variants are also seen (Figure 87.2). These respond to enucleation or conservative excision.

Malignant ameloblastoma and ameloblastic carcinoma

Rarely, an ameloblastoma may develop malignant changes and show metastases. **Malignant ameloblastoma** shows histopathological features of ameloblastoma, both in the primary as well as metastatic lesions. Ameloblastic carcinoma shows histopathological features of malignancy in a primary, recurrent or metastatic lesion.

Adenomatoid odontogenic tumour

These tumours develop from the epithelium of enamel organ or dental lamina and are mainly seen in younger patients (10–19 years) with a female predilection. The anterior part of the maxilla is the most common site and it usually presents as an asymptomatic lesion. It may cause delayed eruption of involved teeth, prompting radiographic investigations (Figure 87.3). Radiographically, it presents as a well-circumscribed radiolucency, often with scattered foci of calcification. The histopathological picture is marked by tubular epithelial structures simulating preameloblasts with a central space, foci of calcification (dentinoid or cementum) and a fibrous capsule. Treatment involves a conservative enucleation. Peripheral variants are reported.

Calcifying epithelial odontogenic tumour

Also known as **Pindborg** tumour, this develops from the epithelium of dental lamina. It is an uncommon lesion and is mainly seen in mature adults with no gender predilection. The posterior of the mandible is the most common site and it usually presents as a painless swelling. Radiographically, it presents as a multilocular or unilocular radiolucency interspersed with varying amounts of calcified structures. Histopathological picture is marked by islands of polyhedral epithelial cells with a fibrous stroma. Large areas of eosinophilic, amyloid-like material may be present extracellularly and display foci of calcification. Treatment involves a marginal resection with a narrow rim of normal bone. Peripheral variants are reported.

Other odontogenic tumours of epithelial origin include squamous odontogenic tumour and clear-cell odontogenic carcinoma.

Mixed odontogenic tumours

This group includes odontomas, ameloblastic fibroma, ameloblastic fibro-odontoma, ameloblastic sarcoma, odontoameloblastoma and odontomes.

Odontoma

Odontomas constitute the most common type of odontogenic tumours and are better termed dental hamartomas. They develop from odontogenic epithelium and mesenchyme, resulting in formation of dental tissues. They are usually asymptomatic but may prevent tooth eruption in the involved area. Most are discovered following dental radiographs to investigate missing teeth. **Compound odontomas** are composed of multiple small tooth-like structures and tend to involve the anterior maxilla. **Complex odontomas** appear as a radiopaque mass of disorganised dental tissue and are more common in the posterior area of the jaws. Odontomas are treated by conservative surgical removal.

Ameloblastic fibroma

Ameloblastic fibroma is an uncommon lesion and is mainly seen during the first two decades of life. The posterior part of the mandible is the most common site and it is usually asymptomatic. Radiographically, it presents as a well-defined unilocular or multilocular radiolucency. Small lesions can be treated with curettage but marginal resection is warranted for recurrences.

Tumours of odontogenic mesenchyme

This group includes odontogenic fibroma, granular cell odontogenic tumour, odontogenic myxoma and cementoblastoma.

Odontogenic myxoma

Odontogenic myxoma develops from odontogenic mesenchyme and is mainly seen in young adults (20–30 years) with no gender predilection. The posterior of the mandible is the most common site and it is usually asymptomatic or presents as a painless jaw expansion. Radiographically, it presents as a unilocular or multilocular radiolucency and may cause root resorption of adjacent teeth. Histopathological features include spindle-shaped or round cells in a loose, myxoid stroma. Myxomas may be treated with curettage but recurrence warrants marginal resection.

Cementoblastoma

Cementoblastoma is uncommon but is the only true neoplasm of cementum (Figure 87.4). It is mainly identified in children and young adults with no gender predilection. The posterior mandible is the most common site and the tumour classically involves the lower first permanent molar. It may present with jaw swelling and pain but can also be asymptomatic. Radiographically, it presents as a radiopaque mass attached to the root of an involved tooth. The histopathological picture simulates an osteoblastoma and is marked by mineralised deposits with irregular lacunae and prominent basophilic reversal lines. Treatment options include surgical removal of the calcified mass combined with either extraction or root amputation (after endodontics) of the involved tooth.

88 Odontogenic cysts

Figure 88.1 OPG showing a dentigerous cyst associated with an impacted left mandibular third molar; note the root resorption of the LL7

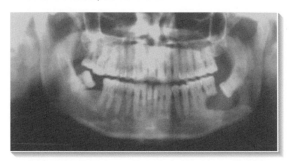

Figure 88.2 A section of OPG showing a dentigerous cyst associated with an impacted upper left maxillary canine
Source: Courtesy of Professor MU Akhtar.

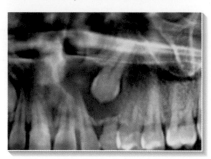

Figure 88.3 OPG showing a dentigerous cyst involving the right mandibular canine; the impacted canine has been displaced close to the lower border of the mandible

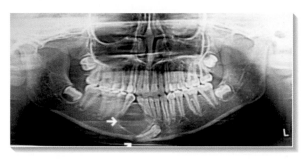

Figure 88.4 OPG showing bilateral mandibular radicular cysts in a patient with neglected dentition and multiple decayed roots; note the goblet-shaped outline of the lesions

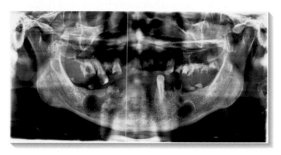

Figure 88.5 OPG showing a large radicular cyst involving the lower anterior teeth following trauma
Source: Courtesy of Professor MU Akhtar.

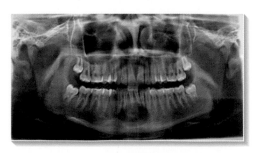

Dentistry at a Glance. First Edition. Edited by Elizabeth Kay. © 2016 John Wiley & Sons, Ltd. Published 2016 by John Wiley & Sons, Ltd.
Companion website: www.ataglanceseries.com/dentistryseries/dentistry

Introduction

A cyst is a pathological cavity containing fluid, semifluid or gaseous material other than pus. Cysts are frequently but not always lined by epithelium. Odontogenic cysts are derived from odontogenic epithelium and develop within the jaw bones. They are classified as developmental or inflammatory.

Developmental odontogenic cysts

Dentigerous cyst

Dentigerous cyst is the commonest developmental cyst (Figures 88.1 and 88.2). It forms as a result of fluid collection between reduced enamel epithelium and the crown of an unerupted tooth. The most commonly involved teeth are the mandibular third molars followed by maxillary canines; other teeth may also be involved. Small cysts may be asymptomatic while larger ones can cause jaw expansion and facial asymmetry. Pain and swelling may develop with infected cysts. Radiographically, it presents as a unilocular radiolucency. Displacement and root resorption of the involved and adjacent teeth can occur (Figure 88.3). Histopathological features are a thin lining composed of flat, non-keratinised epithelial cells and a fibrous connective tissue wall. Treatment consists of enucleation of the cyst along with extraction of the involved tooth. Larger cysts may require a period of marsupialisation prior to enculeation. Rarely, dentigerous cyst may be complicated by the development of an ameloblastoma, squamous cell carcinoma or intraosseous mucoepidermid carcinoma.

Eruption cyst (eruption haematoma)

Eruption cyst is a soft tissue analogue of the dentigerous cyst due to fluid collection between the tooth and dental follicle and appears as a bluish swelling on the gingiva overlying an erupting tooth. Most cysts rupture spontaneously and do not require any treatment.

Odontogenic keratocyst

Odontogenic keratocyst is a developmental cyst that develops as a result of degeneration of the enamel organ before dental hard tissue formation. The most commonly involved teeth are the mandibular third molars followed by maxillary canines; although other teeth may also be involved. Small cysts may be asymptomatic while larger ones can cause pain, swelling and discharge. Keratocysts grow through intramedullary space without causing significant jaw expansion. Radiographically, it presents as a well-circumscribed unilocular radiolucency; however, lesions in the posterior mandible sometimes appear multilocular. Root resorption of adjacent teeth is relatively uncommon. Histopathological features consist of a thin, friable lining composed of stratified squamous parakeratinised epithelial cells. The epithelial lining has a uniform thickness of six to eight cells and shows a wavy pattern on the luminal aspect and palisading of the basal layer. The lumen may contain a clear or cheesy fluid. Treatment consists of enucleation and bone curettage. The recurrence rate is particularly high as the cyst's friable lining makes it difficult to enucleate it in one piece. Use of Carnoy's solution may facilitate enucleation and also help prevent recurrence. Other options include marsupialisation followed by enucleation.

Nevoid basal cell carcinoma (Gorlin–Goltz) syndrome is an inherited (autosomal dominant) disorder characterised by multiple basal cell carcinomata of the skin, skeletal abnormalities (bifid rib, frontal and temporal bossing, kyphoscoliosis) and multiple odontogenic keratocysts of the jaws.

Gingival cyst of the newborn

Gingival cyst of the newborn develop from remnants of the dental lamina and present as small keratin-filled swellings on the alveolar mucosa. Similar non-odontogenic lesions may develop on median palatal raphe due to inclusion of epithelium along the line of fusion of palatal shelves (**Epstein's pearls**) or from minor salivary gland epithelium, and appear as multiple scattered lesions on the hard palate (**Bohn's nodules**). Although common, alveolar and palatal cysts in newborns are self-limiting, drain spontaneously and do not require any treatment.

Lateral periodontal cyst

Lateral periodontal cyst is an uncommon cyst that develops from the remnants of the dental lamina and usually presents in mature adults as a well-circumscribed radiolucency along the lateral aspect of a tooth root. The lower premolar and canine regions are the most common sites and the involved tooth is vital. The histopathological picture is characterised by a thin lining composed of squamous or cuboidal cells and a fibrous connective tissue wall. Treatment consists of careful enucleation of the cyst and preservation of the involved tooth.

Lateral periodontal cyst may present as a soft tissue lesion and is termed gingival cyst of the adult.

Inflammatory odontogenic cysts

Radicular cyst

Also known as an apical or periapical cyst, radicular cyst is by far the most common cyst of the jaws (Figure 88.4 and 88.5). It is an inflammatory lesion, which develops from epithelial cell rests of Malassez as a result of periradicular inflammation. The cyst usually develops in a pre-existing chronic periapical lesion and may remain asymptomatic. Acute inflammatory exacerbation is usually marked by pain, swelling and discharge. The involved tooth is non-vital. It has significant growth potential and may involve adjacent teeth. Movement and mobility of involved teeth may occur over time.

Radiographically, the lesion appears as a radiolucency, usually encompassing the root apex of the involved tooth and loss of the lamina dura. Root resorption of involved teeth may also be evident. However, radiographic features alone are insufficient to differentiate a radicular cyst from a periapical granuloma. Occasionally, the radicular cyst may present along the lateral root surface, simulating a lateral periodontal cyst. Evaluation of periodontal status and tooth vitality are helpful in diagnosing these lesions.

The histopathological picture consists of a cyst lining composed of stratified squamous epithelium, which may show linear calcifications (Rushton bodies). The lumen may be fluid filled or may contain cellular debris. The cyst wall demonstrates dense fibrous tissue with inflammatory changes.

Treatment consists of conventional endodontics of the involved tooth. Larger lesions (>2 cm) may require marsupialisation or enucleation of the lesion following endodontics. Teeth that are deemed unrestorable may require extraction, at which point the lesion will usually resolve.

Residual cyst

A residual cyst develops from inflammatory periapical lesions retained at the site of a tooth extraction. While most lesions may regress or resolve completely over a period of time, surgical intervention may be required for patients experiencing persistent symptoms.

89 Other bone diseases

Figure 89.1 (a) A large central giant cell granuloma involving the right mandible in an adult male; (b) OPG demonstrates a multilocular radiographic appearance

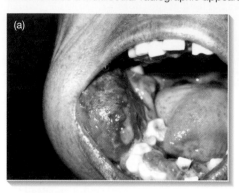 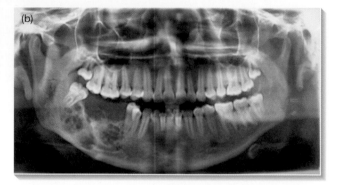

Figure 89.2 (a) A 6-year-old child with a slow-growing, painless bilateral facial swelling; (b) OPG demonstrates multilocular radiolucencies involving the mandibular angle and ramus bilaterally. These findings are consistent with a diagnosis of cherubism

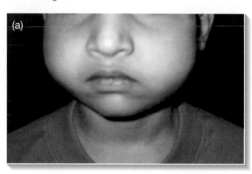 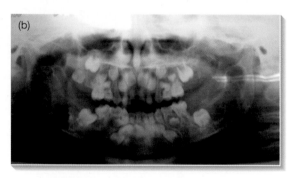

Figure 89.3 Torus palatinus
Source: Courtesy of Professor MAO Lewis.

Figure 89.4 Clinical photograph showing extensive bilateral mandibular tori
Source: Courtesy of Professor MAO Lewis.

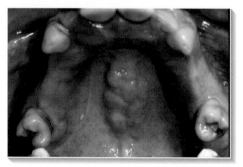 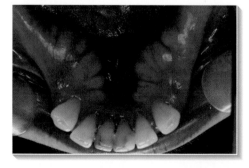

Fibro-osseous lesions

Fibro-osseous lesions involve replacement of normal bone by a fibrous tissue followed by deposition of variable amounts of mineralised tissue (woven bone, lamellar bone or cementum). Early lesions are radiolucent, attain a mixed appearance with time and tend to become radiopaque as they mature. This process occurs in a variety of conditions and diagnosis of a specific condition requires the establishment of a clinical, radiographic and histopathological correlation. The following sections describe recognised fibro-osseous lesions of the jaws.

Fibrous dysplasia

This is a developmental condition caused by a gene mutation, and manifests in a variety of ways:

• **Monostotic:** Presents as slow, painless, unilateral swelling of the jaw. Maxillary lesions are more common. Radiographically,

Dentistry at a Glance. First Edition. Edited by Elizabeth Kay. © 2016 John Wiley & Sons, Ltd. Published 2016 by John Wiley & Sons, Ltd.
Companion website: www.ataglanceseries.com/dentistryseries/dentistry

the lesions are classically described as poorly demarcated 'ground glass' opacities.

- **Polyostotic**: Involves multiple bones. When seen with *café au lait* patches it is termed **Jaffe–Lichtenstein syndrome**. When these features occur with endocrinopathies it is termed **McCune–Albright syndrome**.

Treatment is generally conservative. Functional and aesthetic problems may warrant surgical correction.

Cemento-osseous dysplasia

Cemento-osseous dysplasia (COD) affects the tooth-bearing regions of the jaws, originates from periodontal tissue and manifests first as multiple radiolucent lesions related to the apices of teeth. These then calcify to become radiopaque.

- **Focal COD** usually affects white females in the third to sixth decades. The posterior mandible is involved in majority of cases and lesions are usually asymptomatic.
- **Periapical COD** typically affects black females, usually in the third to fifth decades. Periapical regions of anterior mandibular teeth are the commonest site and involved teeth are vital, allowing differentiation from inflammatory apical lesions.
- **Florid COD** involves multiple areas of the jaws and affects middle-aged black females. Bilateral, symmetric involvement of all four quadrants may be seen.

COD are usually managed conservatively. Symptomatic patients may require operative intervention.

Ossifying fibroma

This is a benign neoplasm affecting mature adults with a female predilection. The posterior mandible is the commonest site of involvement and lesions may cause a painless expansion of the jaw. Lesions are well demarcated and respond to conservative surgical excision.

Paget disease of bone

The condition typically affects white, elderly males. It is characterised by resorption of healthy bone and deposition of primitive vascular (osteoid) bone, resulting in enlargement, distortion and weakening of affected bones. Involvement of vertebrae, limbs and craniofacial skeleton is common. Progressive enlargement of the skull and maxilla sometimes manifests as increasing hat size and the need for maxillary denture replacement. Compression of cranial nerves and osteosarcoma are recognised complications. Skull involvement may lead to a 'cotton wool' appearance on radiographs. High alkaline phosphatase levels are characteristic. Treatment involves medical management with calcitonin and bisphosphonates, and the development of osteosarcoma is a recognised complication.

Giant cell lesions

Giant cell lesions are characterised by the presence of multinucleated giant cells on histopathology and include a variety of conditions of diverse aetiopathogenesis. Diagnosis requires establishing a clinical, radiographic, and histopathological correlation. The following are recognised giant cell lesions of the jaws:

- **Central giant cell granuloma**: This is a reactive lesion mostly seen in subjects younger than 30 years with a female predilection. The anterior mandible is the most common site. It may be asymptomatic or present with jaw pain, swelling, jaw bone perforation and paraesthesia (Figure 89.1). Radiographically, it presents as a unilocular or multilocular bone defect. Non-aggressive lesions respond to curettage while medical management using corticosteroids, calcitonin and interferon α-2a may hold promise for more aggressive lesions.

- **Peripheral giant cell granuloma**: This is discussed in Chapter 86.
- **Cherubism**: This is a developmental condition (autosomal dominant) characterised by bilateral swelling in the posterior mandible, leading to chubby cheeks. It manifests in childhood between 6 and 10 years old. Radiographically, the lesions appear as multilocular defects (Figure 89.2). It is usually managed conservatively as many lesions tend to regress. However, surgical intervention may be used sparingly.
- **Aneurysmal bone cyst**: This is an intraosseous lesion filled with blood and is mostly encountered in the posterior mandible. Radiographically, it appears as a radiolucent, multilocular defect. Treatment involves curettage and enucleation.
- **Simple (traumatic) bone cyst**: This is a fluid-filled bony cavity, mostly seen in the posterior mandible. Radiographically, it appears as a radiolucent defect which may be multilocular. Treatment consists of surgical exploration and curettage.
- **Brown tumour of hyperparathyroidism**: Jaw lesions typically involve the mandible and may appear as unilocular or multilocular radiolucent defects.

Benign lesions and tumours

- **Trori**: These are benign bony growths, most commonly seen on the midline of the palate (Figure 89.3) and mandibular premolar regions, usually bilaterally (Figure 89.4).
- **Osteoma**: These are composed of mature bone and may involve the mandibular body or condyle in young adults. **Gardner syndrome** (autosomal dominant) is characterised by multiple osteomas, supernumerary teeth, epidermoid cysts and colorectal polyposis.
- **Osteoblastoma**: These tumours arise from osteoblasts and typically affect young adults. They tend to involve the posterior mandible.
- **Cementoblastoma**: This is discussed in Chapter 87.

Malignant tumours

- **Osteosarcoma (osteogenic sarcoma)**: This is the most common primary bone malignancy characterised by production of osteoid directly by malignant mesenchymal cells. Jaw involvement is uncommon compared to other sites and primarily affects mature adults with a slight male predilection. Lesions tend to involve the posterior mandible or the alveolar ridge and palate in the maxilla. Pain, swelling, mobility of teeth and paraesthesia are common presenting features but equally sarcomas can be asymptomatic. Radiographically, it presents as a poorly defined radiolucent, radiopaque or mixed lesion. The classic 'sunburst' appearance due to osteophyte deposition may sometimes be evident. Symmetric widening of periodontal ligament space involving several teeth indicates tumour infiltration. The histopathological picture includes malignant mesenchymal cells, with varying degree of differentiation producing osteoid. Chondroid and fibrous tissue deposition may predominate. Management involves a combination of preoperative radiotherapy, chemotherapy and radical surgery.
- **Ewing sarcoma**: This is a primary bone malignancy composed of undifferentiated mesenchymal cells, possibly of neuroectodermal origin. Jaw involvement is rare and mainly involves the mandible. Management involves a combination of surgery, radiotherapy and chemotherapy.
- **Metastatic tumours**: Jaws may be involved by metastases from carcinoma of the breast, lung, thyroid, kidney and prostrate through haematogenous spread. Lesions may manifest with pain, swelling, tooth mobility or paraesthesia.

90 Temporomandibular joint disorders

Figure 90.1 Anterior disc displacement (a) leading to difficulty in translation of condyle (b), which manifests clinically with clicking and trismus

(a)

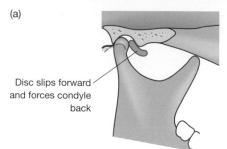

Disc slips forward and forces condyle back

(b)

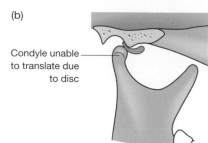

Condyle unable to translate due to disc

Figure 90.2 Severe mandibular micrognathia and facial asymmetry associated with childhood trauma and consequent long-standing bilateral TMJ ankylosis

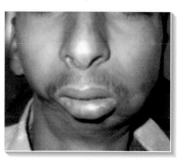

Figure 90.3 Intraoperative image showing right TMJ arthroplasty with silastic following a condylectomy

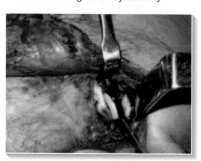

Figure 90.4 Surgical closure following right condylectomy and silastic interpositional arthroplasty using prolene and black silk

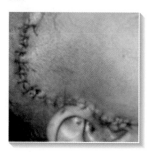

Table 90.1 Differential diagnosis of limited mouth opening

Origin	Common disorders
Intra-articular disorders	Traumatic arthritis Intracapsular fractures Disc displacement (internal derangement) Osteoarthritis Ankylosis Neoplasia (Rheumatoid arthritis, systemic lupus erythematosus) Psoriatic arthritis

Extra-articular disorders	*Muscular disorders*
	   Myofascial pain
	   Fibrosis of masticatory muscles and adjacent soft tissues
	      Burns
	      Radiation therapy
	      Oral submucous fibrosis
	      Systemic sclerosis
	      Fibrosis of pterygomandibular raphe (cleft palate surgery)
	Adjacent Inflammation or infection
	   Pericoronitis
	   Mumps
	   Submandibular abscess
	   Haematoma of pterygomandibular space (IAN block, 3M surgery)
	   Otitis externa
	Extracapsular fractures (condyle, zygoma, maxilla)
	Hyperplasia of coronoid process
	Invading neoplasm from adjacent structures
	Miscellaneous
	   Hysteria
	   Epilepsy
	   Malingering

Temporomandibular joint dysfunction

Temporomandibular joint (TMJ) dysfunction is a common condition, which may result from macrotrauma (e.g. blow to the chin) or microtrauma (e.g. bruxism, jaw clenching). Stress, anxiety and occlusal disturbances are also important factors. It presents with restricted and painful jaw movements, TMJ sounds (clicking or crepitation) and jaw tenderness. It is one of the common causes of limited mouth opening (Table 90.1). However, use of the term TMJ dysfunction does not distinguish between muscle and joint problems; it may be better to describe symptoms either as myofascial pain or an internal derangement (although the two may occur in combination).

Myofascial pain is characterised by diffuse, cyclic pain involving multiple sites, especially the masticatory muscles. It is usually worse in the mornings. However, imaging studies of TMJ are unremarkable. Myofascial pain may have several presentations including: **myositis** (acute painful inflammation secondary to overuse, trauma or infection); **spasm** (acute contraction from overstretching); **contracture** (fibrosis following spasm); and **fibromyalgia** (presence of circumscribed regions within the muscle or 'trigger points', which elicit pain on palpation). Diagnosis: Clinical evaluation and absence of joint pathology on imaging. Treatment: Conservative measures including reassurance, patient education, non-steroidal anti-inflammatory drugs (NSAIDs), muscle relaxants, physiotherapy, occulsal rehabilitation and splints. Alternative therapies can also provide short-term improvements.

Internal derangement of TMJ is characterised by displacement of TMJ disc (meniscus), leading to an abnormal relationship to both the glenoid fossa and the articular eminence. It presents mainly with joint symptoms, including continuous pain, tenderness and clicking (single loud sound) or crepitus (multiple grating sounds). There may be deviation of the mandible on joint movements and the condition may show unilateral or bilateral involvement. Imaging studies provide evidence of disc displacement and damage. Internal derangement exhibits two major patterns:

- **Anterior disc displacement with reduction:** The posterior band of the meniscus is displaced anterior to the condyle. As the meniscus translates anteriorly, the posterior band remains in front of the condyle and the bilaminar zone (retrodiscal lamina) becomes abnormally stretched (Figure 90.1). At some point in the opening movement the slack in the discal attachment is taken up and the condyle slips under the disc with a pop or click being produced. On the closing movement, the disc again slips off the condyle and a closing click is elicited usually softer).
- **Anterior disc displacement without reduction:** The meniscus remains anteriorly displaced at full opening and may lead to significant limitation of mouth opening (<30 mm). Grinding noises in the joint are present initially but disappear later. If the displaced disc is pressing against the inner ear, it may cause subjective hearing loss and tinnitus. Long-term, it may cause a tear or perforation of the meniscus followed by osteoarthritic changes.

Diagnosis: Clinical and radiographic evaluation and the use of magnetic resonance imaging (MRI) scan (disc pathology), computed tomography (CT) scan (bone pathology) and arthroscopy. In the early stages, management is conservative, using measures similar to those used for treatment of myofascial pain. Disc displacement without reduction may be managed with arthrocentesis (joint lavage and manipulation without viewing the joint space) and arthroscopy (diagnostic as well as therapeutic). Surgical management is reserved for advanced cases showing no improvement and options include meniscoplasty or meniscectomy.

Osteoarthritis

Osteoarthritis is a common degenerative joint disease, mainly affecting individuals older than 50 years. Chronic mechanical stress and limited repair capability leads to degenerative changes in the affected joints. It commonly involves multiple joints of limbs and spine but TMJ may also be involved leading to pain, swelling and a reduction of jaw movements. A crackling noise or 'crepitus' may be audible on jaw joint movement. Radiographic changes manifest as narrowing of the joint space, osteophyte formation and radiolucent defects involving the articular surfaces. CT scans, MRI and arthrography are invaluable in the diagnosis. The condition is usually managed conservatively with a reliance on paracetamol (acetaminophen), NSAIDs, occlusal splints and physiotherapy. Advanced disease with severe joint changes may necessitate operative intervention.

Ankylosis

Ankylosis refers to fibrous or bony union of various joint components, leading to reduced mobility. Ankylosis of the TMJ is mainly seen in young children and adolescents. Common causes include trauma and infections of the TMJ. Ankylosis following condylar fractures is common in underdeveloped countries, primarily because of poor trauma management. Haemarthrosis of the joint following trauma leads to progressive ankylosis of TMJ, unilaterally or bilaterally. Most cases present after complete bony ankylosis leads to severe limitation of mouth opening. It may cause arrest of mandibular growth and interfere with nutritional intake (Figure 90.2). Diagnosis is based on clinical and radiographic (orthopantomogram, OPG) evaluation. CT scans are invaluable in determining the extent and severity of ankylosis. Treatment primarily involves surgical arthroplasty to remove the fibrous or osseous tissue and interpositional arthroplasty with temporalis muscle, fascia or synthetic materials (Figures 90.3 and 90.4). Costochondral bone grafts are also indicated in young children to facilitate mandibular growth. Aggressive postoperative physiotherapy is required to prevent recurrences.

Dislocation of TMJ

Dislocation of TMJ occurs when the condyle translates anterior to the articular eminence (unilateral or bilateral). It may occur spontaneously following wide mouth opening (e.g. yawning, eating or dental treatment). It leads to an inability to close the mouth and soon becomes painful due to muscle spasm. It can be reduced with digital manipulation but may require anaesthesia with or without sedation. Recurrent dislocations often require surgical management with eminectomy, or augmentation of articular eminence (Dautrey procedure).

91 Mucosal diseases

Recurrent aphthous ulcers

Recurrent aphthous ulceration (RAU) is one of the most common oral mucosal conditions (Box 91.1). The exact cause of RAU is unknown but mucosal destruction represents a T-lymphocyte-mediated immunological reaction triggered by a variety of agents. These include stress, allergies, genetic predisposition, nutritional deficiencies, hormonal factors and haematological abnormalities. RAU is also observed in association with a number of systemic diseases such as Behçet syndrome, coeliac disease, inflammatory bowel disease, cyclic neutropenia, HIV etc. RAU manifests in three forms:

• Minor aphthous ulcers: These account for approximately 80% cases of RAU and involve the lining mucosa. Ulcers are usually 3–10 mm in size and one to five lesions may be present at a given

time. They heal without scarring in 1–2 weeks and may recur once every few years or up to twice per month.

• Major aphthous ulcers: These account for 10% cases of RAU and may involve the masticatory mucosa, soft palate as well as faucial regions. They are usually 1–3 cm in size and one to ten lesions may be present at a given time. They take 2–6 weeks to heal and may cause scarring.

• Herpetiform ulcers: These represent a unique pattern of RAU and account for 10% cases. A large number of ulcers (up to 100) may be present at a given time, each measuring 1–3 mm. Multiple small ulcers may coalesce to form larger ulcers. The ulcers usually heal in 7–10 days. The clinical presentation simulates primary herpes simplex virus infection and hence the name. Herpetiform ulcers usually involve the lining mucosa and tend to reoccur more often than the minor or major types.

Management: RAU is diagnosed on clinical grounds. A full blood count, serum ferritin and folate levels may help to identify any underlying haematological abnormalities. Additional investigations may be required to rule out an underlying systemic disease. Treatment is primarily symptomatic and involves topical analgesics and antiseptics as well as corticosteroids. Maintenance of a meticulous oral hygiene is crucial to facilitate healing and prevent secondary infection. Intralesional and systemic corticosteroids may be used in resistant cases.

Box 91.1 Differential diagnosis of oral ulceration

Traumatic
• Mechanical
• Chemical
• Thermal
• Electric
• Radiation

Recurrent
• Aphthous
  • Minor (most common)
  • Major
  • Herpetiform
  • Behçet syndrome

Infective
• Bacterial
  • Syphilis
  • Acute necrotising ulcerative gingivitis
  • Tuberculosis
  • Cancrum oris
  • Scarlet fever
  • Diphtheria
  • Gonorrhoea
• Viral
  • Herpes simplex
  • Herpes zoster
  • Herpangina
  • Hand, foot and mouth disease
  • HIV (HSV, CMV, mycobacterium, neutropenia)
• Fungal
  • Candidosis
  • Histoplasmosis
  • Cryptococcosis
  • Zygomycosis
  • Aspergillosis
  • Paracoccidiomycosis
• Protozoal
  • Lieshmaniasis

Neoplastic
• Squamous cell carcinoma
• Lymphoma
• Others (e.g. intraoral melanoma)

Systemic conditions
• Blood dyscrasias
  • Anaemia
  • Leukaemia
  • Neutropenia
  • Hypereosinophilic syndrome
• Gastrointestinal diseases
  • Coeliac disease
  • Crohn's disease
  • Ulcerative colitis
• Immune/autoimmune
  • Pemphigus vulgaris
  • Bullous pemphigus
  • Cicatricial pemphigoid
  • Erosive lichen planus
  • Lupus erythematosus
  • Reiter disease
  • Behçet syndrome
• Hereditary
  • Epidermolysis bullosa
• Idiopathic
  • Lichen planus
  • Erythema multiforme
  • Sarcoidosis
• Malnutrition
  • Scurvy
  • Pellagra
• Connective tissue disease
  • Periarteritis nodosa
  • Vasculitides
  • Giant cell arteritis
  • Wegener granulomatosis

Drugs
• Non-steroidal anti-inflammatory drugs, e.g. aspirin, phenylbutazone, indomethacin
• Cytotoxic drugs, e.g. bleomycin, dactinomycin, daunorubicin, cytosine arabinoside, methotrexate, 5-flurouracil
• Others, e.g. nicorandil, allopurinol, penicillamine

Behçet syndrome

Behçet syndrome represents an immune-mediated multisystem disorder characterised by recurrent oral and genital ulcers, similar to RAU, along with cutaneous and ocular inflammatory lesions. Arthritis and central nervous system involvement is also reported but the disease may affect other systems. Treatment depends on the severity of the disease but often requires a combination of immunosuppressive agents (corticosteroids, cyclosporine, azathioprine, interferon α-2a, methotrexate and dapsone).

Vesiculobullous disorders

Vesiculobullous disorders represent a range of diseases of diverse aetiopathogenesis characterised by blister formation due to fluid collection within the epithelium (vesicles) or connective tissue (bullae).

Viral infections

A variety of oral viral infections may present with intraepithelial vesiculation. These include herpes simplex, varicella zoster, measles and infection with coxsackievirus (herpangina, hand, foot and mouth disease).

Autoimmune diseases

Pemphigus: This disease is caused by production of autoantibodies directed against desmosomes resulting in intraepithelial vesiculation. The disease has several forms but pemphigus vulgaris is the commonest variety. Oral mucosal involvement often precedes skin lesions and the disease is typically seen in adults. Blister formation may be induced with firm lateral pressure (Nikolsky's sign).

Benign mucous membrane pemphigoid: This is caused by production of autoantibodies directed against the basement membrane, resulting in subepithelial vesiculation. It affects elderly adults with a female predilection. Apart from oral mucosal involvement, ocular involvement forms an important component of the disease with a risk of blindness. Ocular disease can lead to multiple lesions, which heal with significant and progressive scarring, hence the name cicatricial pemphigoid (cicatrix = scar). Cutaneous and genital lesions may be observed.

Bullous pemphigoid: This is caused by production of autoantibodies directed against the basement membrane, resulting in subepithelial vesiculation. It is the commonest autoimmune blistering condition and affects elderly adults without any gender predilection. Cutaneous involvement is the primary feature and lesions heal without scarring. Oral mucosal involvement occurs less frequently.

Hereditary disorders

Epidermolysis bullosa: This comprises a heterogeneous group of hereditary disorders characterised by blistering mucocutaneous ulceration. Common varieties include simplex, junctional and dystrophic. Oral involvement is more common with the dystrophic type with subepithelial vesiculation. Other dental anomalies like anodontia, enamel hypoplasia and neonatal teeth may be seen.

Idiopathic disorders

Erythema multiforme: This is an immune-mediated condition characterised by mucocutaneous ulceration.

- **Erythema multiforme minor:** This may be preceded by herpes simplex virus infection and presents with flat, dusky red, rounded cutaneous lesions with necrotic centres (target lesions). Haemorrhagic crusting of lips may be seen.
- **Erythema multiforme major (Stevens–Johnson syndrome):** This is often triggered by drug exposure and may present with cutaneous, ocular, genital and oral mucosal lesions.

Angina bullosa haemorrhagica: This condition is characterised by blood blisters on the soft palate and tongue. Trauma, corticosteroid inhalers and hypertension may play a part but the exact cause is unknown. Lesions heal without scarring.

Lichen planus: This is a common dermatological disease with frequent oral involvement. Clinically, it manifests in a reticular or ulcerative variety. The latter may sometimes involve subepithelial vesiculation.

Orofacial granulomatosis

Orofacial granulomatosis represents a group of immune-mediated disorders characterised by histopathological evidence of non-specific granulomatous inflammation in the oral mucosa. It may manifest as persistent, painless swelling of the lips, termed **cheilitis granulomatosa** (of Miescher). When lip lesions are seen in combination with a fissured tongue and recurrent facial paralysis, the presentation is termed **Melkersson–Rosenthal syndrome**. Intraoral involvement may also be seen and manifests as ulceration, oedema, fissuring and papules. Diagnosis of the condition requires a biopsy to rule out other granulomatous diseases like sarcoidosis, tuberculosis and Crohn's disease, or a foreign body. Management is variable but often involves corticosteroids and other immunosuppressive agents.

92 Oral cancer and precancer

Figure 92.1   Reticular lichen planus involving the right buccal mucosa with characteristic Wickham striae

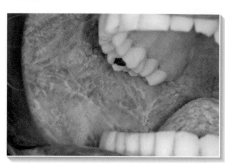

Figure 92.2   Erosive lichen planus on the right buccal mucosa; also note melanin pigmentation of tongue dorsum

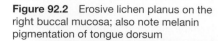
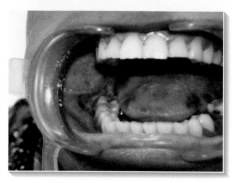

Figure 92.3   Diffuse thick homogenous leukoplakia involving the ventral aspect of tongue

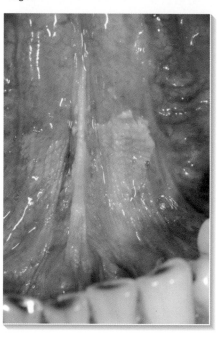

Figure 92.4   Widespread thick homogenous leukoplakia with interspersed nodular changes involving the dorsum of tongue

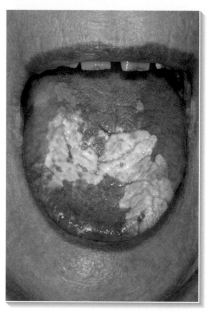

Figure 92.5   Leukoplakia of the labial gingival mucosa in a 60-year-old adult patient

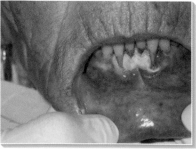

Figure 92.6   A lesion involving the left ventrolateral aspect of tongue; the lesion shows erythroplakic changes in the centre while the peripheral margins of the lesion show leukoplakic changes

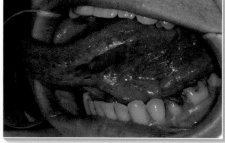

Figure 92.7   Squamous cell carcinoma manifesting as a noduloulcerative growth involving the right ventrolateral border of the tongue; note the hairy change on the tongue dorsum resulting from smoking

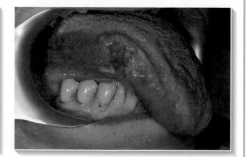

Source: Figures 92.1–92.7, courtesy of Professor MAO Lewis.

Dentistry at a Glance. First Edition. Edited by Elizabeth Kay. © 2016 John Wiley & Sons, Ltd. Published 2016 by John Wiley & Sons, Ltd.
Companion website: www.ataglanceseries.com/dentistryseries/dentistry

Introduction

A **premalignant lesion** denotes a morphologically altered tissue that has a greater than normal risk of malignant transformation. Oral premalignant lesions include: leukoplakia, erythroplakia, palatal changes associated with reverse smoking and actinic cheilosis.

A **premalignant condition** denotes a disease or patient habit that does not necessarily alter the clinical appearance of local tissue but is associated with a greater than normal risk of precancerous lesion or cancer development in that tissue. This group includes conditions causing mucosal atrophy (oral submucous fibrosis, Plummer–Vinson syndrome and glossitis of tertiary syphilis), erosive lichen planus (Figures 92.1 and 92.2), discoid lupus erythematos, inherited cancer syndromes (dyskeratosis congenita, xeroderma pigmentosum and Fanconi anaemia) and immunosuppression (immunosuppressive therapy for organ transplants, graft versus host disease following stem cell transplantation and HIV).

When there is a suspicion of a premalignant or malignant lesion, a prompt or an urgent referral to a maxillofacial surgeon is mandatory. An incisional biopsy is usually the initial investigation, which dictates future management. Long-term, periodic follow-up in a specialist setting is mandatory.

Leukoplakia

Leukoplakia denotes a white patch that cannot be diagnosed clinically or pathologically as any other disease (Figures 92.3–92.5). The diagnosis of the lesion is based on exclusion rather than a definable appearance. Aetiological factors include tobacco smoking, ultraviolet (UV) radiation (lip) and microorganisms (*Candida albicans, Treponema pallidum*). Generally, it is identified in adults (>40 years) with a male predilection. Common sites for leukoplakia include lip vermilion, buccal mucosa and gingivae. Common variants include: mild (thin), homogenous (thick), nodular, verrucous, proliferative verrucous or speckled leukoplakia. Histopathological features include hyperkeratosis and acanthosis, and it is these which mask the underlying vasculature and impart the white colour. More importantly, up to 25% of lesions may demonstrate varying degree of dysplasia (mild, moderate or severe). Dysplasia is most likely in lesions affecting the oral floor, ventral tongue and lip vermilion. Treatment is dictated by the severity of the dysplasia on an incisional biopsy. The goal is to achieve complete excision of dysplastic lesions with a scalpel, or destruction with electrocautery, cryotherapy or lasers (including photodynamic laser therapy). Medical treatment has also been tried successfully with bleomycin.

Erythroplakia

Erythroplakia denotes a red patch that cannot be diagnosed clinically or pathologically as any other disease (Figure 92.6). The aetiology of erythroplakia is similar to leukoplakia. Generally, it is identified in elderly (>65 years) with a marked male predilection. It usually appears as a flat or raised, well-demarcated red patch, often with a velvety texture. However, it is asymptomatic otherwise. Common sites include the oral floor, ventral tongue and soft palate. Multiple lesions may also be seen. Histopathological features include epithelial atrophy and lack of keratin production, making the underlying vasculature show through and it is this which gives the red appearance. More importantly, most lesions demonstrate severe dysplasia or a carcinoma *in situ*. Treatment is dictated by the severity of the dysplasia as with leukoplakia.

Actinic cheilosis

Actinic cheilosis is a premalignant lesion associated with long-term exposure to UV radiation and involves the lower lip vermilion. It is usually seen in people <45 years with a marked male predilection. It causes mucosal atrophy, leady to rough scaly areas on the lip vermilion. Focal ulceration may indicate progression to a squamous cell carcinoma. Prevention includes the use of lip balms with sunscreens. Surgical excision (vermilionectomy) is required for lesions displaying a premalignant change.

Oral submucous fibrosis

Oral submucous fibrosis is a high-risk premalignant condition associated with the use of betel quid or 'paan', mainly in South East Asian populations. Betel quid contains areca nut, which causes chronic and progressive mucosal scarring due to excessive production and cross-linking of collagen fibres. Nutritional deficiencies, ingestion of spicy food, genetic and immunological factors may also play a contributory role. Oral submucous fibrosis may be seen in young adults (18–25 years) with a female predilection. Initial presenting complaints include a burning sensation on oral mucosa, accompanied by vesicles and petechiae. Characteristically, mucosal rigidity results in moderate to severe trismus. Buccal mucosa is the primary site displaying palpable fibrous bands but tongue, soft palate and gingivae may also be involved. Histopathological features include epithelial atrophy and deposition of dense, avascular connective tissue; 10–15% of lesions demonstrate dysplasia or a carcinomatous change. Treatment options include intralesional corticosteroids, surgical splitting of fibrous bands with nasolabial flap reconstruction and intralesion interferon-γ. Unfortunately, lesions seldom regress with habit cessation.

Oral squamous cell carcinoma

Oral cancer accounts for approximately 3% of all cancers and is also the sixth most common cancer (Figure 92.7). The aetiology of oral squamous cell carcinoma (OSCC) is multifactorial and includes extrinsic (tobacco, alcohol, syphilis and UV radiation) as well as intrinsic (malnutrition and iron-deficiency anaemia) factors. OSCC is mainly found in elderly males but in recent years it has also been reported in young people. Common sites include lip vermilion, tongue (posterolateral and ventral aspect) and oral floor. However, it can also affect the soft palate, buccal mucosa and hard palate. It may present as an exophytic (mass-forming) or endophytic (ulcerated) lesion and may be preceded by a leukoplakic or erythroplakic patch. Clinical evaluation of OSCC is most commonly based on the tumour size and extent of lymph node/ distant metastasis (TNM staging). Histopathological features include sheets or islands of anaplastic epithelium with invasion of underlying connective tissue. Depending on the degree of differentiation, OSCC is classified as well differentiated, moderately differentiated, poorly differentiated or undifferentiated. This histopathological classification is called grading. Treatment depends on the stage and site of the disease but primarily consists of radical surgical excision of the lesion along with neck dissection, with or without radiotherapy. Adjuvant chemotherapy is also used.

Verrucous carcinoma is a low-grade variant of OSCC, often caused by the use of smokeless tobacco. It has a deceptively benign histopathological appearance and clinical correlation is crucial. Metastasis is rare and the overall prognosis is generally good.

93 Salivary gland disorders

Figure 93.1 A mucocele involving the mucosal aspect of right lower lip in a 26-year-old male

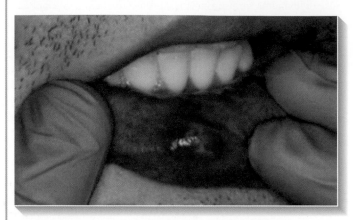

Figure 93.2 Mucous extravasation cyst (ranula) in the oral floor

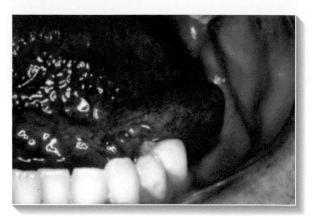

Figure 93.3 Bilateral sialosis involving the parotid glands in an elderly woman

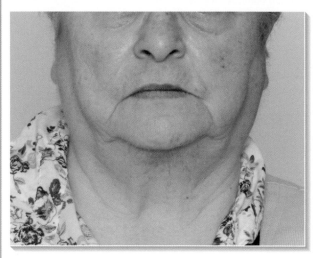

Figure 93.4 Intraoral view of a patient with xerostomia; note multiple teeth with evidence of root caries, thick viscous saliva can also be observed

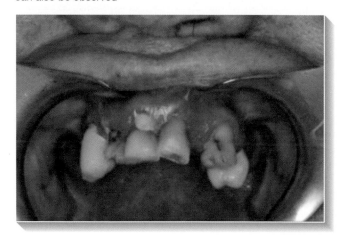

Source: Figures 93.2, 93.3 and 93.4, courtesy of Professor MAO Lewis.

Dentistry at a Glance. First Edition. Edited by Elizabeth Kay. © 2016 John Wiley & Sons, Ltd. Published 2016 by John Wiley & Sons, Ltd.
Companion website: www.ataglanceseries.com/dentistryseries/dentistry

Non-neoplastic disorders

Mucocele is a common lesion caused by rupture of salivary gland ducts leading to extravasation of mucin into the soft tissues. It may be caused by trauma (lip biting) or may be idiopathic. It can present at any age and the lower lip (lateral to the midline) is the most common site (Figure 93.1). Other sites include buccal mucosa, ventral tongue and soft palate. The lesion commonly appears as a painless, soft, fluctuant mucosal swelling with recurrent variation in size. Surgical excision is the treatment of choice.

Ranula is a mucocele that develops in relation to the sublingual gland and appears in the oral floor, usually lateral to the midline (Figure 93.2). It presents as a painless fluctuant swelling often with a bluish hue. Removal of the feeding sublingual gland is the treatment of choice.

Sialadenitis is an inflammatory disorder. It may be caused by paramyxovirus (mumps, endemic parotitis). It is transmitted via urine, saliva or respiratory droplets and is characterised by inflammatory involvement of the parotid glands, usually bilaterally. It may be complicated by epididymo-orchitis. MMR vaccine is used for prevention and treatment is primarily symptomatic. Bacterial sialadenitis is mostly caused by *Staphylococcus aureus* and may be associated with ductal obstruction or decreased flow. Surgical mumps develops following a recent surgery and is often related to dehydration. Non-infectious causes include Sjögren syndrome, radiation therapy and sarcoidosis.

Sialadenosis (sialosis) refers to a painless, non-inflammatory and non-infectious enlargement of salivary glands (Figure 93.3). It may be associated with diabetes mellitus, acromegaly, pregnancy, alcoholism, bulimia, malnutrition and drugs (antihypertensives, antipsychotics). It is often bilateral and most commonly involves the parotid gland.

Sialolithiasis is stone formation within the ductal system. The submandibular gland is the most common site and it presents with recurrent meal time swelling and discomfort. Often the stone is palpable along the course of the submandibular duct. Radiographs, ultrasound, sialography, computed tomography and magnetic resonance imaging (MRI) may all aid the diagnosis. Treatment options include surgical removal of the stone, lithotripsy and salivary endoscopy.

Sialorrhoea is an uncommon condition characterised by excessive salivation. It may be associated with local irritation (aphthous ulcers, dentures), gastroesophageal reflux disease, drugs (lithium, parasympathomimetics), heavy metal poisoning and rabies.

Sjögren syndrome is an autoimmune disorder characterised by dry eyes (xerophthalmia) and dry mouth (xerostomia), and may be classified as primary (no associated autoimmune disorder) or secondary (associated with other autoimmune disorders). It is primarily seen in middle-aged adults with a female predilection. The major oral feature is xerostomia with its associated symptoms and complications. The histopathological picture is dominated by glandular damage caused by lymphocytic infiltration. The condition is associated with an increased risk (up to 40 times) for lymphoma. Diagnosis is based on salivary and tear flow rates, haematology, serum immunology, sialography, biopsy, and MRI. Treatment is mainly symptomatic based on artificial saliva and tears and sometimes sialogogues (e.g. pilocarpine).

Xerostomia is a subjective sensation of a dry mouth. It may transient (fluid loss, dehydration) or chronic (Sjögren syndrome, diabetes mellitus, diabetes insipidus, sarcoidosis, HIV, radiation therapy and medications, especially antihistamines, antihypertensives, antipsychotics, parasympatholytics). Clinically, patients have difficulty in mastication, swallowing and demonstrate atrophy of filiform papillae. Complications include oral candidiasis, rampant tooth decay and sometimes taste disturbances (Figure 93.4). Treatment is based on symptomatic relief and addressing any underlying cause.

Frey syndrome may follow surgery involving the parotid or temporomandibular joint and is related to damage to the auriculotemporal nerve. Regeneration of the nerve (6 months–2 years) may lead to innervation of the local sweat gland and salivation is accompanied by preauricular sweating, hence the name **gustatory sweating**

Neoplastic disorders

Salivary gland tumours account for over 1% of all neoplastic disease. The majority (60–80% occur in the parotid gland and a large proportion of these are benign. This is followed by tumours of minor salivary glands with the palate being the most common site. Tumours of sublingual glands are rare but a vast majority of these are malignant. Surgical removal is the treatment of choice for salivary gland tumours.

Pleomorphic adenoma is the most common benign neoplasm and the parotid gland is the most common site followed by the palate. It usually presents as a painless swelling in middle-aged adults with a female predilection. The histopathological picture consists of a mixture of glandular epithelium and myoepithelial cells in a mesenchymal background.

Adenolymphoma (Warthin tumour) is a benign neoplasm that exclusively occurs in the parotid. It may develop from heterotropic glandular tissue within parotid lymph nodes or from ductal epithelium with secondary lymphoid tissue formation. It presents as a painless mass in elderly males and may show fluctuance. Bilateral metachronous Warthin tumours are also reported. The histopathological picture is characterised by a mixture of ductal epithelium (enclosing cystic spaces) and a lymphoid stroma.

Mucoepidermoid carcinoma is the most recognised malignant tumour and usually presents as a slow-growing painless mass. The parotid gland is the most common site and may occur any time between the second and seventh decade. Pain and facial nerve involvement may also occur. The histopathological picture is consists of a mixture of mucus and epithelial cells.

Adenoid cystic carcinoma commonly involves minor glands, usually on the palate as well as the parotid in middle-aged adults. Although slow-growing, pain may be a prominent symptom. The histopathological picture consists of myoepithelial and ductal cells arranged in a cribriform, tubular or solid pattern. Perineural invasion is a prominent feature.

Acinic cell adenocarcinoma also primarily develops in the parotid gland. The age range of patients varies between the second and seventh decade with a female predilection. It usually presents as a slow-growing painless mass. The histopathological picture consists of a well-circumscribed proliferation of serous acinar cells with a granular basophilic cytoplasm and darkly staining eccentric nuclei. The tumour shows an infiltrative growth pattern and may be solid or cystic.

94 Pigmented lesions

Figure 94.1 Amalgam tattoo
Source: Scully C et al. (2010). *Oral Medicine and Pathology at a Glance*. Reproduced with permission of John Wiley and Sons, Ltd.

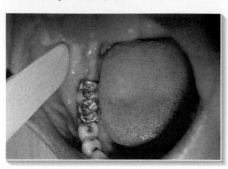

Figure 94.2 Racial pigmentation: diffuse pigmentation involving the labial gingival mucosa in an adult of Afro-Caribbean origin

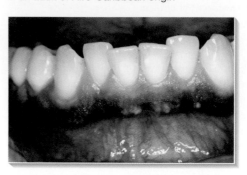

Figure 94.3 Pigmented naevi on the left upper and lower lips

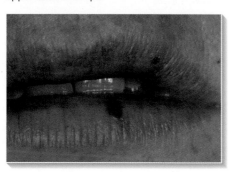

Figure 94.4 Melasma; diffuse hyper pigmentation of facial skin in a pregnant subject, depicting 'mask of pregnancy'

Figure 94.7 Hairy tongue; marked brown-black staining of tongue dorsum

Figure 94.5 An asymmetrical pigmented lesion on the right maxillary alveolar ridge; the lesion was diagnosed as a melanoma on histopathology

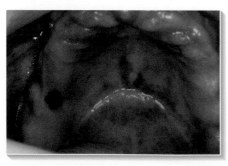

Figure 94.6 Hairy tongue; widespread yellow-brown staining of tongue dorsum associated with elongation of filiform papillae in a smoker

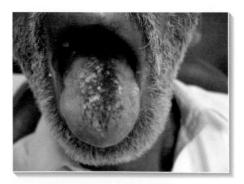

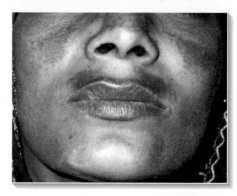

Source: Figures 94.3, 94.5 and 94.7, courtesy of Professor MAO Lewis.

Dentistry at a Glance. First Edition. Edited by Elizabeth Kay. © 2016 John Wiley & Sons, Ltd. Published 2016 by John Wiley & Sons, Ltd.
Companion website: www.ataglanceseries.com/dentistryseries/dentistry

Introduction

Pigments are coloured substances, some of which are normal constituents of cells (e.g. melanin), whereas others are abnormal and collect in cells only in special circumstances. Pigments may be exogenous or endogenous and differ greatly in origin, chemical constitution and biological significance. Oral pigmentation does not represent a specific disease and may be associated with a variety of developmental and acquired disorders. It needs to be emphasised that many oral lesions may exhibit a distinct colour, for example leukoplakia, erythroplakia, varicosities, haemangioma, and mucocele, etc., but these are not related to accumulation of pigments and should not be labelled as such. This section discusses some of the common and well-recognised disorders.

Exogenous pigmentation

Exogenous pigmentation of oral mucosa may result from implantation of a variety of coloured substances. The most common amongst these is dental amalgam (**amalgam tattoo**). Amalgam may be incorporated into the oral mucosa during operative dental procedures and trauma. Amalgam tattoos often appear as gray or black macular lesions and are most common on the gingival, alveolar and buccal mucosa (Figure 94.1). Periapical radiographs may help to localise radiopaque amalgam deposits. Amalgam tattoos do not require any treatment but suspicious lesions may warrant a biopsy.

Other foreign bodies responsible for oral pigmentation may result from intentional tattooing, graphite from lead pencils (hard palate) and other foreign bodies implanted due to trauma. Superficial staining of oral mucosa may result from foods, beverages and medications but is often temporary. Use of betel quid or 'paan', which is common in South Asia, causes a brownish staining of teeth and oral mucosa.

Intentional occupational or accidental exposure to heavy metal salts not only leads to oral pigmentation but more importantly may result in systemic metallic intoxication with significant systemic and oral abnormalities. Systemic metallic intoxication is well recognised with ingestion of lead, mercury, silver, gold, bismuth and arsenic.

Endogenous pigmentation

Racial pigmentation: Racial melanin pigmentation is most common and is seen in dark-complexion individuals (Figure 94.2).

Ephelides (freckles): Ephelides are small (<0.5 cm) brown cutaneous macules associated increased melanosomes. They appear in early childhood after sun exposure in a cyclic fashion in fair skinned people. They do not require any treatment.

Pigmented naevi: Pigmented naevi are common and represent a benign proliferation of melanocytes (Figure 94.3). These tend to develop with age and white adults may have approximately 10–40 nevi per person. Intraoral nevi typically occur on the lip vermilion and palate. Although benign themselves, a substantial proportion of melanomas develop from pre-existing nevi.

Peutz–Jeghers syndrome (hereditary intestinal polyposis syndrome): It is a relatively rare condition and is usually inherited as an autosomal dominant trait but new mutations may be responsible for up to one-third of cases. It is characterised by hyperpigmented melanin spots on the skin of extremities and perioral region. Oral pigmentation may involve vermilion border, labial and buccal mucosa, and the tongue. Also there are generalised hamartomatous multiple polyps of the intestinal tract, which may lead to intestinal obstruction. Patients need to be monitored for their visceral polyps and genetic counselling is advisable.

Melasma: Melasma is characterised by melanin hyperpigmentation of the facial skin and may appear as symmetric brown macular lesions in sun-exposed areas (Figure 94.4). It is an acquired condition and is most commonly seen in adult dark-skinned women during pregnancy but may also be associated with oral contraceptives containing both oestrogen and progesterone. Melasma is a benign condition and may resolve after delivery or discontinuation of contraceptive medication.

Melanoma: Melanoma is an aggressive cutaneous malignancy of melanocytes; <1% of melanomas may occur intraorally, mainly on the hard palate or maxillary alveolus. It appears as a dark brown to black lesion with irregular borders (Figure 94.5). Ulceration and bleeding may also be seen and with further growth, the lesion may transform into an exophytic mass with destruction of the underlying bone. Radical surgical excision remains the treatment of choice. Mortality is primarily related to distant metastasis.

Café au lait pigmentation: *Café au lait* (coffee with milk) pigmentation is a characteristic pattern of cutaneous pigmentation and is well recognised in neurofibromatosis. It can also be seen in association with polyostotic fibrous dysplasia (**Jaffe–Lichtenstein** syndrome). When polyostotic fibrous dysplasia is associated with *café au lait* patches and endocrinopathies it is termed **McCune– Albright** syndrome.

Endocrine disorders: Addison disease (primary hypoadrenocorticism) is associated with brown or black pigmentation of buccal mucosa, tongue or gingivae. Other conditions include adrenocorticotropic hormone (ACTH) therapy and ACTH-producing tumours (e.g. lung cancer) and Nelson syndrome (enlargement of a pituitary adenoma after bilateral adrenalectomy).

Medications: A variety of drugs may enhance oral mucosal pigmentation. These include antimalarials (chloroquine, hydrochloroquine, quinidine, quinacrine), cytotoxics (busulfan, cyclophosphamide, doxorubicin, 5-fluorouracil, cisplatin), oral contraceptives, minocycline, zidovudine, phenothiazines (chlorpromazine), ketoconazole and clofazimine.

Smoker's melanosis: Tobacco smoking is associated with increased melanin pigmentation and is frequently seen on the anterior facial gingivae (cigarette users) and buccal mucosa (pipe smokers).

HIV: Hyperpigmentation of skin, nails and oral mucosa is reported in HIV and may be related to medications (e.g. zidovudine, ketoconazole) and adrenocortical damage but may also be a direct consequence of HIV infection.

Miscellaneous: Increased melanin pigmentation may develop as a secondary phenomenon in chronic inflammation (gingivitis, periodontitis), hyperkeratosis and lichen planus. **Hairy tongue** is characterised by elongation of filiform papillae with increased keratin deposition on the tongue dorsum (Figures 94.6 and 94.7). It leads to a yellow, brown or black discoloration of tongue mucosa due to the activity by pigment-producing bacteria or staining from tobacco and food. It is a benign condition and resolution may be achieved by improving oral hygiene and avoiding smoking.

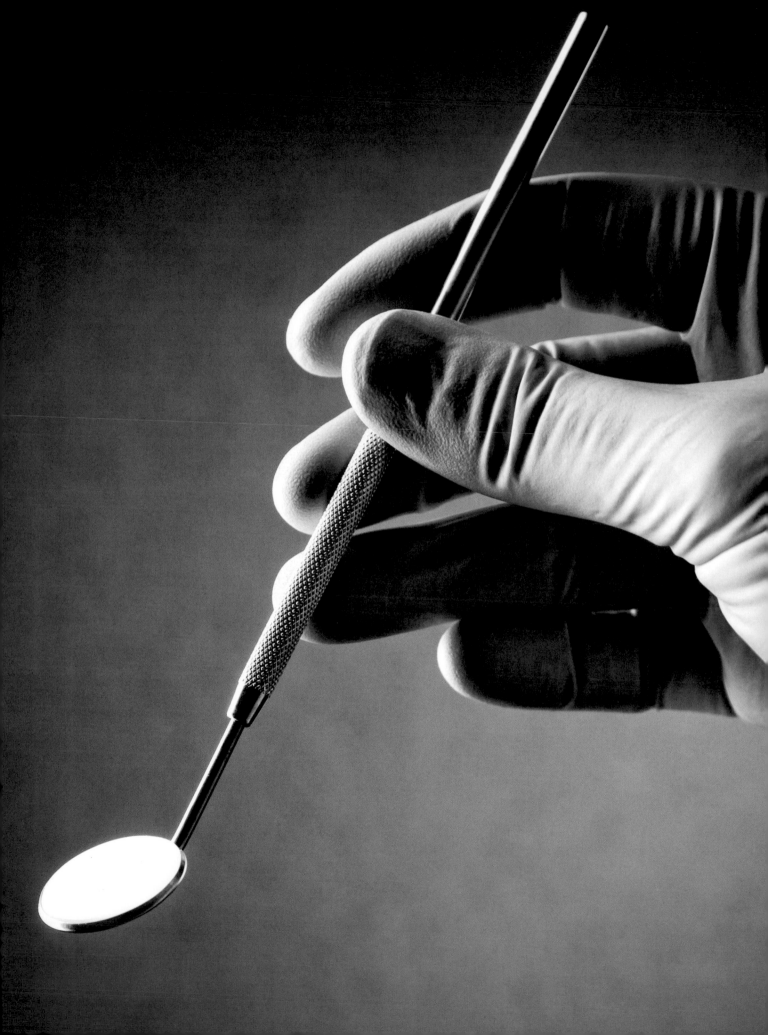

The Medically Compromised Patient

Part 3

Chapters

95 Haematological disorders

Figure 95.1 Recurrent aphthous stomatitis

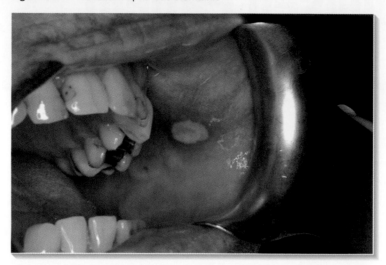

Figure 95.2 Angular cheilitis

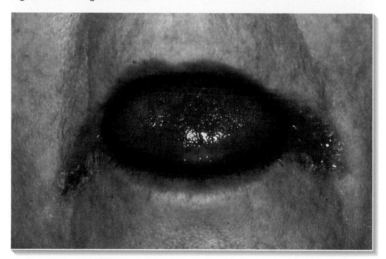

Figure 95.3 Candidosis in acute leukaemia

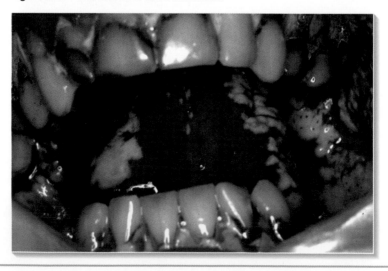

Dentistry at a Glance. First Edition. Edited by Elizabeth Kay. © 2016 John Wiley & Sons, Ltd. Published 2016 by John Wiley & Sons, Ltd.
Companion website: www.ataglanceseries.com/dentistryseries/dentistry

The normal adult has approximately 5 litres of blood, comprising 44% cells and 56% fluid plasma. Red cells (erythrocytes) are the most numerous cells with lower numbers of white cells (leucocytes) and platelets.

Anaemia

Anaemia is defined as either a reduced number of red blood cells or reduced level of haemoglobin (less than 135 g/L for men, less than 115 g/L for women) detected in a full blood count (FBC). A number of forms of anaemia, usually related to mean (red cell) corpuscular volume (MCV), are recognised and additional haematological tests are required to determine the exact cause in an individual patient. Iron-deficiency anaemia, associated with reduced MCV (microcytic), and pernicious anaemia, associated with increased MCV (macrocytic) are two of the more frequently encountered forms of anaemia. Both of these conditions may first present with orofacial signs and symptoms, in particular recurrent aphthous stomatitis, angular cheilitis and glossitis (Figures 95.1 and 95.2).

Iron deficiency can arise due to lack of intake, such as vegetarian or vegan diet, poor absorption due to bowel disease, increased requirement during pregnancy or blood loss as a result of heavy periods or gastrointestinal ulceration/ malignancy. It is essential to determine the cause of any iron deficiency prior to providing replacement therapy. Failure to identify the cause can result in delay in the diagnosis of gastrointestinal malignancy.

Although deficiency of vitamin B_{12} can occur due to poor intake (vegan diet), it is most frequently due to reduced absorption from the gastrointestinal tract. Pernicious anaemia represents low vitamin B_{12} due to lack of secretion of intrinsic factor (required for absorption of vitamin B_{12}) by gastric parietal cells and/or poor absorption of vitamin B_{12} in the terminal ileum. Diagnosis is made by the Schilling test. Treatment of vitamin B_{12} deficiency involves provision of replacement by intramuscular injections.

Haemolytic anaemia

These conditions are characterised by an increased rate of red cell destruction and shortened life span of erythrocytes (normal lifespan is 120 days). A range of conditions, hereditary or acquired, can cause haemolytic anaemia. Sickle cell anaemia is a specific form of haemolytic anaemia that can lead to an acute crisis and death if the patient experiences a low oxygen environment, such as during general anaesthesia. Sickle cell patients should be treated under local anaesthesia.

Bleeding disorders

A number of conditions can result in abnormal haemostasis and blood clotting. Haemophilia is an inherited disorder that is characterised by low levels of clotting factors, in particular factor VII (haemophilia A) and factor IX (haemophilia B, Christmas disease). There is obviously a potential for excessive bleeding during dental treatment, such as subgingival scaling or tooth extraction.

Anticoagulant therapy
Warfarin

The oral use of the coumarin, warfarin, is widespread in medicine for its anticoagulant properties. Warfarin is a vitamin K antagonist and targets factors II, VII, IX and X and proteins C and S in the clotting cascade. It is prescribed for the prevention and treatment of pulmonary embolism, venous thrombosis (including deep vein thrombosis), thromboembolic complications (in particular atrial fibrillation) and reduction of thromboembolic events, especially stroke. A patient taking warfarin requires regular monitoring of their level of coagulation by measurement of the International Normalises Ratio (INR) to avoid any potential bleeding problems. The INR is a measure of the patient's prothrombin time (PT) compared to a normal control. A warfarinised patient's INR is typically between 2.0 and 4.5.

Disadvantages: Warfarin has a relatively long half-life (20–60 hours), which means its effects are still present for 2–3 days after discontinuation of the drug. In addition, warfarin has many drug interactions, including some that are used in dentistry; specifically, miconazole (even topical use), fluconazole, erythromycin, azithromycin and non-steroidal anti-inflammatory drugs (NSAIDs) (see Chapter 104). All these drugs should be avoided in patients taking warfarin because they could result in significant bleeding. In addition, carbamazepine induces enzymes that metabolise warfarin and if given can result in clots.

Benefits: It is cheap to prescribe and it has a reversal agent available (vitamin K). There may be better compliance in taking warfarin due to the regular monitoring of the INR.

Dabigatran and rivaroxaban

Due to the problems associated with warfarin, alternative oral anticoagulants, namely dabigatran and rivaroxaban, have recently been developed. Both these new drugs target specific sites in the coagulation cascade. Dabigatran, is a direct thrombin inhibitor. Rivaroxaban acts by binding and inhibiting factor Xa, thereby preventing thrombin from being produced.

Haematological malignancy
Leukaemia

Leukaemia is a condition that is characterised by an overproduction of non-functional blood-forming (haemopoietic) cells. Two forms of acute leukaemia are recognised, depending on the type of stem cell involved, namely myeloid (acute myeloid leukaemia, AML) or lymphoid (acute lymphoblastic leukaemia, ALL). AML tends to occur in adulthood whilst ALL is most frequently seen in children. Diagnosis of leukaemia is made from FBC, blood film and examination of bone marrow. Treatment consists of chemotherapy and possible bone marrow transplantation.

Oral symptoms, in particular candidal infection, gingival bleeding, oral ulceration or failure of extraction sockets to heal, may be the initial presenting features of acute leukaemia (Figure 95.3).

There are two chronic forms of leukaemia, namely chronic myeloid leukaemia (CML) and chronic lymphoblastic leukaemia (CML), both of which tend to affect adults. Chronic leukaemia is often asymptomatic and discovered when a full blood count is taken for other reasons.

Lymphoma

Lymphoma may be defined as either Hodgkin lymphoma or non-Hodgkin lymphoma, depending on the lymphoid tissue or cells involved. Treatment involves a combination of chemotherapy and radiotherapy, depending on the type and stage of the disease. The dental importance of lymphoma is that it may first present as painless swelling of the cervical lymph nodes in the neck.

Myeloma

Myeloma is a plasma cell malignancy that produces defective immunoglobulins and osteoclastic factors, causing bone lesions and pain. The dental features include root resorption and deposition of amyloid in the soft tissues. Treatment is based on the use of chemotherapy.

96 Immune disorders

Figure 96.1 Oral candidosis

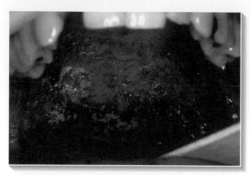

Figure 96.2 Erythematous candidosis

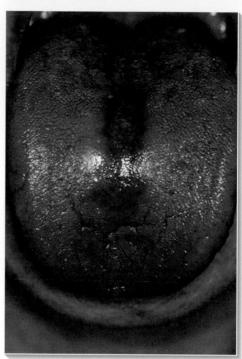

Figure 96.3 Herpes labialis

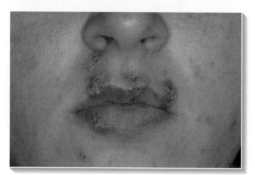

Figure 96.4 Human papilloma viral lesion

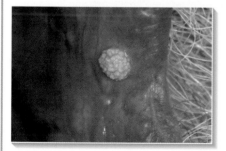

Figure 96.5 Hands in rheumatoid arthritis

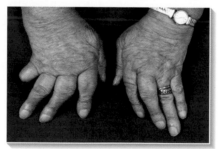

Figure 96.6 Dry mouth in Sjögren's syndrome

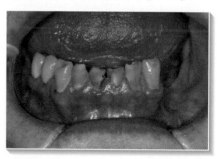

Introduction

The immune system is concerned with recognising foreign material and protecting the individual from infection. The components of the immune system can be classified into the innate or adaptive immune response.

The **innate** (inborn) response is the natural immunity that exists prior to sensitisation from an antigen. It is the first defence encountered by a pathogen and is mostly non-specific. When a microorganism penetrates a host, receptors are activated, which trigger different responses. These include phagocytosis of bacteria by macrophages and neutrophils, activation of the complement system, the release of antiviral interferons and the production of inflammation.

The **adaptive** response provides specific protection after exposure to an antigen. It is composed of T and B lymphocytes. B cells are activated to secrete antibody, which is the humoral element of adaptive immunity. T cells can be divided into cytotoxic T cells, which detect and destroy infected cells, and helper T cells, which are essential for most antibody and cell-mediated responses. The adaptive response needs to be activated therefore can be delayed before a response is seen. Adaptive responses can function on their own but mostly act by interaction with the innate mechanisms.

Dentistry at a Glance. First Edition. Edited by Elizabeth Kay. © 2016 John Wiley & Sons, Ltd. Published 2016 by John Wiley & Sons, Ltd.
Companion website: www.ataglanceseries.com/dentistryseries/dentistry

Allergy

Allergy can be defined as a hypersensitivity reaction initiated by immunological mechanisms. The allergic response can be broken down into two stages. Firstly, the induction phase where IgE antibodies are formed in response to contact with the allergen. Secondly, the reactive phase where the degranulation of mast cells releases histamine, inducing the clinical symptoms of allergy. This most common mechanism of hypersensitivity is called type I. Refer to table of classification of hypersensitivity reactions (Table 96.1).

Asthma

The main allergens are house dust mite, grass pollen and pet dander. Less commonly chemicals, foods and drugs can cause allergic asthma. (See Chapter 98 for more details.)

Angioedema

Angioedema is swelling at the dermal level caused by inflammation and oedema. In the orofacial region it can lead to lip, tongue and facial swelling. Common allergens include drugs, food, cosmetics and insect stings. Angioedema can also be triggered by other stimuli such as stress, vibration, cold and heat. It can be hereditary and caused by dysfunction or reduction in C1 esterase inhibitor, causing a problem with the complement cascade.

Treatment for mild angioedema is avoidance of the allergen. To treat a mild reaction and non-threatening oedema, oral antihistamines can be prescribed. In a major reaction and upper airway involvement the patient should be treated as for anaphylaxis (see below).

Eczema

This is a local erythematous inflammation of the skin and can be induced in foods such as cow's milk and egg in children. A delayed local inflammation after skin has been in contact with various metals is known as contact dermatitis.

Anaphylaxis

This is a severe allergic reaction that is life-threatening and can lead to death if adrenaline is not promptly administrated when required. The clinical features include erythema, urticaria, angioedema, bronchospasm, tachycardia, hypotension and shock. Anaphylaxis is a medical emergency and needs prompt recognition and removal of the precipitating cause. First-line treatment includes management of airway and breathing difficulties and administration of oxygen. For severe reactions and life-threatening airway, breathing and circulation problems, intramuscular adrenaline (0.5 mL adrenaline injection 1 : 1000) should be administrated. The dose can be repeated at 5-minute intervals, if necessary.

Immunodeficiency and disorders

These patients can have absent or defective parts of the immune system either due to a genetic cause or an acquired disease causing immunodeficiency. The problems caused by a defective immune system include: recurrent infections, autoimmune disease and malignancy. Recurrent infections may be diagnosed in dental practice, such as oral candidosis (Figure 96.1) or severe gingivitis, and may be difficult to treat, or may present with rare infections, indicating potential immunodeficiency as a cause.

Autoimmune disease

This is when the balance between the body recognising self-molecules and possible pathogens becomes disrupted. In autoimmune diseases the body's immune system recognises these self-molecules as pathogens and attacks them. This can be restricted to certain organs or be systemic disease. Examples of organ-specific diseases include: type 1 diabetes mellitus, Addison disease, coeliac disease and the vesiculobullous disorders. Systemic autoimmune conditions include: rheumatoid arthritis, Sjögren's syndrome, systemic lupus erythematous and scleroderma. The treatment of autoimmune disease commonly involves an immunosuppressant.

Immunosuppressants

Immunosuppressant drugs are used to deliberately induce immune suppression in autoimmune disease, post-transplant and after graft surgery. Generally, patients on immunosuppressive drugs are more at risk of opportunistic infections and malignancy. The infections can be fungal or viral. Candidal infections are common in immune suppression and can present clinically as acute pseudomembranous candidosis, acute erythematous candidosis (thrush), chronic erythematous candidosis (denture stomatitis) and chronic hyperplastic candidosis (Figure 96.2). Treatment with systemic fluconazole is generally required. Viral infections are usually caused by the herpes virus and can present as severe recurrent herpes labialis (Figure 96.3) or herpetic ulceration. The papilloma virus can present intraorally with multiple papillomatous lesions in these patients, and affecting the skin (Figure 96.4).

Rheumatoid arthritis

Rheumatoid arthritis is a chronic autoimmune inflammatory condition that principally affects synovial joints, resulting in destruction of cartilage and bone. The most frequently involved joints are the small joints of the hands (Figure 96.5), feet and cervical spine. Diagnosis is made on a combination of clinical signs and symptoms, haematological findings and radiographic features. Treatment is based on provision of anti-inflammatory and immunomodulating drugs.

It is essential to support the neck of a patient with rheumatoid arthritis during dental treatment because some patients are at risk of dislocation of the atlantoaxial joint. In severe cases, the patient may have difficulty attending a dental practice. In addition, changes in the hands causes reduced manual dexterity and ability to maintain oral hygiene. Rheumatoid arthritis may be the connective tissue component in secondary Sjögren's syndrome (dry eyes, dry mouth and connective tissue disease) (Figure 96.6).

Table 96.1 Types of hypersensitivity reaction

Classification	Effector mechanism	Example of clinical condition
Type I immediate	IgE	Anaphylaxis
Type II cytotoxic	IgM, IgE, complement, phagocytosis	Nephritis
Type III immune complex	IgM, IgE, complement, precipitins	Vasculitis
Type IV delayed	T-Lymphocytes	Contact dermatitis
Other idiopathic	Varies	Non-specific rash

97 Cardiovascular disorders

Figure 97.1 Gingival overgrowth caused by a calcium channel blocker

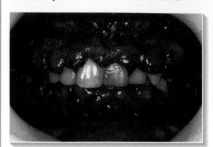

Figure 97.2 Dry mouth caused by diuretic therapy

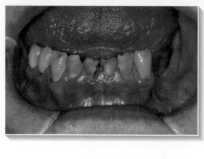

Figure 97.3 Lichenoid drug reaction

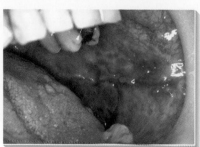

Figure 97.4 Oral ulceration – nicorandil-induced ulcer

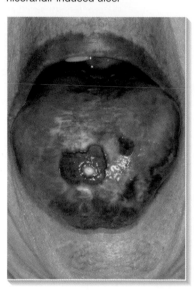

Table 97.1 Antihypertensive drugs and oral manifestations

Drug group	Examples	Oral manifestation
Diuretics	Furosemide	Dry mouth, lichenoid reactions
β-blockers	Atenolol, propanol	Dry mouth, lichenoid reactions
ACE inhibitors	Ramipril, lisinopril, enalapril	Dry mouth, glossitis, lichenoid reactions, angioedema
Angiotensin II receptor blockers	Losartan, candesartan	Altered taste
Calcium channel blockers	Amlodipine, nifedipine	Gingival hyperplasia

Hypertension

A patient with a blood pressure (BP) recording in excess of 140/90 mmHg on at least three separate occasions in a relaxed atmosphere is defined as having hypertension. Raised BP is associated with an increased risk of heart disease, stroke and renal failure (Box 97.1). More than 90% of cases of hypertension have no known cause and this is termed as 'primary' or 'essential' hypertension. Secondary hypertension can be caused by renal disease, endocrine disorders, coarctation of the aorta, pre-eclampsia in pregnancy and drugs. Hypertension is mainly asymptomatic.

General management involves life-style modification, in particular loss of excess weight, limited alcohol, low-salt diet and regular exercise. In addition, drug therapy has a role, including the use of diuretics, angiotensin converting enzyme (ACE) inhibitors, angiotensinogen II receptor blockers, β-adrenergic blockers and calcium channel blockers.

Antihypertensive medication can cause a range of adverse effects within the oral tissues (Figures 97.1, 97.2 and 97.3; Table 97.1). Severe hypertension can result in prolonged postoperative bleeding.

Box 97.1 Risk factors for cardiovascular disease

- Smoking
- Hypertension
- Excess alcohol
- Diet
- Family history
- Diabetes mellitus
- Obesity
- Hypercholesterolaemia

Angina

Angina is a descriptive name given to chest pain caused by myocardial ischaemia. Patients describe the symptoms as a tightness, compression or even crushing central chest pain that comes on with cold, stress and exercise. The pain can also radiate to the left arm or neck and include pain in the mandible that may mimic toothache. Symptoms are relieved by rest.

General management includes minimising known risk factors, such as smoking, hypertension and hypercholesterolaemia.

Dentistry at a Glance. First Edition. Edited by Elizabeth Kay. © 2016 John Wiley & Sons, Ltd. Published 2016 by John Wiley & Sons, Ltd.
Companion website: www.ataglanceseries.com/dentistryseries/dentistry

Preventative therapies include the daily use of aspirin and lipid-lowering drugs (statins). Acute attacks are treated with sublingual glyceryl trinitrate (GTN). If angina attacks become frequent, long-term nitrates and β-blockers are often given.

It is important to be able to recognise the signs and symptoms of an angina attack because these may be precipitated by anxiety immediately prior to and during dental treatment. GTN medication should be readily available to be given promptly, if required. Nicorandil, a drug that is used for the long-term management of angina, may cause a characteristic adverse effect of persistent oral ulceration (Figure 97.4).

Myocardial infarction

A myocardial infarction (MI) occurs as a result of ischaemic necrosis of the myocardium due to thrombus occlusion of a coronary artery (Box 97.2). An MI characteristically presents as central crushing chest pain lasting longer than 20 minutes, usually occurring at rest and is not relieved with nitrates. The pain is also associated with sweating, vomiting, breathlessness and restlessness.

Box 97.2 Definitions used in cardiovascular disease

- **Thrombus:** A solid mass of blood constituents which can form in an artery or vein
- **Embolus:** Material that is carried by the blood from one point in the circulation to lodge at another point
- **Ischaemia:** An inappropriate reduction in blood supply to an organ or tissue
- **Infarction:** Death of tissue due to ischaemia
- **Atheroma:** Accumulation of cholesterol and lipids in the arterial intimal surface

---

An ambulance and emergency services must be called immediately if an MI is suspected. Following acute management the patient will need prompt transfer to a coronary care unit (Box 97.3). Initial treatment should include GTN, aspirin (300 mg chewable), high-flow oxygen and, if available, relative analgesia (50% oxygen, 50% nitrous oxide). Cardiopulmonary resuscitation must be initiated if the patient goes into cardiac arrest.

A patient who has recently suffered an MI is at an increased risk of a further attack and therefore stressful situations, such as dental treatment, are best deferred for at least 3 months and preferably 1 year. MI sufferers are likely to be on a number of forms of medication to prevent further infarcts and manage any underlying hypertension, many of which can produce adverse

---

Box 97.3 Investigations in cardiovascular disease

- Electrocardiogram (ECG), including exercise ECG and 24-hour ECG
- Echocardiogram
- Blood pressure monitoring
- Angiography

---

effects in the oral tissues (Table 97.1). Other relevant drug therapy includes daily aspirin, which will increase postoperative bleeding time, and statins, some of which interact with antifungal agents used for oral infections, including miconazole and fluconazole.

Valvular disease

Infective endocarditis

Infective endocarditis (IE) represents an infection predominantly involving the heart valves. IE can develop on normal, defective or prosthetic heart valves. The bacterial species most frequently recovered in cases of IE are viridians-group streptococci (*Streptococcus mutans* and *Streptococcus sanguis, Enterococcus faecalis* and *Staphylococcus aureus*). The tissue changes are diverse and result from the complications of infection, valve destruction, embolic damage of organs and immune complex deposition at distant body sites.

The initial treatment of IE is provision of intravenous bactericidal antibiotic therapy, choice of which will be informed by the results of blood culture and antibiotic susceptibility. Surgery may be required in cases of severe heart damage or infection of prosthetic valves.

Relevance to dentistry: Historically, dental treatment has been implicated in the onset of IE because the bacterial species recovered are also frequently encountered as members of the commensal oral microflora. In the past therefore, antibiotic prophylaxis was routinely given to patients thought to be at a risk of developing IE following dental treatment. However, clinical guidelines were published by the National Institute for Health and Clinical Excellence (NICE) in March 2008 advising that the administration of prophylactic antibiotic therapy was no longer justified at the time of invasive dental procedures. This recommendation has been the subject of considerable debate with cardiologists and some still recommend prophylaxis for high-risk patients, such as those with a previous history of IE.

Rheumatic fever

Rheumatic fever is an inflammatory disease occurring in children and young adults. It is caused by infection with Group A β-haemolytic streptococcal species, usually occurring 2–3 weeks after a sore throat. Symptoms of rheumatic fever include fever, joint pain and loss of appetite. Inflammatory changes due to immune complex deposition may involve all three layers of the heart (carditis) resulting in cardiac murmurs, regurgitation and even failure. Heart involvement may produce permanent damage and even death. Otherwise, rheumatic fever is mostly self-limiting although some patients have recurrent attacks.

The treatment of rheumatic fever is penicillin to eradicate the streptococcal infection.

A history of rheumatic fever increases the risk of developing infective endocarditis. As mentioned above, the historic need to provide prophylactic antibiotic during invasive dental treatment to such patients has been revised by NICE.

98 Respiratory disorders

Figure 98.1 Candidosis in the soft palate

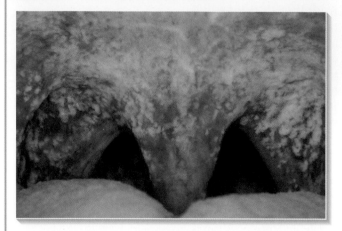

Table 98.1 Oral manifestations of respiratory disease

Oral manifestations	Associated respiratory disease or treatment
Dry mouth	Inhalers, medications, high-flow oxygen
Oral pseudomembranous candidosis	Inhalers
Oral ulceration	Tuberculosis
Gingival swelling	Sarcoidosis
Oral pigmentation	Lung cancer

Figure 98.2 Ulceration of the tongue due to tuberculosis

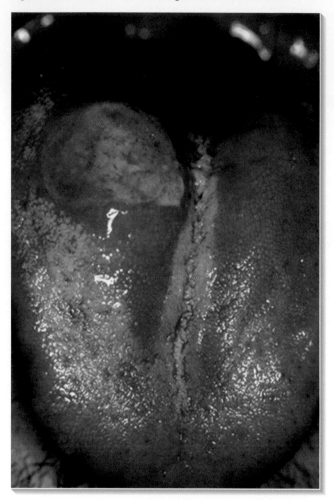

Sinusitis

Sinusitis is the result of infection and inflammation of the paranasal air sinuses. The most frequent symptoms are headache, nasal congestion and facial pain, which become more severe on bending over. Onset of sinusitis is often related to the common cold.

Treatment should initially be symptomatic and involve steam inhalation, decongestants and anti-inflammatory medication. Antibiotics are only indicated if symptoms persist following first-line treatment.

It is important to make an accurate diagnosis because sinusitis can be confused with inflammatory pain of dental origin due to infection in maxillary teeth.

Asthma

Asthma, which is a chronic inflammatory condition, represents a reversible airway obstruction that affects between 10 and 15% of the population. The symptoms comprise a combination of cough, wheeze, breathlessness and/or chest tightness. The symptoms of asthma are typically worse at night and early morning. Interestingly, the prevalence of asthma appears to be increasing. Many trigger factors are recognised, the most frequent being house dust, animal dander, pollen, drugs, cold air, exercise and emotion.

Patient education on the avoidance of trigger factors and provision of drug treatment are important in effective asthma management. Bronchodilators, such as Beta-2 agonists (salbutamol), anticholinergic bronchodilators (ipratropium) and inhaled corticosteroids (beclomethasone and fluticasone) are the mainstay of specific drug treatment. In acute exacerbations, a short course of systemic corticosteroids and antibiotics may be required.

It is important to record the severity of asthma in an individual patient. A good guide of the severity is the number of hospital admissions caused by acute episodes and frequency of the need for medication. If the condition is well controlled then an asthmatic patient can be treated routinely under local anaesthesia. However, patients should have their regular inhalers with them before undertaking treatments to use if an acute attack develops. Oral adverse effects of inhaler therapy include dry mouth, particularly with Beta-2 agonist preparations, and pseudomembranous candidosis (thrush) (Table 98.1). Candidosis is characteristically seen in the soft palate (Figure 98.1), which can be minimised if the patient rinses with water after using the inhaler. Non-steroidal ant-inflammatory drugs and aspirin should be avoided as they may trigger an asthma attack.

Chronic obstructive pulmonary disorder

The acronym COPD is used to describe a chronic progressive airways obstruction, most frequently a combination of bronchitis and emphysema. The main symptoms are a slowly progressive cough, sputum production, wheeze and breathlessness. COPD is strongly associated with smoking.

It is essential that a patient with COPD stops their smoking habit. Specific treatment will depend on the severity of symptoms but is likely to involve bronchodilators, inhaled steroids (if significant reversibility is established) and antibiotics (in acute infective exacerbations). Patients with chronic respiratory failure may require long-term oxygen therapy.

A patient with COPD may have difficulty lying flat and therefore needs to have dental treatment sitting upright. The use of rubber dam may be difficult due to reduced airway. Intraoral pseudomembranous candidosis may be present due to the use of steroid inhalers. It is important to avoid the prescription of any medications that may cause respiratory depression (in particular benzodiazepines). The strong association with smoking puts such patients at an increased risk of mouth cancer.

Sarcoidosis

Sarcoidosis is a multisystem disease characterised by the presence of non-caseating granulomas in affected organs. The presentation depends on the organs involved although it is most frequently thoracic with erythema nodosum, bilateral hilar lymphadenopathy and arthralgia.

The prognosis of sarcoidosis is good and no treatment is given. In symptomatic chronic sarcoid, oral steroids and chloroquine may be given and this pattern carries a worse prognosis.

There may be parotid or gingival enlargement along with lip swelling related to the underlying granulomatous disease. The patient may complain of a dry mouth associated with secondary Sjögren's syndrome.

Tuberculosis

The incidence of tuberculosis (TB) is increasing in almost all parts of the world. The initial infection with *Mycobacterium tuberculosis*, which is spread by respiratory droplets, is known as primary tuberculosis. Characteristically, primary infection affects the lungs but can occasionally be extrapulmonary within the central nervous system, kidneys or gastrointestinal tract. Primary TB is usually symptomless or non-specific but can result in malaise, weight loss, fever and cough.

All cases of TB must be reported to the public health authorities so that contact tracing and screening can be organised. A range of antituberculous drugs are available and one or more need to be taken regularly for extended periods. Failure to adhere to drug regimens has resulted in the emergence of multiple-resistant forms of TB.

Infection can be transmitted as a result of the aerosols that are generated during the provision of dental care. This is particularly relevant in a patient with active pulmonary TB. Aerosols should be kept to a minimum with use of high-volume aspiration and general anaesthetics avoided. TB can occasionally initially present as persistent oral ulceration (Figure 98.2) or swelling in the neck.

Lung cancer

Lung cancer is the leading cause of death in the UK. Smoking is the most important cause, being associated with 90% of cases, and there is a higher incidence in urban areas. The main features are cough, chest pain, haemoptysis and breathlessness. Non-specific features include malaise, lethargy and weight loss. Bronchial cancer can be divided into either small cell lung cancer (SCLC) or non-small cell lung cancer (NSCLC). As a generalisation, SCLC grows more rapidly and metastasises early than NSCLC.

Treatment will depend on an individual patient and nature of the tumour but will involve a combination of surgery, radiotherapy and chemotherapy. Management is often limited to palliative care and cure is rare. The 5-year survival rate is extremely poor at 6%.

These patients will have an associated increased risk of oral cancer due to their smoking history. As with all smokers, support for smoking cessation should be given.

99 Gastroenterology and nutritional disorders

Figure 99.1 Lip swelling

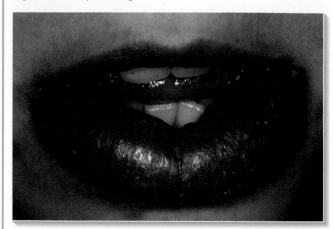

Figure 99.2 Full-thickness gingivitis

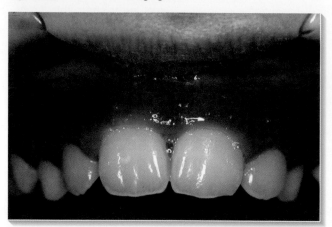

Figure 99.3 Aphthous stomatitis

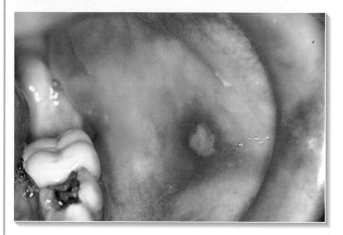

Figure 99.4 Angular cheilitis

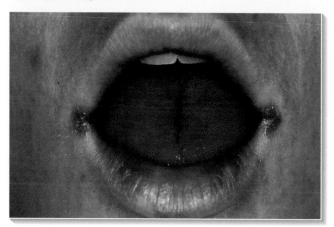

Dentistry at a Glance. First Edition. Edited by Elizabeth Kay. © 2016 John Wiley & Sons, Ltd. Published 2016 by John Wiley & Sons, Ltd.
Companion website: www.ataglanceseries.com/dentistryseries/dentistry

Crohn's disease

Crohn's disease is a chronic granulomatous bowel disorder that can arise anywhere within the gastrointestinal tract but principally affects the terminal ileum. Symptoms are abdominal with pain, distension and diarrhoea. A range of other symptoms, including weight loss and skin rashes, may be present. Diagnosis is made by a combination of findings of colonoscopy and biopsy demonstrating granulomata.

Crohn's disease can be the underlying cause of recurrent aphthous stomatitis. In addition, there are a number of other orofacial signs, in particular lip swelling (Figure 99.1), full-thickness gingivitis (Figure 99.2) and mucosal tags, that are associated with this condition. When these signs are limited to the mouth and in the absence of gut involvement the condition may be referred to as orofacial granulomatosis.

Ulcerative colitis

Ulcerative colitis is a chronic inflammatory bowel disorder of the colon. The condition causes a mucus bloody diarrhoea. Diagnosis is made by direct examination using colonoscopy. Treatment is based on systemic corticosteroids and other immunomodulating drugs, particularly sulphasalazine and azathioprine.

Ulcerative colitis can be an underlying factor in recurrent aphthous stomatitis (Figure 99.3).

Coeliac disease

Coeliac disease is an autoimmune inflammatory bowel disorder that arises due to hypersensitivity to alpha gliadin fraction of gluten found in wheat, rye, oats and barley. The presentation mainly involves abdominal pain, altered bowel movements, with increased frequency or constipation, and greasy stool. Malabsorption results in weakness and weight loss. In childhood, this will cause short stature. Once diagnosed, by detection of anti-tTG antibodies in the blood, the patient must strictly adhere to a gluten-free diet.

The presence of coeliac disease should be excluded in dental patients complaining of recurrent oral ulceration, glossitis or angular cheilitis (Figure 99.4).

Carcinoma

Carcinoma, in the form of squamous cell carcinoma, can develop at any site within the gastrointestinal tract. Mouth cancer and oesophageal cancer are of specific relevance to dentistry because the patient may first present in the dental surgery with a compliant of difficulty or pain on swallowing. Carcinoma lower in the gut will produce abdominal symptoms, weight loss and passage of blood in the stools. Diagnosis involves a combination of biopsy and imaging techniques such as computed tomography scanning and magnetic resonance imaging. Late presentation is associated with a poor prognosis.

Gastro-oesophageal reflux disease

Gastro-oesophageal reflux disease (GORD) is a condition that represents acid reflux from the stomach due to abnormal relaxation of the lower oesophageal sphincter. Repeated exposure of the teeth to acid results in erosion of the palatal surfaces of the upper anterior teeth. Patients also complain of altered or unpleasant taste, particularly on wakening.

Peptic ulceration

Ulceration can occur at any site within the gastrointestinal track but is most frequent in stomach and duodenum. Causative factors that have been implicated include stress, increased gastric acid production and infection involving *Helicobacter pylori*. The presenting symptom is pain. Diagnosis is made from the history, supplemented with radiographic examination (barium meal). Treatment involves advice on life style and the provision of antacid medication, usually ranitidine or omeprazole. Antibiotic therapy can be given to eradicate *Helicobacter pylori* infection. From a dental perspective it is essential to avoid prescription of non-steroidal anti-inflammatory drugs (NSAIDs) because these are acidic and likely to cause further irritation or bleeding of the gut mucosa.

Irritable bowel syndrome

A relatively high percentage of the population complain of recurrent abdominal symptoms and altered bowel movements, in particular episodes of diarrhoea. This situation is commonly referred to as irritable bowel syndrome (IBS). Whilst there is no direct dental relevance, the presence of IBS is a frequent feature in patients with atypical facial pain or burning mouth syndrome.

Vitamin C deficiency

Deficiency of vitamin C (ascorbic acid) results in the condition of scurvy. The basis of scurvy is lack of adequate intake of vitamin C in the diet. The condition is relatively rare as long as a balanced diet containing fruits and vegetables is maintained. Early symptoms include malaise and tiredness. Gingivitis and periodontal disease are well-recognised oral manifestations.

Vitamin D deficiency

A deficiency of vitamin D is termed rickets. Causes of rickets include poor diet, lack of exposure to sunlight, malabsorption and renal disease. The clinical manifestations are based on the effects on bone due to low calcium, with bow leg deformity and bone pain. Diagnosis is made by haematological investigations that show low calcium, low phosphate and raised alkaline phosphatase.

Dental manifestations are rare but can include delayed eruption of teeth and radiolucency of the bones of the jaws.

Other deficiencies

See Chapter 95 for details of deficiency of iron, vitamin B_{12} (pernicious anaemia) or folic acid.

100 Endocrine disorders

Figure 100.1 Pregnancy epulis.
Source: Courtesy of Professor MAO Lewis.

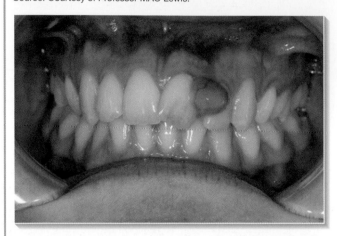

Figure 100.2 Oral lichenoid reaction to metformin

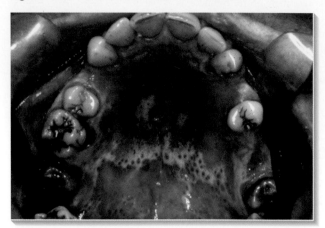

Figure 100.3 Brown tumour

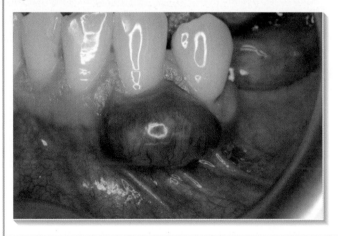

Figure 100.4 Mucosal pigmentation due to Addison's disease

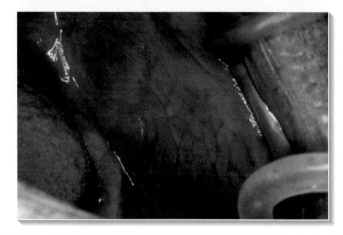

Pregnancy

Routine medical history should include the possibility of a patient being pregnant. If possible, any treatment should be avoided in the first 3 months, due to possible effects on the developing foetus, and in the third trimester, due to comfort of the patient in the dental chair. Certain drugs, including a number of analgesics and antimicrobial agents, must not be prescribed during pregnancy and, as a general rule, any prescribing should be limited to essential drugs only. The use of local anaesthetics containing vasopressin is contraindicated. In addition, radiographs should not be taken.

Hormonal changes associated with pregnancy can predispose to the development of a generalised gingival swelling or a localised oral lesion known as pyogenic granuloma, which if present on the gingival margin is commonly referred to pregnancy epulis (Figure 100.1). The granuloma can be removed under local anaesthesia but may recur until after childbirth. Interestingly, some women who suffer from recurrent aphthous stomatitis do not experience episodes of ulceration whilst pregnant.

Puberty

Hormonal changes occurring in puberty have been implicated in generalised gingival swelling in a similar way to that seen in pregnancy.

Diabetes mellitus

Diabetes is caused by an altered secretion or action of insulin resulting in raised blood glucose. The incidence of diabetes is increasing dramatically and poses one of the greatest health problems in the Western world. The aetiology of diabetes is usually either autoimmune destruction of the pancreatic cells that manufacture insulin (type 1 diabetes, onset in childhood) or impaired function of insulin due to obesity (type 2 diabetes, onset in adulthood). Lack of appropriate glycaemic control results in raised blood glucose, the presence of which can be detected in either the blood or urine. High glucose levels cause increased urine production, so the patient becomes thirsty due to dehydration. Undiagnosed or poorly controlled diabetes produces a range of oral manifestations, including dry mouth, burning mouth syndrome, advanced periodontal disease and candidosis.

Type 1 diabetes is treated by provision of insulin by daily injection whilst type 2 diabetes usually involves the use of drugs (such as sulphonylureas or biguanides), given orally, and dietary advice. Oral hypoglycaemic drugs, such as metformin or gliclazide, are generally recognised to be a cause oral lichenoid drug reactions (Figure 100.2).

Thyroid disease

The thyroid gland secretes two thyroid hormones, (thyroxine, T3, and tri-iodothyronine, T4), which control body metabolism. Excessive production of these hormones is termed hyperthyroidism whilst under production is referred to as hypothyroidism. Diagnosis of altered thyroid function is made by measurement of serum levels of both thyroid hormones and thyroid-stimulating hormone (TSH), which is secreted by the pituitary gland. Hyperthyroidism is characterised by increased pulse rate, heat intolerance and weight loss. In contrast, hypothyroidism is associated with reduced pulse rate, dislike of cold and weight gain.

Hyperthyroidism is caused by immune disease (Grave disease), goitre and thyroid tumours. Treatment involves provision of antithyroid drugs (such as carbimazole), radioiodine therapy or surgery. Increased severity of periodontal disease and premature eruption of teeth have been described in hyperthyroid patients. Protrusion of the eyes (exophthalmos) is a characteristic feature of hyperthyroidism that may be noticed in the dental surgery.

Causes of hypothyroidism include autoimmune conditions, drugs, surgery and neoplasia. Treatment is based on the provision of thyroxine. Delayed tooth eruption has been described in hypothyroidism.

Parathyroid disease

The parathyroid glands, which are situated adjacent to the thyroid gland, secrete a hormone (parathyroid hormone, PTH) that controls calcium levels.

The most frequent cause of over secretion of PTH is benign neoplasia of the gland. There are few symptoms of parathyroidism but raised levels of calcium (hypercalcaemia) can result in stone formation in the kidneys. A specific lesion of dental relevance is the development of a localised giant cell swelling of the jaws, known as a brown tumour due to its coloration (Figure 100.3). Radiographs will show a radiolucency in the underlying bone due to osteoclast activity.

Low levels of calcium in hypoparathyroidism result in altered nerve and muscle function. Facial twitching and tingling are presenting symptoms. The most frequent cause of hypoparathyroidism is previous surgery of the thyroid gland, because parathyroid glands are intimately associated with the thyroid gland. Diagnosis is based on haematological findings of reduced plasma calcium, raised plasma phosphate and reduced response to PTH stimulation. Treatment consists of providing parathyroid replacement therapy along with calcium supplements and vitamin D. Dental manifestations include structural defects, short roots and dentine dysplasia, and delayed eruption of the teeth.

Pituitary disease

The pituitary gland secretes a number of hormones (Box 100.1) and therefore the presence of a tumour in the gland can produce a range of clinical signs and symptoms due to either excessive secretion or deficiency of hormones. Excessive secretion of growth hormone produces a condition known as acromegaly, which can present in the dental surgery as enlargement of the jaws and spacing of the teeth. There is also enlargement of the hands and feet.

Adrenal disease

The adrenal glands, which are sited on top of the kidneys, secrete a number of hormones that regulate metabolism, fluid balance and immune function (glucocorticoids), sodium and potassium balance and male sexual characteristics (androgens). Tumours in the adrenal glands can result in overproduction or underproduction of a number of hormones, with a wide range of clinical effects.

There are two important conditions that are related to altered adrenal function, namely Addison's disease, which is a reduced secretion state due to destruction of the adrenal tissue, and Cushing's syndrome, which is a situation that results from prolonged high levels of glucocorticoids.

Addison's disease can be diagnosed by detecting a low level of plasma cortisol. Treatment is provision of glucocorticoid and mineralocorticoid replacement. A specific dental manifestation of the disease is increased pigmentation of the oral mucosa (Figure 100.4).

Cushing's syndrome is most frequently caused by prolonged intake of steroid drugs. Rare causes include adrenal tumour and pituitary tumour. The clinical presentation is characteristic and involves moon face, acne, bruising, central weight gain, peripheral muscle wasting and hypertension. Diagnosis is made by monitoring levels of cortisol. Treatment involves eliminating the predisposing cause.

Box 100.1 Hormones secreted from the pituitary gland

Anterior lobe
- Growth hormone (GH)
- Thyroid stimulating hormone (TSH)
- Adrenocorticotropic hormone (ACTH)
- Beta-endorphin
- Prolactin
- Lutenising hormone (LH)
- Follicle stimulating hormone (FSH)
- Melanocyte stimulating hormone (MSH)

Posterior lobe
- Oxytocin
- Antidiuretic hormone (vasopressin)

Renal disease

The most prevalent diseases of the kidney and urinary tract are urinary tract infection (UTI) in women and benign prostatic hypertrophy in men. The most relevant renal disorders to dental practice are renal failure and renal transplant.

Renal failure

Renal failure can be classified as acute or chronic depending on its speed of onset.

Acute renal failure

Acute renal failure (ARF) is a sudden and rapid decline in renal function that is usually reversible. It usually lasts days to weeks. The causes can be divided into prerenal, renal or postrenal, or a combination of these. Prerenal causes include: hypovolaemia, decreased cardiac output, severe liver failure and renal artery obstruction. Intrinsic renal failure can have a variety of causes but about 90% are due to acute tubular necrosis secondary to ischaemia or nephrotoxins. Postrenal failure occurs when there is obstruction of the urinary outflow tracts. The management of ARF can be a medical emergency and is unlikely to be encountered at the dental practice. The correction of fluid balance, hyperkalaemia and pulmonary oedema require emergency resuscitation.

Chronic renal failure

Chronic renal failure (CRF) usually develops slowly over months or years and tends to be irreversible in nature. Common causes include: diabetes mellitus, hypertensive nephropathy, inflammation of the glomeruli (glomerulonephritis), recurrent renal infections and drug exposures. The symptoms and signs of CRF are often insidious and may present late with haematuria, urinary tract infections, renal pain or oedema.

The management of CRF is initially to correct the underlying cause if possible. This may involve diabetes control, immunosuppression in glomerulonephritis and antibiotics for recurrent UTI. This is followed by control of the complications such as high blood pressure, anaemia and acidosis. In the majority of patients with CRF there is progression to end-stage renal failure, which will require a form of renal replacement. This may be dialysis or renal transplantation. Dialysis is the removal of toxins from the blood by diffusion across a semipermeable membrane. It can be one of two forms: haemodialysis or continuous ambulatory peritoneal dialysis. The complications of dialysis and renal transplant related to dentistry are discussed in the following section.

Dental aspects of renal disease

This can be related to the co-morbidities of the renal disease or secondary to the medications or dialysis used to control the disease.

The three main systemic complications of chronic renal failure are cardiovascular, bleeding tendency and immunosuppression. The cardiovascular problems relevant to dentistry include hypertension, congestive heart failure and calcification of the heart valves. In oral surgery procedures, it is essential that good haemostasis is achieved as these patients are at increased risk of bleeding because of hypertension and a possible platelet dysfunction. This platelet dysfunction can cause purpura and widespread bruising. Uraemia can lead to increased risk of infection and immunosuppression. Dental infections need to be managed promptly with the appropriate dosage of antibiotic.

Oral manifestations of renal disease include xerostomia, altered taste, glossitis, oral candidosis and oral ulcers related to the underlying anaemia. The medications relevant to dentistry used in treating the underlying renal disease include: ciclosporin potentially causing gingival hyperplasia, bisphosphonates and corticosteroids. If the patient is undergoing renal dialysis, dental treatment is best carried out the following day as the renal function will be optimal. In dialysis patients an arteriovenous fistula may be created in the antecubital fossa to facilitate vascular access and it is important not to use this arm for blood pressure monitoring or by the dentist for vascular access.

In end-stage renal failure renal transplant is considered, which offers improved survival. The complications are rejection of the transplant, increased atheroma risk, hypertension, susceptibility to infection and malignancy due to the immunosuppressive drugs. This may present to the dentist as cutaneous cancer (basal cell carcinoma) on the lip or oral cancer (squamous cell carcinoma).

Prescribing in renal failure

Medications routinely used in dental practice need to be carefully considered before prescribing to patients in renal failure. They can cause problems because of a reduction in renal excretion and failure to excrete the metabolites leading to toxicity in patients. Side effects of the drugs are often poorly tolerated in patients with renal disease. The medications and appropriate dose adjustment in patients with renal impairment are listed in the prescribing in renal impairment in the guidance on prescribing section of the British National Formulary (BNF).

The main groups of drugs that are used in dentistry and need to be reduced in patients with kidney disease include antimicrobials and aciclovir. Non-steroidal anti-inflammatory drugs (NSAIDs) should be avoided in moderate and severe renal impairment and only used at the lowest effective dose in mild renal disease.

Dentistry at a Glance. First Edition. Edited by Elizabeth Kay. © 2016 John Wiley & Sons, Ltd. Published 2016 by John Wiley & Sons, Ltd.
Companion website: www.ataglanceseries.com/dentistryseries/dentistry

102 Intellectual impairment

Impairment, disability and handicap are often inter-related. The terms used to describe these conditions vary widely between countries, although there is an International Classification system, which helps differentiate between each. Intellectual impairment can be defined as having an intelligence quotient (IQ) of less than 70 on a standard IQ test or having a formal diagnosis of mental retardation. Management of intellectual impairment depends on the individual person and severity of the underlying condition. A specific concern is the ability to obtain informed consent. From a dental perspective, maintenance of oral hygiene and good diet are major issues. All efforts should be made to provide routine dental treatment under local anaesthesia, although extra time and special facilities may be required. Unfortunately, the use of sedation or general anaesthesia is sometimes required. Individuals with intellectual impairment also often have a number of medical conditions, in particular cardiac abnormalities, that complicate general anaesthesia.

Down syndrome

Down syndrome is a genetic chromosomal disorder caused by the presence of a third chromosome 21 (trisomy 21). In addition to the characteristics short stature and flat/ broad facial features, all Down syndrome individuals have learning disability. There is a wide range of other clinical signs and symptoms, a number of which have implications for the provision of dental care. Cardiac, immunological and neurological conditions are frequently present. Dental features include an enlarged tongue (which is exaggerated by a small mouth), delayed tooth eruption, malocclusion and recurrent aphthous stomatitis. Given appropriate support, many patients with Down syndrome can undergo a successful education and most can be treated in general dental practice.

Autism

Autism is caused by an abnormal neural development that produces altered social interaction and communication such that an autistic individual often lives in their own isolated world. Characteristic signs include repetitive, compulsive and ritualistic behaviour. The condition is believed to have a genetic cause although the basis of this is complex. Diagnosis is usually made in early childhood. Autistic individuals prefer steady surroundings with routine in daily life. A visit to the unfamiliar environment of a dental surgery can precipitate altered and erratic behaviour, which will complicate the delivery of dental treatment.

Asperger syndrome

Asperger syndrome is a similar disorder to autism in that it affects social interaction but differs in that language remains normal, the onset is later in life and patients have particularly high IQ.

Cerebral palsy

Cerebral palsy is a term used to describe a range of abnormalities of motor control that are due to damage to the brain either before, during or within the first few months of birth. The damage may have been caused by low oxygen levels, infection, trauma, hyperbilirubinaemia biochemical factors or genetic predisposition. The clinical presentation is characterised by abnormalities of movement and posture along with a range of other disabilities, including deafness, altered vision, impaired speech and epilepsy. Although learning impairment may be present, many patients with cerebral palsy have high IQ. Diagnosis is made from clinical presentation. Although any brain damage is permanent treatment should be aimed at minimising the impact of associated defects.

A prominent dental feature is drooling, probably as a result of impaired swallowing rather than excess salivation. Other dental implications include malocclusion, attrition of tooth surfaces, periodontal disease and delayed eruption of teeth. An individual assessment of a patient with cerebral palsy should be made prior to delivery of dental care to take into consideration access difficulties due to a wheelchair, ability to sit in the dental chair, uncontrollable movements and level of co-operation.

Stroke

Stroke is a focal neurological deficit lasting longer than 24 hours caused by blockage or rupture of cerebral blood vessel. If the symptoms resolve in less than 24 hours, such a situation is referred to as a transient ischaemic attack (TIA). Risk factors for stroke include age, smoking, hyperlipidaemia, hypertension, diabetes and cardiac arrhythmias. Modification or elimination of risk factors is an essential component of treatment and prevention. Management may include medications, physiotherapy, occupational therapy and speech therapy. Dental care of a stroke patient may be complicated by communication difficulties. The patients may need help with oral care and their gag reflex may be affected. Such patients are likely to be taking aspirin, anticoagulant or antihypertensive medications, all of which have an impact on the delivery of dental treatment.

Parkinson disease

Parkinsonism is a syndrome of tremor, rigidity, bradykinesia and loss of postural reflexes. Parkinson disease is one cause of parkinsonism and results from the depletion of dopamine-containing neurones in the subtantia nigra and increased acetylcholine. Features important in dentistry include the difficulty in initiating movement, therefore getting in and out of the dental chair may be a problem. In addition, a patient may complain of excess saliva (sialorrhoea), drooling and dysphagia. The medications used to treat Parkinson disease also have a range of dental adverse effects: dopaminergic medications produce dry mouth, altered taste and oral ulceration and antimuscarinic medications can also cause dry mouth.

103 Neurological disorders

Figure 103.1 Unshaven area due to presence of a 'trigger spot' in trigeminal neuralgia

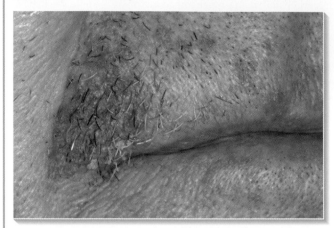

Figure 103.2 Loss of function of the right facial nerve due to Bell's palsy. Source: Courtesy of Professor MAO Lewis.

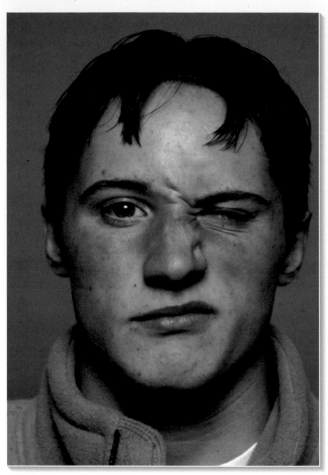

Cranial nerve disorders/palsies

Knowledge of the function of the 12 cranial nerves is essential for the dental clinician (Table 103.1).

Trigeminal neuralgia

The classical features of trigeminal neuralgia are a unilateral electric-shock like pain that is rated as '10 out of 10' within one branch of the trigeminal nerve. Factors that trigger the pain include, eating, touching or washing the face. In males this may prevent shaving a particular area of the face (Figure 103.1). Causes of dental pain, such as pulpitis, cracked tooth syndrome or dentine hypersensitivity, should be excluded. Diagnosis is made on clinical symptoms. However, an magnetic resonance imaging (MRI) scan should be performed in patients under the age of 40 years to exclude multiple sclerosis or in cases where there are other signs and symptoms. An MRI scan may reveal the presence of an aberrant artery adjacent to the trigeminal nucleus. Trigeminal neuralgia responds well to carbamazepine therapy. A minority of patients taking carbamazepine will develop a skin rash. Alternative drugs are phenytoin, amitriptyline, gabapentin or pregabalin.

Alternatively, surgical approaches include local injection of absolute alcohol, cryotherapy or surgical section. Neurosurgical approaches are also available, in particular microvascular decompression (MVD) and radiofrequency ablation (RFA).

Multiple sclerosis

Although the exact cause of multiple sclerosis (MS) is unknown, it is generally accepted that it represents an immune-mediated demyelination of areas of the brain and spinal cord. It usually follows a relapsing and remitting course, although it may enter into a progressive phase. There is a wide variation in the clinical signs and symptoms and sufferers may present with eye pain, numbness/ tingling in the limbs, leg weakness or ataxia. Diagnosis is based on clinical findings and evidence of lesions disseminated in time and space. MRI is extremely helpful.

Table 103.1 Cranial nerves and clinical signs of dysfunction

Number	Cranial nerve	Clinical sign of dysfunction
I	Olfactory	Loss/decreased sense of smell
II	Optic	Loss of visual acuity, visual field defects
III	Oculomotor	Ptosis, dilated pupil, eye faces down and out
IV	Trochlear	Diplopia
V	Trigeminal	Sensory: decreased corneal reflex, sensory loss Motor: weakness of masseter muscles
VI	Abducens	Diplopia: eye cannot turn inwards
VII	Facial	LMN (lower motor neurons): weakness of all the muscles of facial expression (same side as lesion) UMN (upper motor neurons): weakness of the muscles of the lower part of the face (on the side opposite the lesion)
VIII	Vestibulocochlear	Sensorineural deafness, tinnitus, vertigo
IX	Glossopharyngeal	Impaired gag reflex
X	Vagus	Difficulty swallowing, soft palate asymmetry on saying 'ah'
XI	Accessory	Wasting of sternomastoid and trapezius muscles resulting in difficulty turning head and shrugging shoulders
XII	Hypoglossal	Tongue deviates to affected side on protrusion

The relevance of MS to dentistry is that it can first present as facial pain in the dental surgery due to trigeminal neuralgia. MS should be suspected in any patient who develops symptoms consistent with trigeminal neuralgia below the age of 40 years. Treatments include steroids and disease-modifying agents, such as interferon.

There have been unsupported claims that MS is associated with dental amalgam and these have resulted in patients having their restorations removed in an attempt to halt the condition.

Epilepsy

Epilepsy is a neurological condition characterised by the tendency to have continuing seizures. An epileptic seizure is a result of paroxysmal discharge of cerebral neurons causing an abnormal event or convulsion. Seizures can be classified into generalised (tonic–clonic, absence or myoclonic) or partial (simple or complex). Tonic–clonic seizures are also known as grand mal seizures and they usually have an aura before a sudden onset of a rigid phase followed by the clonic/ convulsion phase. The patient may have signs of marked bruxism, tongue biting and urinary incontinence. In a situation where the seizure lasts longer than 5 minutes, then this is classed as status epilepticus and requires immediate treatment as a medical emergency. According to the UK Resuscitation Guidelines, medication should only be given if seizures are prolonged (convulsive movements lasting 5 minutes

or longer) or recur in quick succession. In this event an ambulance should be summoned urgently. If a patient continues to fit after an ambulance has been called, then the emergency administration of buccal midazolam to assist in terminating the seizure is warranted. The dose of midazolam is 10 mg for an adult and an appropriately reduced dose for a child. Factors that should raise concern about the possibility of an epileptic seizure are a previous history of poor seizure control and a recent change in medication.

Recognition of the onset of a seizure and ability to manage the situation is important because stress related to dental care may precipitate an attack. In addition, an important aspect of epilepsy that is relevant to dentistry is the gingival hyperplasia associated with phenytoin drug therapy.

Giant cell arteritis

This granulomatous inflammatory disease was previously termed 'temporal arteritis' due to its location within the temporal artery. However, recognition that it may occur within vessels at other locations in the head and neck has resulted in the use of the more general term of giant cell arteritis. The condition is aged related and occurs far more frequently in patients over 55 years old. The condition presents with symptoms of malaise, weight loss, jaw claudication and headache. In some cases there may be superficial tenderness in the temporal region. Diagnosis can be difficult but raised levels of haematological inflammatory markers may be an indication, especially erythrocyte sedimentation rate (ESR) and C-reactive protein (CRP). Historically, an attempt to establish a definitive diagnosis involved arterial biopsy. However, it is now recognised that this investigation can give a false-negative result due to the presence of areas of non-inflamed vessel (skip lesions). The treatment of giant cell arteritis involves provision of high doses of systemic steroids. Failure to control the inflammatory process may result in blindness.

Motor neuron disease

This results from destruction of the upper motor neurons and anterior horn cells in the brain. Presenting features include muscle cramps, loss of strength, weakness in the legs with altered gait and difficulty speaking. There is no sensory loss. There is no effective treatment and the condition is usually fatal as a result of respiratory failure within 5 years. It most frequently affects men in middle age.

Bell's palsy

Facial nerve palsy can occur either because of a stroke (upper motor lesion) or Bell's palsy (lower motor lesion). Bell's palsy is caused by inflammatory pressure on the facial nerve during pregnancy, viral infection or presence of a tumour. The presentation is characterised by the absence of voluntary movements of the facial muscles resulting in the inability to furrow the forehead, raise the eyebrow, close the eye or smile on the affected side (Figure 103.2).

The condition needs to be treated promptly with high-dose corticosteroid therapy (40–50 mg oral prednisolone) and systemic antiviral therapy, such as aciclovir. An eye patch should be provided to protect the eye. Most cases resolve within 3–4 weeks.

104 Drugs and dental care

Figure 104.1 Drug-induced xerostomia.
Source: Courtesy of Professor MAO Lewis.

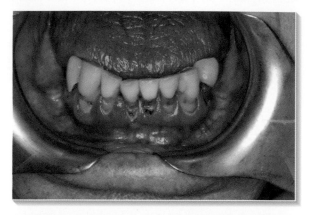

Figure 104.2 Lichenoid drug reaction presenting as erosions on the tongue

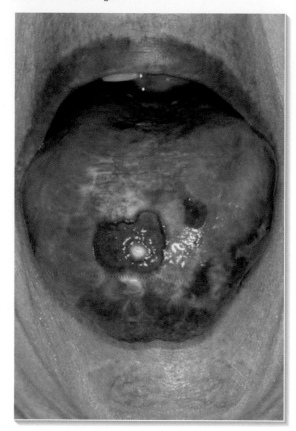

Figure 104.3 Oral candidosis (thrush) in the palate

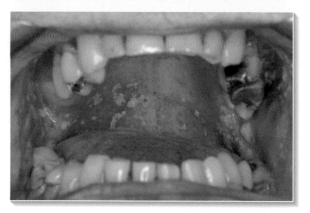

Figure 104.4 Widespread gingival hyperplasia induced by phenytoin

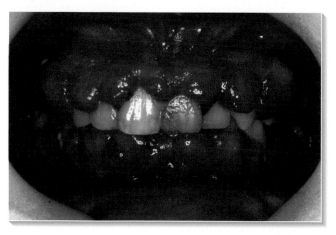

An increasing number of individuals are taking regular medication. It is not unusual for patients to be taking numerous drugs for conditions such as hypertension, diabetes, pain and depression. This situation is sometimes described as polypharmacy and is most often seen in patients over the age of 65 years. An example of polypharmacy would be the treatment regimen following a myocardial infarction, consisting of a statin, angiotensin-converting (ACE) inhibitor, beta-blocker, aspirin and possibly an antidepressant. Many patients now routinely carry with them a print out of their current medication and this is invaluable to clinicians.

Dentistry at a Glance. First Edition. Edited by Elizabeth Kay. © 2016 John Wiley & Sons, Ltd. Published 2016 by John Wiley & Sons, Ltd.
Companion website: www.ataglanceseries.com/dentistryseries/dentistry

Drugs prescribed in female patients that are pregnant or breast-feeding need to be prescribed with care and only if the benefit to the mother is thought to be greater than the risks to the foetus or breast-feeding infant.

Special care is also required in prescribing to dental patients with liver disease or renal disease and drug doses may need to be reduced or certain drugs avoided.

The impact of drugs can be divided into (1) the impact on delivery of dental treatment; (2) potential drug interactions; and (3) adverse effects of drug therapy that produce oral lesions.

Impact on delivery of dental treatment
Warfarin

Patients who have or had deep vein thrombosis, pulmonary embolism, atrial fibrillation and metal prosthetic heart valves are likely to be taking warfarin to decrease blood coagulation (see Chapter 95). As any dental treatment involving bleeding, most frequently tooth extraction, can result in prolonged bleeding, the patient's INR (International Normalised Ratio) should be measured. The current guidelines in the BNF are that to ensure that it is below 4 before carrying out routine extractions. Local measures for haemostasis control may be required, such as suturing. Stopping warfarin exposes the patient to a risk of thrombosis and outweighs the risk of oral bleeding complication.

Antiplatelet drugs

Long-term administration of antiplatelet monotherapy is widely used to prevent myocardial infarction or stroke. Dual antiplatelet therapy, aspirin and clopidogrel, is used in patients with stents. From a dental point of view in patients on antiplatelet monotherapy, the medication should not be stopped before dental treatment, including extractions. Local haemostatic measures may be required to control postoperative bleeding. Patients on dual therapy may need referral to a local oral surgery or maxillofacial unit.

Potential drug interactions

Drugs prescribed by the dental practitioner for dental disease may potentially interact with a drug that the patient may be already taking. The latest edition of the British National Formulary (BNF) is an important source of information and includes an appendix detailing drug interactions. It is strongly advised that this is referred to for any potential drug interactions before any drugs are prescribed.

Interactions that the dentist may frequently come across include the following drugs.

Azole antifungals

These include topical miconazole and fluconazole tablets. If these antifungal agents are prescribed in a patient on warfarin it can cause the INR to be raised and the increased anticoagulation may lead to life-threatening bleeding. They can also interact with statins causing muscle pain and can cause an increased anticonvulsant action of phenytoin.

Antibiotics

There is evidence that antibiotics can affect the absorption of oral contraceptives; therefore it is advisable to warn patients of this so they can use other methods of contraception. This includes the antibiotics amoxicillin, co-amoxiclav and metronidazole, amongst others. Antibiotics can also increase the anticoagulant effect of warfarin and frequent testing of the INR is advised.

Analgesics

In dental practice, aspirin, ibuprofen and paracetomol may be prescribed for pain relief. Aspirin should be avoided in patients on warfarin as there is an increased risk of impaired haemostasis. It can also increase gastric irritation and ulceration in combination with non-steroidal anti-inflammatory drugs (NSAIDs) and corticosteroids and ideally this combination should be avoided.

Adverse effects of drug therapy that produce oral lesions
Reduced salivary function (xerostomia)

A number of drugs can cause reduced production of saliva (Figure 104.1) due to blockage of the parasympathetic nervous stimuli within the salivary glands. This is a side effect of many different drug categories, including anticholinergics, antidepressants, antipsychotics, antihypertensives, antihistamines, antimigraine, anti-HIV, diuretics and neuroleptics. It is often difficult to substitute the medication and often the patient is managed by diet and fluoride advice, saliva stimulants and replacements.

Increased salivary function (ptyalism)

Drugs with a cholinergic effect can result in an increase in salivary production. The antipsychotic drug clozapine also has a side effect of hypersalivation and can result in a complaint of drooling.

Lichenoid reactions

Drugs that may cause lichenoid reactions (Figure 104.2) include: antihypertensives, hypoglycaemics, antimalarials, antiepileptics and NSAIDs. The oral lesion may start within a few weeks of implementing the new medication and then consideration should be given to changing the drug. Lichenoid reactions need to be differentiated between ones with a local cause, lesions with a direct contact of a restorative material and ones caused by systemic drugs.

Candidosis

Different types of oral candidosis can be caused by medications. Pseudomembranous candidosis (Figure 104.3) and acute erythematous candidosis typically can occur on the soft palate after corticosteroid inhaler use. It also may be more generalised in the oral cavity following broad-spectrum antibiotic use and systemic immunosuppression.

Gingival swelling

The drugs that have been found to cause gingival hyperplasia (Figure 104.4) are phenytoin, ciclosporin, nifedipine and amlodipine. Being a young patient and poor plaque control are both risk factors that can increase the risk of drug-induced gingival hyperplasia. The management of these patients is firstly to see if the medication can be changed; however, in some cases there is no alternative medication and gingival surgery is required.

Altered taste

There are many factors that may lead to a disturbance of taste. Medications are one of these main causes, either by drug-induced xerostomia leading to an altered taste or by causing changes to the taste bud receptors. Drugs that deplete serum zinc levels, such as diuretics, can also result in an altered taste. Drugs such as penicillamine, captopril, antithyroid drugs, lithium, cytotoxic agents and rifampin are all thought to lead to taste disturbance.

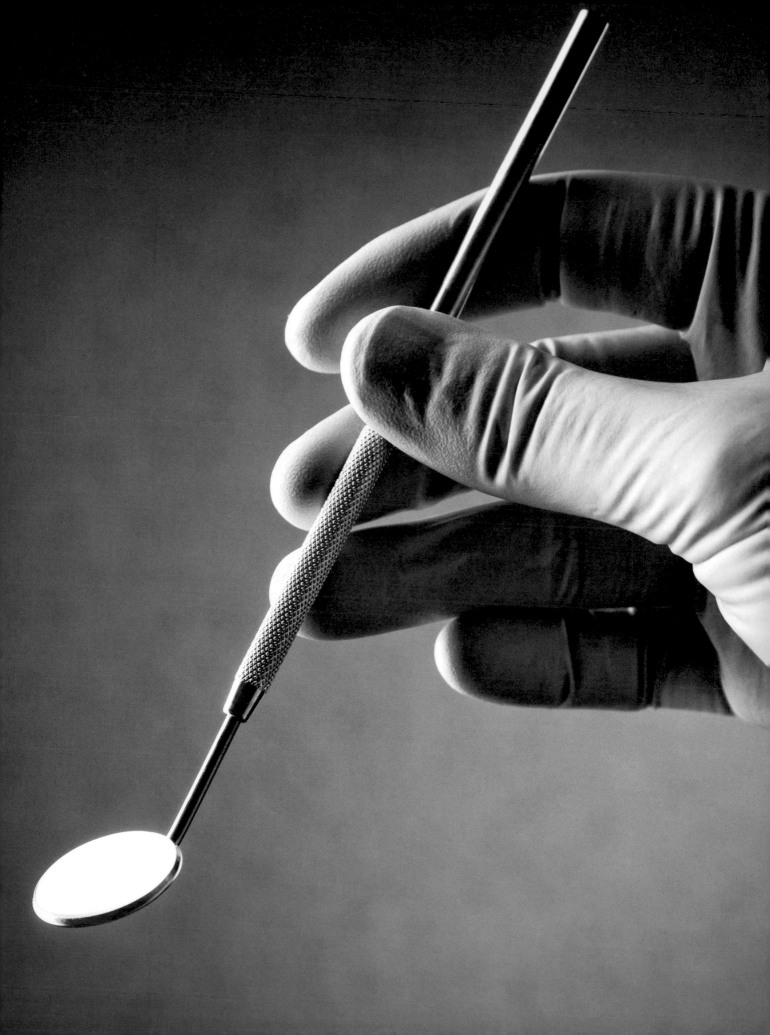

Orthodontics

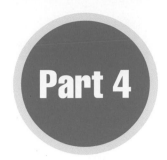
Chapters

105 The developing dentitions

Figure 105.1 Stages of tooth development. The tooth germ passes through the characteristic bud, cap and bell stages, followed by hard tissue formation and eruption. (A,B) Highlights of the crown stage tooth germ. dl, dental lamina; df, dental follicle; eee, external enamel epithelium; sr, stellate reticulum; iee, inner enamel epithelium; dp, dental papilla; cl, cervical loop; d, dentine; e, enamel; a, ameloblasts; hers, Hertwig's epithelial root sheath; o, odontoblasts; p, pulp.

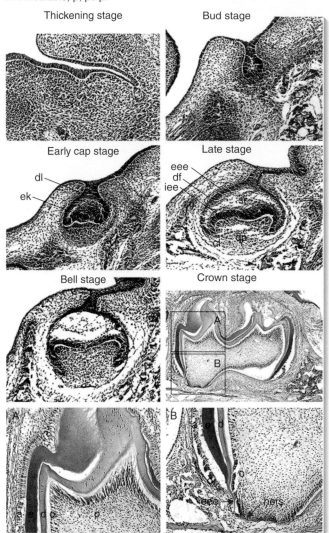

Figure 105.2 Eruption of the primary incisor teeth

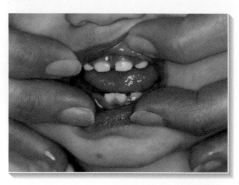

Figure 105.3 The complete primary dentition

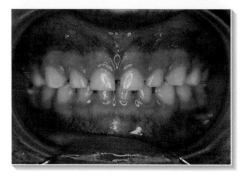

Figure 105.4 Establishing a class I molar occlusal relationship in the mixed dentition

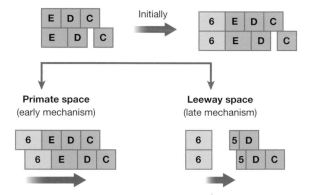

Figure 105.5 The early mixed dentition, the first permanent molars and incisors have erupted

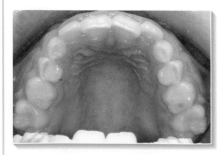

Figure 105.6 Eruption of the premolar and canine dentition

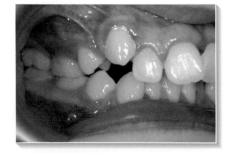

Figure 105.7 Eruption of the third molars in a 17-year-old girl

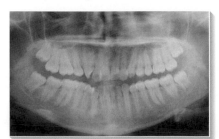

Dentistry at a Glance. First Edition. Edited by Elizabeth Kay. © 2016 John Wiley & Sons, Ltd. Published 2016 by John Wiley & Sons, Ltd.
Companion website: www.ataglanceseries.com/dentistryseries/dentistry

Development of the dentitions

Humans develop two dentitions in their lifetime; the primary dentition erupts between the ages of 6 months and 2.5 years, whilst the permanent dentition appears at the age of around 6 years and is completed in the late teens.

The primary dentition

Tooth development begins in the embryo at around 6 weeks *in utero* and is achieved through molecular signalling between ectoderm of the frontonasal process and first pharyngeal arch and neural crest cells in the underlying mesenchyme. These interactions take place at multiple stages of tooth development, including early initiation, during the acquisition of shape within the tooth germ and later, during hard tissue formation (Figure 105.1).

At birth the tooth-bearing regions of the maxilla and mandible are covered by thickened mucous membranes called gum pads, which facilitate suckling. Within the early jaws, development of the primary teeth is well advanced at birth, with the crowns of all the teeth complete by the age of 1 year.

Occasionally, a child is born with teeth already present within the mouth, these so-called natal teeth are usually poorly formed primary incisors, which are usually lost fairly early.

During normal development of the primary dentition, the incisors are usually the first to erupt between 6 and 12 months of age (Figure 105.2), followed by the primary first molars at around 15 months, the canines at around 18 months and, finally, the second molars at 2–2.5 years. The complete primary dentition (Figure 105.3) is said to have four ideal features, although these are rarely all seen together:

- Spaced, upright incisors with a positive overjet and overbite
- Anthropoid spaces are present mesial to the maxillary Bs and distal to the mandibular Cs
- The distal edges of the second molars are flush in the terminal plane
- The molar relationship is class I.

The mixed dentition

The mixed dentition period represents a transition from primary to permanent dentitions and is usually present from the age of 6 to around 12 years of age.

The first permanent teeth to erupt are usually the first molars, which appear behind the primary second molars at around 6 years of age (Table 105.1). In an ideal primary dentition, the second molars are in a class I relationship and have a flush terminal plane (because the upper second primary molar is smaller mesiodistally than the lower). In this situation, because of their similar size the permanent molars will erupt into a cusp-to-cusp relationship. In order to establish a class I molar occlusion one of two mechanisms occurs (Figure 105.4):

- Early mesial shift of the mandibular dentition into the primate space (which is distal to the primary canine) or
- Late mesial shift of the mandibular first molar when the primary second molar is exfoliated (this shift will be relatively greater than that in the maxilla because the maxillary second primary molar is smaller than the mandibular).

In reality, the characteristically variable nature of tooth exfoliation and eruption, differential growth of the jaws and variation that is seen in the primary molar relationship will mean that a wide range of molar relationships are seen.

Table 105.1 Chronology of permanent tooth eruption

Tooth	Eruption (years)
Maxilla	
1	7.5
2	8.5
3	11.5
4	10.5
5	11.5
6	6.5
7	12.5
8	19
Mandible	
1	6.5
2	7.5
3	9.5
4	11
5	11.5
6	6.5
7	12.5
8	19

The next phase of the mixed dentition is eruption of the permanent incisors, which replace the primary incisors between the ages of 7 and 9 years old (Figure 105.5). The permanent incisors are larger than their primary predecessors and space to accommodate them without crowding is obtained from:

- The primary incisors being spaced
- The permanent incisors erupting in a more labial position
- Movement of the primary canines distally as the incisors erupt.

The final phase of mixed dentition development is eruption of the permanent premolar, canine and second molars (Figure 105.6). These teeth replace the primary canine, first and second molar, respectively. This in-filling of teeth is aided by the fact that the combined mesiodistal width of the three primary teeth is actually larger than their permanent successors. This difference is known as the leeway space. The order of eruption is variable, but in the mandible the canine often erupts first, whilst in the maxilla the canine is usually last. The second permanent molars usually erupt after the canines and premolars, at around 12 years of age, to establish the permanent dentition.

The early part of the mixed dentition phase is often associated with some characteristic and transient changes in the occlusion:

- The manifestations of a prolonged digit sucking habit (anterior open bite, unilateral crossbite)
- The so-called 'ugly duckling' phase (midline diastema between the permanent central incisors) during eruption of the permanent canines.

The permanent dentition is completed in the late teens with eruption of the third molars, if these teeth are present (Figure 105.7). However, they often fail to appear, either being absent or impacted.

Maturation of the permanent dentition

The permanent dentition does not remain stable with age. A number of variable and unpredictable features are known to be associated with age, with the appearance of late crowding of the mandibular incisor teeth often being seen in the late teenage years and beyond.

106 Orthodontic assessment

Figure 106.1 Frankfort plane

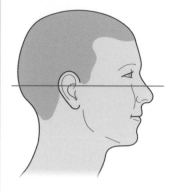

Figure 106.2 Class I, II and III malocclusion according to the position of A-point and B-point, and their relationship to the zero meridian (vertical red line)

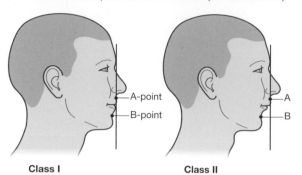

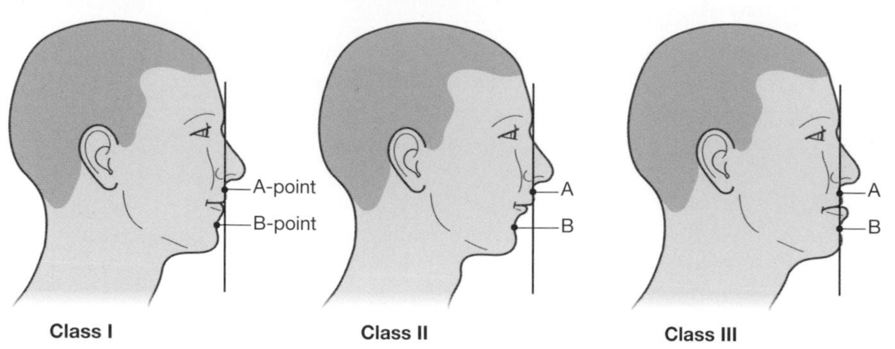

A-point
B-point

Class I

A
B

Class II

A
B

Class III

Figure 106.3 Frankfort-mandibular plane angle (a) and face heights (b)

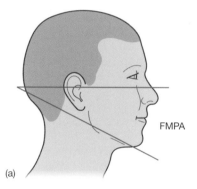

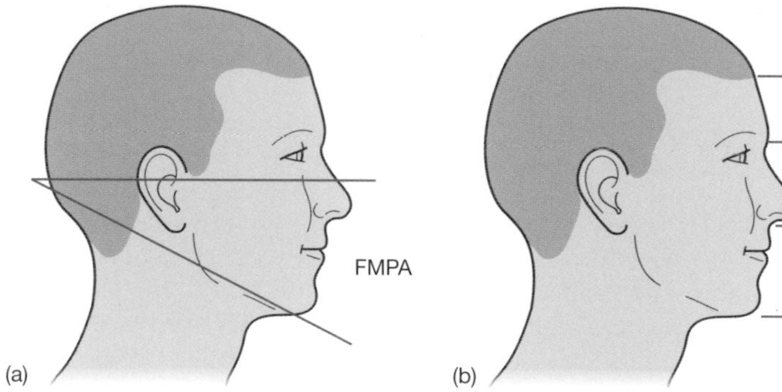

FMPA

(a)

(b)

UFH
MFH
LFH

TFH

Figure 106.4 Facial symmetry

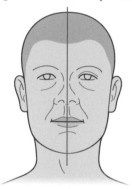

Figure 106.5 Nasolabial angle and lip relationship to E-line

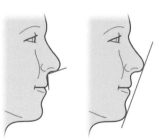

Figure 106.6 Incisor relationship

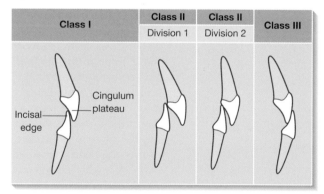

Class I	Class II Division 1	Class II Division 2	Class III

Incisal edge
Cingulum plateau

Figure 106.7 Variation in overbite

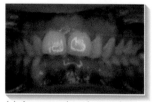

(a) Increased and complete

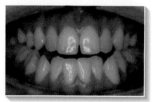

(b) Open bite

Figure 106.8 Molar relationship

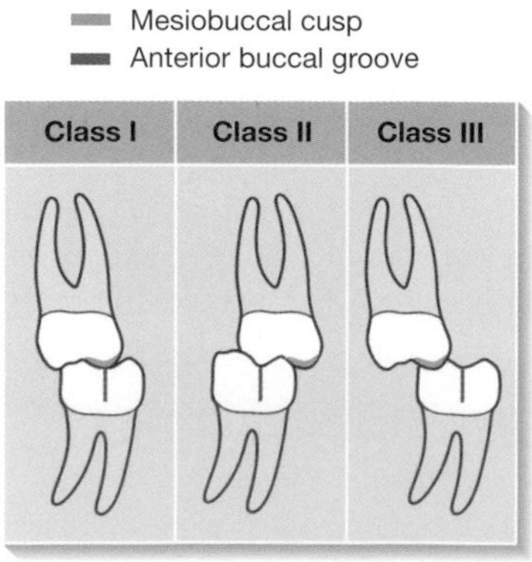

▬ Mesiobuccal cusp
▬ Anterior buccal groove

Class I	Class II	Class III

Figure 106.9 Canine relationship

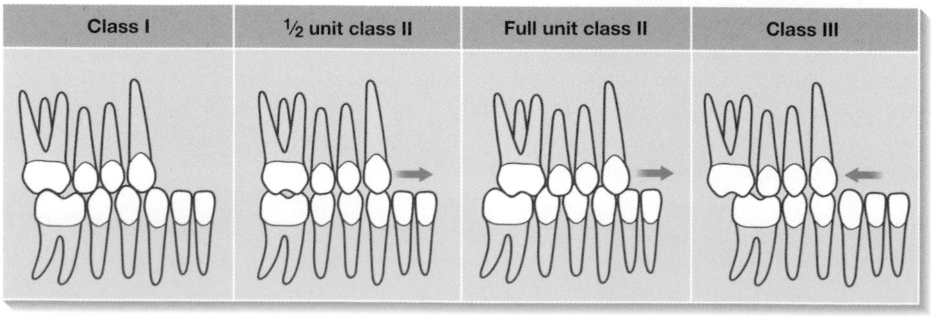

Class I	½ unit class II	Full unit class II	Class III

Dentistry at a Glance. First Edition. Edited by Elizabeth Kay. © 2016 John Wiley & Sons, Ltd. Published 2016 by John Wiley & Sons, Ltd.
Companion website: www.ataglanceseries.com/dentistryseries/dentistry

Clinical assessment in orthodontics

At the initial orthodontic appointment the following information should be ascertained:
- What is the complaint?
- Medical history such as: asthma, epilepsy, diabetes, haemophilia, arthritis, amelogenesis and dentinogensis imperfecta, down syndrome, learning difficulties, temporomandibular joint disorders, nickel allergy and latex allergy
- Habits or trauma
- Previous orthodontic treatment (may indicate possible compliance issues or an increased risk of root resorption).

Extraoral examination
Skeletal assessment

The patient should be examined sitting upright and focussing on the horizon, with the Frankfort plane (a line joining the inferior margin of the orbit with the superior margin of the external auditory canal) parallel to the floor (Figure 106.1).

Anterior–posterior (Figure 106.2):
1 Relationship of soft tissue A and B-point (positions of deepest concavity on maxilla and mandible, respectively):
  a Skeletal class I: A-point palpable approximately 2 mm ahead of B-point
  b Skeletal class II: A-point is palpable >4 mm ahead of B-point
  c Skeletal class III: B-point is palpable <2 mm behind A-point.
2 Relationship of soft tissue A and B-points to zero-meridian: the zero meridian is represented by a vertical line from the soft tissue nasion (bridge of the nose) perpendicular to the Frankfort plane. Soft tissue A-point should lie on this line and soft tissue B-point should lie approximately 2 mm behind it.

Vertical (Figure 106.3):
1 The Frankfort–mandibular plane angle (FMPA) should be approximately 27°.
2 Face heights: the middle face height (MFH) and lower face height (LFH) should be equal. MFH is measured from soft tissue glabella to soft tissue subnasale and LFH from subnasale to soft tissue gnathion. LFH is calculated as a percentage of the total face height (TFH = MFH + LAFH) and should be approximately 55%.

Transverse assessment (Figure 106.4): the patient should also be assessed for any facial asymmetry. When an asymmetry is noted, assess for any mandibular displacement on closing, which might be contributing. A compensatory maxillary cant may also be present.

Soft tissue assessment

The following features should be recorded:
1 Lip relationship:
- Competent: together at rest
- Potentially competent: able to come together once any dental obstruction has been removed
- Incompetent: apart at rest

2 Tongue: the tongue is difficult to assess at rest; however, patients that habitually posture the tongue forwards should be noted (can impact on treatment and long-term stability)
3 Nasiolabial angle (Figure 106.5): the angle formed between the base of the nose and upper lip (94–110°)
4 E-line (Figure 106.5): a line tangential to the tip of the nose and soft tissue pogonion (should lie ahead of both lips, with the lower lip around 2 mm behind).

Intraoral examination

Intraoral examination involves:
Assessment of the teeth present clinically and general dental health (restorations, caries, oral hygiene and periodontal disease)
For each dental arch:
- Crowding or spacing
- Tooth rotations, displacements, impactions
- Position and inclination of canines and labial segments to the dental bases
In occlusion:
- Incisor relationship (Figure 106.6)
  - Class I: the lower incisor edges occlude with or lie below the cingulum plateau of the upper central incisor
  - Class II division 1: the lower incisor edges lie posterior to the cingulum plateau of the upper incisors and the upper incisors are proclined/ average inclination and there is an increased overjet
  - Class II division 2: the upper incisors are retroclined with a normal or occasionally increased overjet
  - Class III: the lower incisor edges lie anterior to the cingulum plateau of the upper incisors.
- Overjet (measured from most proclined upper incisal edge to the corresponding lower incisor)
- Overbite (the upper incisors should overlap the lower incisors by a third to half of their clinical crown height)
  - An increased overbite can be complete to tooth or palate (traumatic when the lower incisors contact the palatal mucosa or the upper incisors contact the lower labial mucosa and cause soft tissue damage (Figure 106.7)
  - An incomplete overbite is positive overbite with no incisal contact
  - An anterior open bite has no vertical overlap between the incisors (Figure 106.7)
- Molar relationship (Figure 106.8)
  - Class I: mesiobuccal cusp of upper first molar occludes with mesiobuccal grove of lower first molar
  - Class II: mesiobuccal cusp of upper first molar occludes anterior to mesiobuccal groove of lower first molar
  - Class III: mesiobuccal cusp of lower first molar occludes mesial to upper first molar mesiobuccal groove
- Canine relationship (Figure 106.9)
- Centrelines: both should be noted in relation to the facial midline and each other
- Crossbites: a transverse discrepancy between the dental arches or a premature contact, resulting in a displacement of the mandible on closing.

Orthodontic records

Clinical examination is supplemented by radiographs, study models, extra- and intraoral photographs.
Radiographic investigations:
- Dental panoramic tomogram: assess dental development, assessment of unerupted teeth, root morphology, pathology
- Lateral cephalogram: assess anterior–posterior and vertical skeletal pattern, incisor inclination and soft tissue profile; can also help with location of unerupted teeth
- Upper standard occlusal: diagnose and assess the presence of supernumerary teeth, impacted teeth, root morphology and pathology

Study models:
- Pretreatment planning, space analysis, treatment progress.

107 Fixed orthodontic appliances

Figure 107.1 Components of a fixed appliance

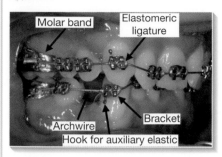

Molar band
Elastomeric ligature
Archwire
Bracket
Hook for auxiliary elastic

Figure 107.2 Preadjusted edgewise brackets have an in-built prescription for tip, torque and in–out

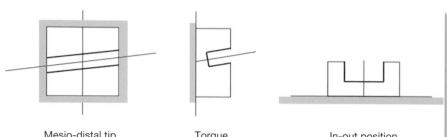
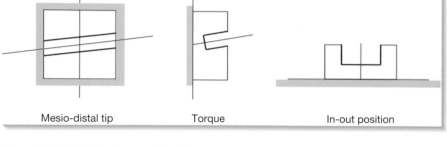

Mesio-distal tip | Torque | In-out position

Figure 107.3 Ceramic preadjusted edgewise brackets

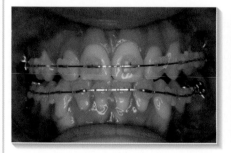

Figure 107.4 Self-ligating preadjusted edgewise brackets

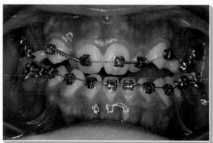

Figure 107.5 Lingual brackets
Source: Courtesy of Dirk Bister.

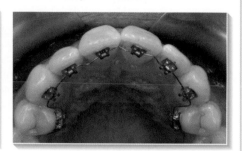

Figure 107.6 Temporary anchorage device

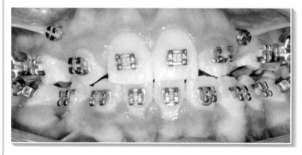

Figure 107.7 Transpalatal arch

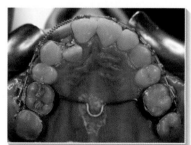

Figure 107.8 Quadhelix

Figure 107.9 Stages of treatment with fixed appliances: (a) treatment of a crowded class III case involved extraction of four first premolars, (b) alignment and levelling, (c) space closure and arch co-ordination to obtain (d) a class I occlusion

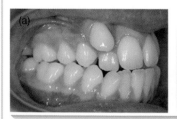
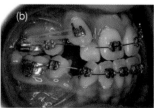
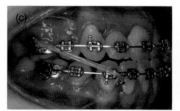
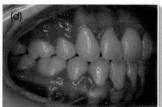

(a) (b) (c) (d)

Fixed appliances

Definition: an appliance that is fixed to the teeth by the orthodontist and cannot be removed by the patient.

Mode of action: fixed appliances apply mechanical forces to the teeth in order to achieve a range of tooth movements.

Advantages and disadvantages of fixed appliances are given in Table 107.1.

Components of a fixed appliance (Figure 107.1) are:
• Brackets – stainless steel preadjusted edgewise bracket systems are the most common type of fixed appliance
• Bands and bonded tubes for the molar teeth
• Archwires, which generate forces that are transmitted to the tooth via the bracket
• Auxiliaries, which are either attached to or work in conjunction with fixed appliances and help control tooth movement.

Dentistry at a Glance. First Edition. Edited by Elizabeth Kay. © 2016 John Wiley & Sons, Ltd. Published 2016 by John Wiley & Sons, Ltd.
Companion website: www.ataglanceseries.com/dentistryseries/dentistry

Preadjusted edgewise brackets

Preadjusted edgewise brackets (Figure 107.1) have a base, a rectangular edgewise slot for the archwire and a mechanism for holding the archwire in the slot (either tie-wings for an elastomeric ligature or a self-ligating mechanism):

- Each bracket has a prescription for each individual tooth position built into it (Figure 107.2)
- The slot produces mesiodistal tooth angulation or tip
- The bracket base inclination provides the necessary torque
- The slot to bracket base distance provides the correct on/out position.

There are a variety of bracket variations available:

- Brackets can be composed of metal (see Figure 107.1), ceramic (Figure 107.3) or a combination of these materials.
- Self-ligating brackets engage the archwire using a gate or clip (Figure 107.4). Self-ligating brackets were introduced in an attempt to reduce friction and clinical time.
- Lingual brackets are bonded to the lingual and palatal aspects of the teeth and provide optimal aesthetics for the patient (Figure 107.5); however, they are expensive, clinically challenging and can cause soft tissue irritation of the tongue.

Archwires

The ideal properties of an archwire will depend upon the stage of treatment and type of tooth movement that is being carried out (Table 107.2). Unfortunately, there is no single type of archwire that can be used throughout treatment; instead, a series of different archwires are used as treatment progresses.

Table 107.1 Advantages and disadvantages of fixed appliances

Advantage of fixed appliances	Disadvantage of fixed appliances
Multiple tooth movements achievable Controlled root movement in three dimensions	Greater risk of iatrogenic damage (soft tissue trauma, root resorption, decalcification) Susceptible to breakages Plaque control more difficult

Auxiliaries

- Separators are used to provide space for band placement on posterior teeth.
- Elastomeric modules or stainless steel ligatures hold the archwire within the bracket slot.
- Elastomeric chain can be attached to move single or multiple groups of teeth.
- Elastic thread can apply traction to individual teeth.
- Closed or open coil springs can be used to hold, create or close space.
- Intermaxillary or intramaxillary elastics can be used to translate groups of teeth.
- Hooks can be attached to the archwire.

Temporary anchorage devices (TADs) are miniscrews inserted intraorally into the bone to provide absolute anchorage (Figure 107.6).

Headgear consists of a head cap or neck strap attached to a fixed appliance using a Kloehn facebow. The inner part of the bow slots into headgear tubes on molar bands. To reinforce anchorage the headgear is worn for 10–12 hours per day with a force of 250–350 g per side. To distalise the buccal segments and restrain maxillary growth headgear should be worn for longer, up to 14 hours per day with a force of 450–500 g delivered per side.

Transpalatal arches (TPAs) (Figure 107.7) are constructed of a 0.9-mm stainless steel wire attached to a molar band, which runs across the roof of the mouth. They are used primarily for anchorage reinforcement or the derotation/ expansion of molar teeth.

A quadhelix (Figure 107.8) is used for maxillary arch expansion and crossbite correction. The appliance sits in the palatal vault and consists of four helices made from 0.9 to 1-mm stainless steel attached to molar bands. The palatal arms apply a lateral force to the buccal segments.

Stages of treatment with fixed appliances

Treatment with preadjusted edgewise fixed appliances involves a number of stages, including alignment and leveling of the arches, space closure and co-ordination of the arches to achieve a class I incisor relationship (Figure 107.9).

Table 107.2 Properties and applications of archwires

Archwire material	Archwire properties	Clinical applications
Nickel titanium	Low modulus of elasticity High springback Low continuous force	Excellent aligning archwire, which is able to engage multiple displaced teeth Exerts low forces with little permanent deformation
Stainless steel	Good resistance to deformation Low springback and stored energy Good joinability and formability, therefore you can weld to the archwire and place bends Low friction	Rectangular stainless steel is used for levelling of the occlusal plane, torque expression and space closure Twistflex (multistrand wires) for fixed retainers
Beta-titanium alloy	Properties midway between those of stainless steel and nickel titanium High yield strength Low elastic modulus Medium springback Good formability and weldability	Used as a finishing archwire as springback allows some deflection of the archwire without permanent deformation Finishing bends can be placed to detail individual tooth position and achieve occlusal settling
Cobalt chromium	High stiffness Good formability Good biocompatability	Can be hardened by heat-treating in the laboratory and used for the construction of auxiliaries, such as a quadhelix
Aesthetic archwires	Coated archwires are metal with a Teflon or epoxy resin coating Poor durability due to failure of the coating and clogging within the bracket slot Composite archwires are constructed from pure silicon dioxide Poor mechanical properties compared with traditional counterparts	Used when patients request less conspicuous appliances

108 Removable orthodontic appliances

Figure 108.1 Acrylic removable appliance design

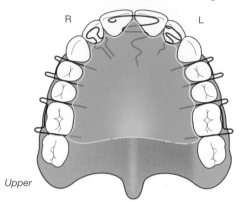

Upper

- Adams cribs (6 4/4 6) 0.7 mm stainless steel (SS)
- T-spring UR2 0.5 mm SS
- Z-spring UL2 0.5 mm SS
- Double cantilever spring (1/1) 0.5 mm SS

Figure 108.2 Hawley retainer appliance design

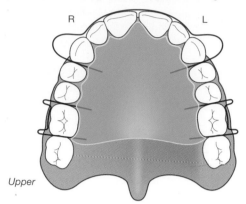

Upper

- Adams cribs (6/6) 0.7 mm SS
- Anterior labial bow (321/123) 0.7 SS

Figure 108.3 Modified twin block appliance design

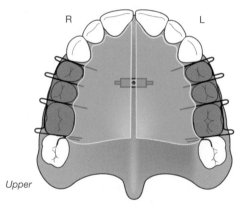

Upper

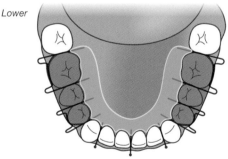

Lower

- Adams cribs $\frac{6\ 4/4\ 6}{6\ 4/4\ 6}$ 0.7 mm SS
- Ball ended clasps $\frac{}{3\ 2\ 1/1\ 2\ 3}$
- Occlusal rests 7/7 0.7 mm SS
- Midline expansion screw
- Posterior acrylic blocks (70°)

Figure 108.4 Twin block functional appliance and then fixed appliances used to correct a class II division 1 malocclusion

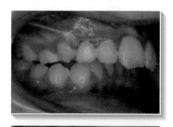

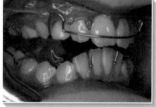

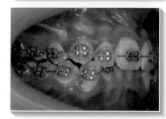

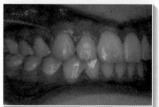

Removable appliances

Definition: Removable appliances can be taken out of the mouth by the patient.

Mode-of-action: Removable appliances apply mechanical forces to the teeth but with a restricted range of movement.

Types of removable appliance are:

- Acrylic
- Retainers
- Functional appliances
- Aligners.

Removable appliances can be used in a number of clinical situations and can achieve:

- Tipping of teeth
- Correction of anterior or posterior crossbites
- Overbite reduction
- Space maintenance
- Vertical anchorage during the extrusion of unerupted teeth
- Maxillary protraction or restraint in conjunction with reverse or conventional headgear, respectively
- Growth modification
- Alignment of mild crowding.

Acrylic appliances

Acrylic removable appliances (Figure 108.1) and some retainers are conventionally made of an acrylic base plate, retentive and active components (Tables 108.1–108.3). Clasps are used anteriorly and posteriorly to stabilise a removal appliance.

Retainers

Retainers (Figure 108.2) are appliances designed to maintain the position of the teeth following orthodontic treatment (Table 108.4).

Functional appliances

Functional appliances are designed to change the postural position of the mandible in growing patients, with the aim of correcting the functional environment of the dentition and influencing the position of the teeth and growth of the jaws. In class II cases, the aim is to encourage mandibular growth, whilst in class III cases mandibular growth is restrained and maxillary growth encouraged. Functional appliances are used very successfully in the management of class II malocclusions (Figures 108.3 and 108.4).

Functional appliances used to treat a skeletal class II patterns have similar effects:

- Retroclination of the upper incisors
- Proclination of the lower incisors
- Distal tipping of the maxillary dentition
- Mesial eruption of the mandibular buccal dentition
- Restraint of maxillary development
- Anterior growth and remodelling of the mandibular condyle and glenoid fossa.

Aligners

Aligners are clear plastic trays that are worn full time by the patient and changed on a regular basis to achieve desired tooth movements.

Fitting a removable appliance

1 Check the appliance is for the correct patient.
2 Feel the fitting surface of the acrylic base plate for any areas of roughness and smooth if indicated.
3 Show the patient the appliance and explain what the aims are.
4 Try the appliance in and adjust accordingly to ensure optimal retention.
5 Demonstrate the mode of insertion and removal and ensure the patient is competent to carry out this unaided.
6 Verbal and written instructions for the following should be provided:

Full-time wear

Remove to clean teeth and appliance

Remove appliance for sport and wear a gumshield if indicated

Initially speech will be affected; however, this will improve with time

Initial wear will result in increased saliva production

Contact the orthodontist if there is any discomfort, breakage or loss.

7 A review should be made in 2 weeks to ensure adaption and compliance.
8 A review should be made in 4 weeks for re-activation of springs and to assess treatment progression.

Table 108.1 Acrylic base plate

Component	Description
Passive acrylic base plate	Complete palatal coverage and extension ensures no undesired tooth movement and vertical anchorage
Flat anterior bite plane	For reduction of an increased overbite in a growing patient. Separation of the posterior occlusion by 1–2 mm encourages the posterior molars to erupt, reducing the overbite
Inclined anterior bite plane	Can encourage and retain musculoskeletal correction of a skeletal II malocclusion following functional appliance treatment
Posterior bite plane	Used to open the bite during correction of anterior and posterior crossbites
Incorporation of a midline screw	Correction of a buccal crossbite through activation of a midline expansion screw (1 turn per week at 0.25 mm per turn)
Addition of prosthetic teeth	As well as offering an aesthetic solution prosthetic teeth can act as a space maintainer following premature loss of a tooth, particularly an incisor, where they prevent drifting of adjacent teeth, loss of space and maintain the centreline

Table 108.2 Retention

Tooth	Diameter of stainless steel wire (mm)	Name of clasp
654|456	0.7	Adams clasp (first molars and premolars)
6E|E6	0.6	Double Adams crib Useful in the late mixed dentition
4|4	0.7	Adams clasp
1|1	0.7	Southend clasp provides increased anterior retention

Table 108.3 Active components

Active component	Diameter of stainless steel wire (mm)	Indication and mode of activation
Z-spring (Figure 108.1)	0.5	To move an incisor labially
Double Z-spring	0.6	To move two anterior teeth labially
T-spring	0.6	To move incisors labially and premolars or molars buccally
Cantilever spring (Figure 108.1)	0.6	To procline an incisor
Palatal finger springs	0.5	To move a canine mesially or distally
Buccal canine retractor	0.5 (with sleeve) or 0.7	For retraction of mesially angulated canines
Roberts retractor	0.5 with tubing	Useful for tipping proclined maxillary incisors
Labial bow	0.7	Can be used to retract incisors or simply provide retention

Table 108.4 Retainers

Type of retainer	Mode of action
Hawley retainer	Retained with Adams cribs on the first molars and an anterior labial bow that can have acrylic added (acrylated) to improve retention and prevent rotation
Begg retainer	A horseshoe-shaped labial bow that extends around the dentition allowing occlusal settling
Vacuum-formed retainer	Clear thermoplastic retainers that fit tightly around the entire dentition Aesthetically pleasing and cost effective

109 Major malocclusions

Figure 109.1 Class I malocclusion with a reduced incomplete overbite and crowding

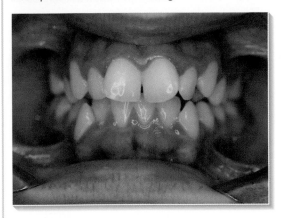

Table 109.1 Treatment of crowding

Degree of crowding	Treatment options
Mild: 1–4 mm per arch	Minor arch expansion, interproximal enamel reduction or extraction (second premolars)
Moderate: 5–8 mm per arch	More significant arch expansion First premolar or second premolar extraction
Severe: >9 mm per arch	First premolar extraction ± anchorage support (which can include headgear, removable appliances and temporary anchorage devices)

Figure 109.2 Crowding: (a) mild, (b) moderate and (c) severe

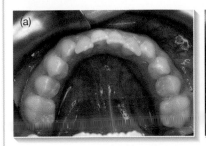 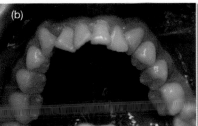 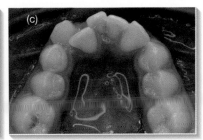

(a)   (b)   (c)

Figure 109.3 Class II division 1 malocclusion

Figure 109.4 Class II division 2 malocclusion

Figure 109.5 Class III malocclusion

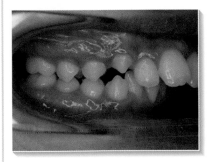 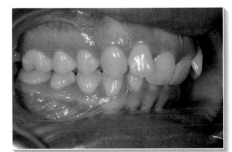 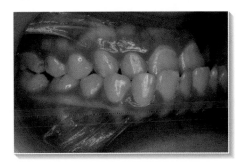

Orthodontic treatment planning

The majority of orthodontic treatment is carried out in the late mixed or permanent dentition in order to utilise any growth potential and maximise compliance.

Objectives of treatment

The fundamental objectives of treatment will differ for each individual case, but often include:

- Overjet and overbite correction
- Relief of crowding
- Levelling and aligning the arches
- Achieving a class I incisor relationship
- Accepting or improving the facial profile
- Achieving Andrew's six keys of static occlusion (Box 109.1)
- Achieving an ideal functional occlusion.

Box 109.1 Andrew's six keys of occlusion

- Class I molar relationship with the distal surface of distobuccal cusp of the upper first molar occluding with the mesiobuccal cusp of the lower second molar
- Correct crown inclination (torque)
- Correct crown angulation (tip)
- No tooth rotations
- Tight contact points
- Flat occlusal plane

Class I malocclusion

Usually patients with a class I occlusion (Figure 109.1) have a normal skeletal base relationship. The profile is generally accepted and the main indications for treatment are:

- Crowding
- Transverse discrepancies (such as crossbite, which might require upper arch expansion to correct).

Crowding and spacing

A space analysis should be undertaken to quantify the extent of the crowding or spacing in each arch (Figure 109.2). The amount and site of crowding and condition of the teeth will influence treatment planning (Table 109.1). Space can generally be created in three ways:

- Arch expansion (including molar distalisation if the molar relationship is class II)
- Tooth extraction
- Interproximal enamel reduction.

Spacing can occur due to microdontia, hypodontia or a combination of both. Treatment will require either space closure or maintenance and will depend upon a number of factors (Box 109.2).

Class II malocclusion

A class II discrepancy presents with:

- Proclined upper incisors and an increased overjet (class II division 1) (Figure 109.3)
- Retroclined upper incisors and an increased overbite (class II division 2) (Figure 109.4).

Treatment of a class II malocclusion will be dependent on:

- Age of the patient (adolescent patients are amenable to growth modification)
- Presence of any digit sucking habit (Box 109.3)

Box 109.2 Treatment of spacing

- **Hypodontia:** maxillary lateral incisors and mandibular second premolars are the most commonly absent teeth, following third molars. There are two treatment options:
  - Close space
  - Open space for prosthetic replacement of the missing teeth.
- **Absent upper lateral incisors and indications for space closure:**
  - Class I malocclusion with crowding in the lower arch necessitating premolar extractions
  - Class II malocclusion with an increased overjet where space closure will help to retract the upper incisors and reduce the overjet
  - When there are several missing teeth a multidisciplinary approach is indicated.
- **Indications for redistribution of space for absent upper lateral incisors:**
  - Class III malocclusion and a well-aligned lower arch
  - The canines have an increased bulbosity and increased chroma making them inappropriate for composite camouflage
  - When the buccal segments are class I with optimal interdigitation and spacing anteriorly.

Box 109.3 Presenting features of a digit sucking habit

- Indentations on the skin of the digit sucked
- Proclined upper incisors
- Retroclined lower incisors
- Incomplete overbite or localised anterior open bite
- Buccal cross-bite ± displacement on closure due to narrowing of the maxilla as a result of tissue pressures exerted when sucking

---

- Underlying skeletal discrepancy.
  Strategies include:
- Orthodontic camouflage (accepting the skeletal discrepancy and creating space to correct the incisor relationship with extractions or molar distalisation)
- Growth modification (using a functional appliance in a growing patient to correct the incisor relationship and improve the skeletal pattern)
- Surgery (using jaw surgery in a non-growing patient to definitively correct the anteroposterior jaw relationship and incisor relationship).

Growth modification

Growth modification involves an initial phase of functional appliance therapy to correct the class II relationship and then, usually, fixed appliances to treat what will now be a class I malocclusion. A functional appliance postures the mandible forwards and utilises structural adaptation of the soft tissues to efficiently reduce the overjet, correct the buccal segment relationship and maximise favourable jaw growth. Where the incisors are retroclined in a class II division 2 malocclusion they first need to be proclined, converting the incisor relationship to a class II division 1 and allowing maximum posture of the mandible by creating an overjet. This can be achieved through placement of an upper sectional fixed appliance or by incorporating springs into the design of the functional appliance.

Orthodontic camouflage

Orthodontic camouflage involves accepting the skeletal discrepancy and correcting the class II malocclusion by tooth movement alone. The ability to treat a patient successfully with orthodontic camouflage will depend on the size of the skeletal discrepancy, the amount of incisor decompensation needed and the soft tissue profile (Box 109.4).

• Orthodontic camouflage often involves distalisation of the upper molars into a class I relationship with headgear or (more commonly) the extraction of two premolar units (usually first premolars) and, depending on the size of the overjet and pre-treatment molar relationship, anchorage reinforcement.

• Extraction of lower premolars is also indicated if there is moderate or severe crowding in the lower arch.

• This extraction pattern when carried out in conjunction with extraction of upper first premolars can aid arch co-ordination and allow for use of class II elastics.

> **Box 109.4 Favourable indicators for orthodontic camouflage**
>
> • Mild to moderate skeletal discrepancy
> • Favourable soft tissue profile
> • An ability to achieve lip competency following overjet reduction
> • Mild crowding lower arch
> • Mild to moderate crowding in the upper arch

Surgery

A combined orthodontic–surgical approach involves fixed appliance therapy in conjunction with orthognathic surgery in order to achieve an optimal skeletal pattern, occlusion and profile (Box 109.5).

> **Box 109.5 Clinical features indicating the need to consider combined orthodontic–surgical correction in class II cases**
>
> • More severe skeletal pattern in a non-growing person
> • Increased vertical proportions
> • Retrusive profile
> • Maxillary excess, with excessive incisor show
> • Incompetent lips, a short upper lip length and obtuse nasiolabial angle

---

Class III malocclusion

The skeletal pattern is usually class III and the severity will be a significant influence on management. The vertical relationship is often average or increased. The incisor relationship is class III with an edge-to-edge relationship or reverse overjet (Figure 109.5). Careful examination of the occlusion in both retruded contact and in the intercuspal position is essential in order to detect any anterior displacement of the mandible. Where a patient can achieve an edge–edge incisor relationship the malocclusion is more amenable to orthodontic correction.

Treatment options are:
• Growth modification
• Camouflage
• Surgery.

Orthodontic growth modification

Growth modification in class III patients involves using protraction headgear and a facemask as an interceptive measure to move the upper jaw and dentition forward in the mixed dentition.

Orthodontic camouflage

Orthodontic camouflage can be achieved in milder cases (Box 109.6):

• Upper removal appliance: to push upper incisors forward and correct an anterior cross-bite (a positive overbite is required for stability)

• Fixed appliances: to correct the incisor relationship. When crowding is present in the lower arch and there is a need to retrocline the lower incisors, first premolar extractions are necessary. The upper arch is often treated non-extraction or with the extraction of second premolars to avoid retroclination of the upper incisors.

Care has to be taken in planning a class III malocclusion for camouflage, particularly if lower arch extractions are required. If further unfavourable facial growth occurs, the extraction of lower premolars can compromise subsequent set-up for jaw surgery.

> **Box 109.6 Favourable factors for class III orthodontic camouflage**
>
> • Mild skeletal class III pattern
> • Positive overbite
> • The patient is able to achieve incisal contact in the retruded contact position
> • Minimal dental compensation
> • Minimal growth remaining

Surgery

Anatomical limitations mean that in the presence of larger skeletal discrepancies and where significant dentoalveolar compensation has already occurred there is less scope for correction with orthodontic camouflage alone. A combined approach will be required, involving fixed appliances in conjunction with orthognathic surgery once mandibular growth cessation has been confirmed (Box 109.7).

> **Box 109.7 Features indicating a combined approach for treatment of class III malocclusion**
>
> • More severe class III skeletal pattern
> • Compensated incisors (proclined upper incisors/ retroclined lower incisors)
> • Unfavourable growth is predicted
> • Increased lower anterior face height and a reduced overbite
> • Poor soft tissue profile
> • Transverse discrepancy resulting in a generalised cross-bite
> • Severe crowding in the upper arch and mild crowding in the lower arch

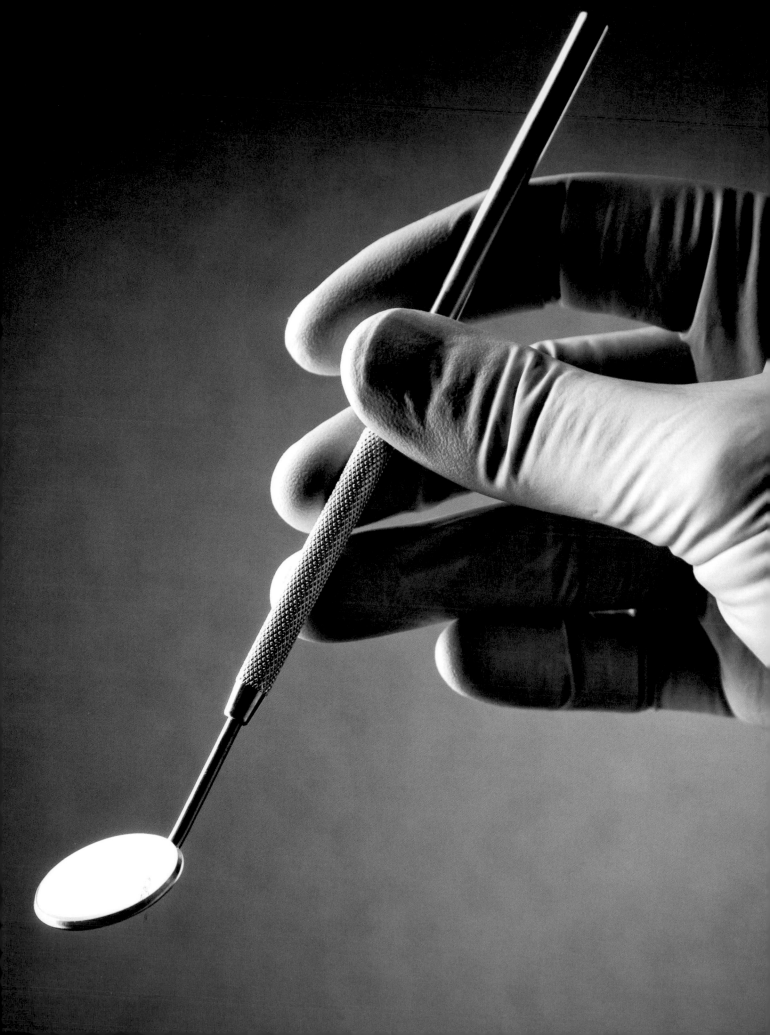

Population sciences and oral health

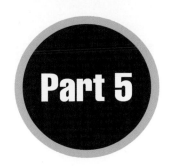

Part 5

Chapters

110 Epidemiology

Figure 110.1 Percentage of the adult population of England, Wales and Northern Ireland who were dentate in 2009

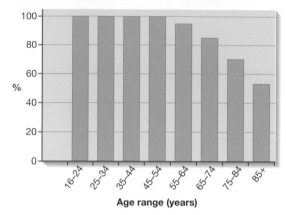

Figure 110.2 Percentage of the dentate adult population of England, Wales and Northern Ireland with any carious teeth in 2009

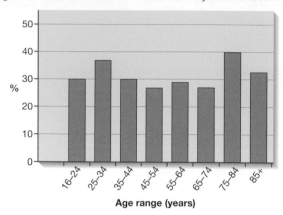

Figure 110.3 Periodontal condition of the dentate adult population of England, Wales and Northern Ireland in 2009

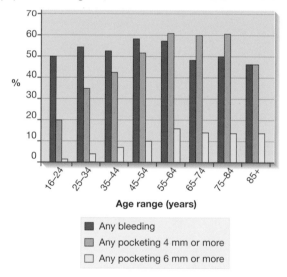

■ Any bleeding
▨ Any pocketing 4 mm or more
□ Any pocketing 6 mm or more

Figure 110.4 Age-specific incidence rates per 100 000 UK population of oral cancer cases in men and women (2007–2009)

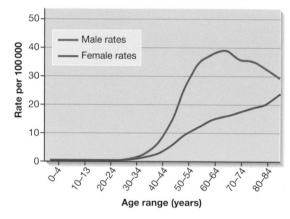

Figure 110.5 Oral cancer rates over time

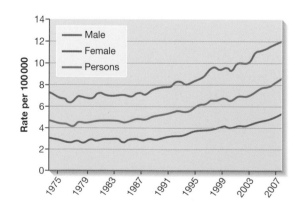

Figure 110.6 Five-year survival rates of oral cancer for patients diagnosed 1996–1999

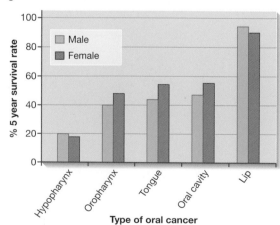

What is epidemiology?

Epidemiology is the study of the distribution and determinants of health-related states or events (including disease), and the application of this study to the control of diseases and other health problems. It is a population-based science that focusses on groups of people rather than individuals.

Descriptive studies can be used to study the distribution of oral diseases in populations (to answer 'who, what and where?' questions). Analytical studies are used to study determinants or possible causes of oral diseases and conditions (to answer 'why and how?' questions). But, as can be seen from the definition, epidemiology is not restricted to just the study of diseases. We can often gain valuable information from studying people who remain healthy too.

Interpreting oral epidemiological data

The two oral diseases that are most commonly encountered by dental practitioners in a clinical setting are dental caries and periodontal diseases. Whilst we may be able to examine a patient's mouth and interpret the findings in relation to a discussion of their dental history in a clinical setting, this option is not usually available to us when dealing with epidemiological data and therefore the interpretation of these data is more complicated. For example, if we note in an epidemiological survey that a tooth is missing, we may not know the reason for this; it could be the result of caries, periodontal disease or even another reason such as trauma or an elective extraction to make space for orthodontic treatment. Thus, we often use epidemiological surveys to describe the current oral health status of a population rather than as a direct record of their caries or periodontal disease experience.

Oral health status of the population

British Adult Dental Health Surveys

The 2009 Adult Dental Health Survey was the fifth national dental survey. They have been carried out once a decade since 1968. Each of these cross-sectional surveys has been used to get a snapshot of the dental health of the adult general population at a particular point in time. Taken together, they can be used to explore how dental health has generally improved in the population over time.

Proportion of people with natural teeth: Within England, the percentage of adults with at least one natural tooth (dentate) was only 72% in 1978 and this had increased to 94% three decades later. Figure 110.1 shows the percentage of adults, by age group, in England, Wales and Northern Ireland in 2009 that were dentate.

Caries: The 2009 survey showed that 31% of dentate adults had obvious caries but that this varied with gender and age. A greater proportion of men (34%) than women (28%) had carious teeth. Regarding age, there was no clear pattern, although the highest percentage of adults with caries among those with teeth was in people aged 75–84 (40%) (Figure 110.2).

Periodontal condition: Overall 54% of adults exhibited gingival bleeding on probing. Pocketing of 4 mm or more was found in 45% of adults and pocketing in excess of 6 mm was found in 8%. Bleeding was more common in men (56%) than women (52%), as was the prevalence of 4-mm pocketing (47% vs. 43%) and 6-mm pocketing (10% vs. 7%). These prevalences also varied by age (Figure 110.3).

British Child Dental Health Surveys

The 2013 national Child Dental Health Survey was the fifth in a series of national surveys carried out every 10 years since 1973. The 2013 survey asked parents to consider whether their children had any problems with their dental health in the previous 6 months as a result of the condition of their teeth and gums. Problems were reported by the parents of 37% of 5 year olds and 55% of 8 year olds.

In addition to the decennial surveys, school-based epidemiological programmes for children of varying age groups are conducted on an approximately annual basis. Children in England aged 12 years old were surveyed in 2008/9. A third of pupils (33.4%) were found to have experience of caries, with an average of 2.21 decayed, missing or filled teeth. Including all the children examined, the average was 0.74 per child.

Oral cancer

Although not as common as caries and periodontal diseases, oral cancer is a very important condition that can be identified by dental practitioners. The main risk factors for oral cancer are tobacco, alcohol, diet and nutrition, sunlight, human papillomavirus and immunosuppression. In 2009, there were more than 6000 new cases (incidence) of oral cancer in the UK. Twice as many men as woman are affected, with 13 new cases per 100 000 men compared to 7 per 100 000 women. Overall, oral cancer accounts for 2% of all new cancer cases in the UK. The lifetime risk of developing oral cancer has been estimated to be 1 in 93 for men and 1 in 186 for women.

Age: Oral cancer incidence is related to age (Figure 110.4). In men the age-specific incidence rates increase dramatically from the age of 45 and peak in the 60s. After age 70 the rates begin to decline. For women the rates also begin to increase from age 45, but the increase is much more gradual and peaks in the over 80s.

Trends over time: Oral cancer rates have been increasing in Britain since the mid-1970s. This increase has been most significant in the last decade, which has seen a 25% increase in rates for men and 28% for women (Figure 110.5).

Survival: Survival from oral cancer varies greatly according to the site of the cancer and the stage of diagnosis, with later-stage cancers having poorer survival than those diagnosed at an earlier stage. Five-year survival rates for people diagnosed between 1996 and 1999 are shown in Figure 110.6, which indicates the best survival is for lip cancers that are easily seen and treated, whereas survival generally decreases with cancers at sites that are less easily seen and tend to be diagnosed later.

111 Social variations in oral health

Figure 111.1 Conceptual framework

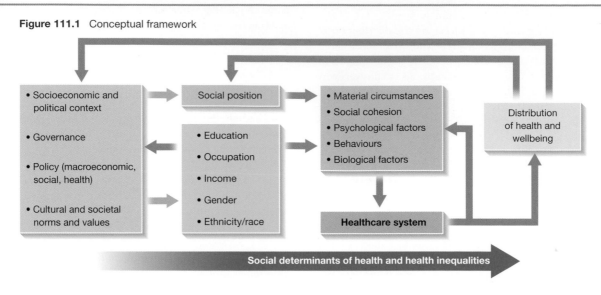

Source: Adapted from CSDH (2008). Closing the GAP in a Generation: Health Equity Through Action on the Social Determinants of Health. Final Report of the Commission on Social Determinants of Health. Reproduced with permission of WHO.

Figure 111.2 Trend in children's admissions to hospital for the extraction of carious teeth 1998–2010 by deprivation

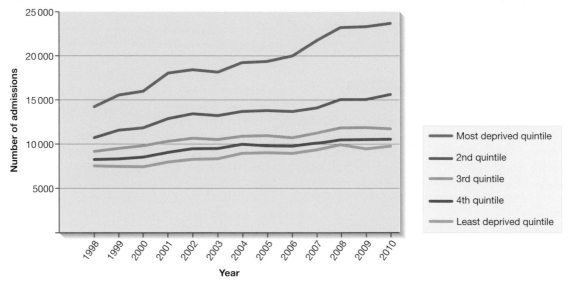

The social gradient of health and disease

Many diseases such as cancers, heart disease, stoke, diabetes and dementia exhibit a social gradient, and are more common among socially disadvantaged groups than those who are relatively more affluent/ advantaged. It is not just that the poorest people experience poor health, but there is a gradient of risk that exists across the whole population, such that the lower a person may be in the social hierarchy, the greater their risk of ill health. This pattern is seen within middle and high income countries of the world irrespective of the overall wealth of a nation and it has been detected across all age groups.

It is not just general health that is affected. Similar social gradients exist with regard to oral health status. This includes caries, periodontal diseases and tooth loss, in both adults and

Dentistry at a Glance. First Edition. Edited by Elizabeth Kay. © 2016 John Wiley & Sons, Ltd. Published 2016 by John Wiley & Sons, Ltd.
Companion website: www.ataglanceseries.com/dentistryseries/dentistry

children. For adults there is also a clear gradient in both oral cancer incidence and survival.

Social determinants of health

Inequalities in health are a consequence of the unequal distribution of health determinants, including the social and physical environment, people's behaviours, biological factors and access to, and effective utilisation of, the healthcare system.

Traditionally, healthcare professionals have attempted to educate people to adopt a healthy lifestyle and to avoid unhealthy behaviours. However, this approach is limited, as those people who are lower in the social gradient tend to have less control over their lives than those who are higher in the social gradient. Thus, whilst this approach is well intentioned, it may perversely actually serve to increase inequalities by being less effective for those in most need.

Poor diet and poor oral hygiene are among the causes of inequalities in oral health. However, in order to deal with these inequalities we need to tackle the underlying reasons why some people have poor diet and poor oral hygiene. The Commission on Social Determinants of Health (CSHD) called this the 'causes of the causes'. The CSHD has developed a conceptual framework that encapsulates the idea of causes of the causes (Figure 111.1).

Social variations in oral health
British Adult Dental Health Surveys

These surveys are described further in Chapter 110.

Proportion of people with no natural teeth: In 2009, 2% of adults living in households classified as being 'managerial and professional occupations' were edentulous. This compared with 5% for those living in households classified as 'intermediate occupations' and 10% for those in 'routine and manual occupations'.

Caries: A greater proportion of adults from manual backgrounds (37%) exhibited caries than those in either intermediate (31%) or managerial/ professional backgrounds.

Periodontal condition: The prevalence of bleeding on probing and the presence of periodontal pocketing across all levels of severity was also found to follow a social gradient in the 2009 Adult Dental Health Survey, as can be seen by Table 111.1.

Table 111.1 Periodontal condition of dentate adults in different socioeconomic classifications, 2009

Classification	Any bleeding (%)	Pocketing of 4 mm or more (%)	Pocketing of 6 mm or more (%)	Pocketing of 9 mm or more (%)
Managerial and professional occupations	49	43	7	1
Intermediate occupations	54	47	9	2
Routine and manual occupations	59	48	11	2

Child dental health

Children from deprived backgrounds are more likely to experience dental caries than those from more affluent backgrounds; this is particularly the case with caries in the primary dentition. There is a pronounced social gradient in the numbers of children being admitted to hospital for the extraction of carious teeth (Figure 111.2), with children in the most deprived quintile of deprivation (i.e. children living in the most deprived 20% of households) accounting for around 40% of the total number of admissions.

Oral cancer

Incidence: The two most significant risk factors for most types of oral cancer are excessive alcohol consumption and tobacco usage (Chapter 110). These health behaviours are socioeconomically linked and, accordingly, oral cancer incidence is also strongly associated with deprivation. Data for England show that rates of head and neck cancer are around 130% higher (i.e. more than double) for men living in the most deprived areas compared with the least deprived, and more than 74% higher for women.

Survival: Not only are the most deprived people more likely to develop oral cancer, but they also have poorer survival rates than those from more affluent backgrounds. Table 111.2 shows the 5-year survival rates for key intraoral sites and illustrates, for example, that half of people from the most affluent backgrounds survive for at least 5 years following a diagnosis of tongue cancer compared to only about one-third of those from the most deprived backgrounds. Although a socioeconomic inequality in survival can be seen for many types of cancers, it is particularly marked for oral cancer.

Table 111.2 Comparison of survival in affluent and deprived patients, 1986–90, in England and Wales

Cancer site	5-year survival % for most affluent	5-year survival % for most deprived	Gap between most affluent and most deprived (%)
Tongue	50.4	34.1	−16.3
Oropharynx	41.9	29.9	−12
Oral cavity	53.9	42.3	−11.6

Social variations in dental attendance and demand for care

Attendance patterns in both adults and children also follow a social gradient in which the most deprived people, and those in most need of dental care, are those least likely to attend a dentist on a regular and asymptomatic basis. The first Adult Dental Health Survey in 1968 indicated that around 40% of adults said that they attended the dentist on a regular basis. By 2009 this figure was 61%. Reported regular attendance from the surveys is associated with more frequent tooth brushing, and lower levels of plaque and calculus.

Psychology and dental care

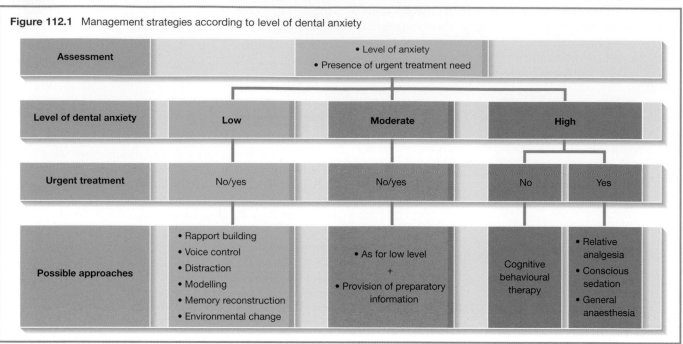

Figure 112.1 Management strategies according to level of dental anxiety

Assessment	• Level of anxiety • Presence of urgent treatment need		
Level of dental anxiety	Low	Moderate	High
Urgent treatment	No/yes	No/yes	No	Yes
Possible approaches	• Rapport building • Voice control • Distraction • Modelling • Memory reconstruction • Environmental change	• As for low level + • Provision of preparatory information	Cognitive behavioural therapy	• Relative analgesia • Conscious sedation • General anaesthesia

Fear of dental treatment and anxiety about dental procedures are very common and are a major reason why people do not attend the dentist or do not enjoy their dental visit. Anxiety can also have an impact on the patient's quality of life, and the quality of dental treatment performed – both in terms of limiting attendance for treatment and in the nature of the dental treatment likely to be performed.

All patients have some level of anxiety about their treatment, which may range from very mild to severely phobic. It follows that it is essential to the clinical management of the patient that the dental team assess the patient's level of anxiety and intervene proportionately. Figure 112.1 provides an overview of possible management strategies according to level of dental anxiety.

Assessment of dental anxiety

There are numerous instruments available for the assessment of dental anxiety, both in children and adults. The most recent Adult Dental Health Survey adopted the Modified Dental Anxiety Scale (MDAS; available at: www.st-andrews.ac.uk/dentalanxiety/), a five-item scale that is reliable and quick to administer. It has cut-offs for mild, moderate and phobic levels of anxiety. While there are more comprehensive measures, which allow for the more specific identification of aspects of the individual's dental anxiety, the MDAS provides a simple, easy to use screening tool. It has been found to be acceptable both to patients and the dental team. A version is also available for use with children (Modified Child Dental Anxiety Scale, MCDAS).

Interventions for individuals with low levels of anxiety

Dental anxiety in young children may be prevented by the avoidance of negative experiences and the promotion of positive experiences for children attending the dental surgery. Examples of such approaches could include encouraging a warm and welcoming child-friendly environment, the provision of acclimatisation visits for children where no invasive dental treatment is performed and the use of fluoride supplements to inhibit caries and thus prevent invasive treatment.

For children attending with low levels of dental fear approaches that can be adopted include:
• **Rapport building:** For example the use of a magic trick. Researchers who used a magic trick to encourage children who on a previous visit to the dental surgery had refused to enter the dental surgery, found that this decreased the time taken for the child to sit in the dental chair and have a radiograph.
• **Voice control:** There are a number of studies to demonstrate that children respond best to a moderately loud voice with a deep tone.
• **Distraction:** Several types of distraction have been reported in the literature, including the use of video-taped cartoons, audio-taped stories and video games. Distraction techniques have been found to be as effective as relaxation-based techniques, and superior to no intervention, but are most effective if the distracting material is made contingent on co-operative behaviour. Children who were shown cartoons that were stopped if they became uncooperative, showed less than half the levels of disruptive behaviour in comparison to children who were shown cartoons regardless of their behaviour.
• **Modelling:** Modelling has been used extensively with children and is generally most effective if the observed child is similar in age, gender and level of dental anxiety to the child watching, if the child enters and leaves the surgery without adverse consequences and if the child is seen to be rewarded for non-anxious behaviour.
• **Memory reconstruction:** Researchers have designed an intervention based on an understanding of the processes of human memory and using positive images to help children reconstruct their memory of dental treatment. The intervention comprises three components. Firstly, the visual component – pictures taken previously of the child smiling during the dental procedure were shown back to the child as a visual reminder about the dental experience. Secondly, verbalisation – the child was asked how he/she would explain to the parents how well they handled the dental appointment. Thirdly, a concrete example – the child was asked to recall a good example of their improved behaviour in the dental setting. The use of this intervention decreases reported anxiety and increases the likelihood that children will re-attend.
• **Environmental change:** These interventions seek to make the dental environment more attractive to children attending the dental surgery. For example decreased dental anxiety was found in children following exposure to positive images of the dental surgery as opposed to neutral images prior to treatment.

For adult patients with low levels of dental fear the following approaches to providing an anxiety reducing environment can be suggested:
• **Enhancing the sense of control**: Uncertainty is anxiety provoking, and can be reduced by providing preparatory information and by enhancing an individuals sense of control over the situation. One widely used technique to do this is the stop signal, which has been shown to be effective in dental settings and a wide variety of other medical settings.
• **Cognitive distraction**, in which the patient is encouraged to think about something other than the dental situation, has been shown to be effective in adults. Evidence suggests that the technique is only useful if the patient is informed that it is likely to reduce anxiety.
• **Environmental change**: The smell of lavender in the dental waiting area has been shown to reduce immediate fear about treatment in adults.

Interventions for individuals with moderate levels of anxiety

The adoption of all the approaches identified for individuals with low levels of anxiety will help to create a calm and welcoming environment. In addition, patients with moderate levels of dental anxiety may benefit from the provision of preparatory information. Information on three aspects of the treatment are important:
• Information about what will happen (procedural information)
• Information about what sensations the individual will experience (sensory information)
• Information about what the individual can do to cope with the situation (coping information).

Interventions for individuals with high levels of anxiety

Where an individual has been identified as having a very high level of dental fear, specialist care is required. This will combine both pharmacological management (sedation or general anaesthetic) with specialist psychological therapies such as cognitive behaviour therapy.

113 Health, illness and behaviour change

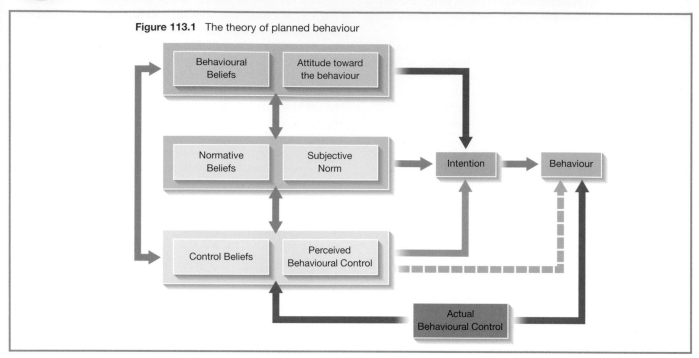

Figure 113.1 The theory of planned behaviour

Improving patients' oral health-related behaviour is an important element of the role of the dentist and the dental team in preventing oral disease. There is a wide range of psychological models and theories to help us understand patient behaviour. Psychologists have developed social cognition models (SCMs) to predict and explain behaviour changes such as screening attendance, dieting and oral hygiene behaviour. 'Social cognitions' are beliefs, thoughts and attitudes concerning behaviours, which are believed to relate to whether or not a person undertakes a particular behaviour. Two social cognition models are:

- Theory of planned behaviour
- Implementation intentions

The reason for this is to highlight an important distinction between motivation and volition. Motivation refers to the intention to engage in a behaviour, whereas volition refers to the processes by which we turn that intention into action. The clinician needs to understand both processes, explore which is most relevant to their patient and implement behaviour change interventions targeted at the appropriate process.

Motivation: the theory of planned behaviour

The theory of planned behaviour states that intention to perform an action is the most immediate predictor of behaviour. This intention, in turn, is determined by attitudes towards the behaviour, perceptions of personal control over the behaviour and beliefs about social norms (Figure 113.1). The concept of 'attitudes' in this theory refers to a general evaluation of the positive and negative aspects of the behaviour. In general, positive attitudes are thought to predict positive intentions to perform the behaviour. Subjective norm refers to the perceived social pressure to perform or not perform the behaviour and is usually assessed as both 'normative beliefs' and 'motivation to comply to social norms'. Normative beliefs are measured with questions such as 'Those important to me think I should do X' whereas motivation to comply with social norms is assessed through questions such as 'It's important to me to do what others think I should do'. According to this theory, an individual is more likely to engage in a given behaviour if he or she perceives that significant others endorse the behaviour and they wish to conform to this pressure. Both attitudes and subjective norm are thought to be direct antecedents of intention. Therefore, intention is the mediating variable between attitudes and subjective norm and behaviour. Perceived behavioural control describes the constraints to behaviour change as perceived by the individual. The general tenet holds that individuals are more disposed to engage in behaviours they feel are achievable and under their personal control. The direct relationship between perceived behavioural control and behaviour is thought to reflect the extent to which measures taken match actual control.

The theory of planned behaviour has been tested in a large variety of settings and populations. The model is a good predictor of intention to engage in a behaviour, but predicts actual behaviour slightly less well.

In order to change motivation, the clinician should target perceived behavioural control by encouraging the patient to think about other situations in which they have successfully changed their behaviour, to consider ways to overcome barriers to change. Also, the clinician should emphasise the positive benefits of behaviour change and the social benefits that may ensue.

Volition: implementation intentions

Implementation intentions promote the initiation and effective execution of a goal-directed activity by stating a specific plan of where, when and how this activity should occur. In order to form an implementation intention, the individual must first identify a goal-directed behaviour and anticipate a suitable situational context to initiate it. For example, the individual might specify 'flossing' as the behaviour and a suitable situation as 'in the bathroom in the evening after brushing my teeth every night'. Alternatively, the patient could be encouraged to associate flossing with a commonly occurring behaviour, for example 'floss after you have washed you hair'.

A systematic review of 63 studies of the effect of implementation intentions on behaviour provides evidence that forming implementation intentions makes an important difference as to whether or not people successfully translate their intentions into actions. This finding was robust across a variety of different behaviours.

To date, three studies have applied implementation intentions to oral hygiene-related behaviour. All three studies found that asking patients to make plans of where, when and how they will floss led to increases in the number of times per week that they reported flossing, and improvements in periodontal health.

Overall conclusions

In conclusion then, the distinction between motivational and volitional stages appears to be important. Clinicians should distinguish between individuals who lack the motivation to change their oral hygiene behaviour, and those who are motivated but require support in planning and maintaining behaviour change. Targets for motivational interventions that appear to be important are placing an emphasis on the benefits of behaviour change and enhancing self-efficacy beliefs about oral hygiene behaviours. For volitional interventions planning where, when and how the individual will engage in the oral hygiene behaviour appears to be a highly effective brief intervention.

114 Special care dentistry

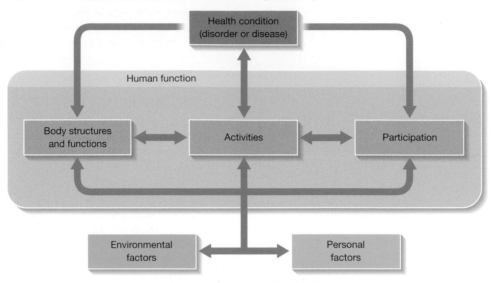

Figure 114.1 International classification of functioning, disability and health

Health condition
(disorder or disease)

Human function

Body structures
and functions ⟷ Activities ⟷ Participation

Environmental
factors ⟷ Personal
factors

Source: Faulks D, Hennequin M (2006). *J Disabil Oral Health* 7: 143.
Reproduced with permission of the British Society for Disability and Oral Health.

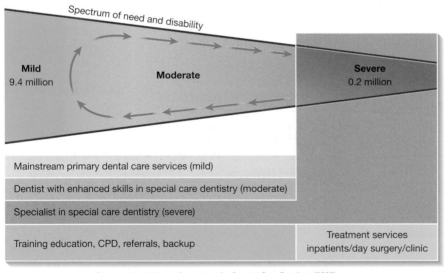

Figure 114.2 The integrated role of the special care dentist

Spectrum of need and disability

Mild
9.4 million

Moderate

Severe
0.2 million

Mainstream primary dental care services (mild)

Dentist with enhanced skills in special care dentistry (moderate)

Specialist in special care dentistry (severe)

Training education, CPD, referrals, backup

Treatment services
inpatients/day surgery/clinic

Source: Joint Advisory Committee for Special Care Dentistry (2003).
A Case of Need: Proposal for a Speciality of Special Care Dentistry. RCS, England.

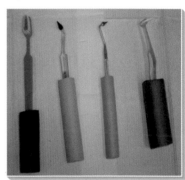

Figure 114.3 Modified toothbrushes

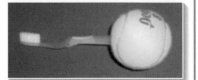

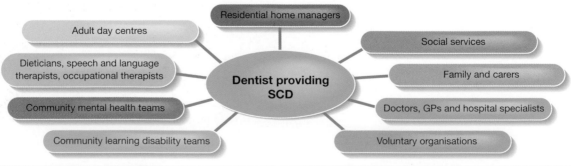

Figure 114.4 Working with others

Residential home managers

Adult day centres

Social services

Dieticians, speech and language
therapists, occupational therapists

Family and carers

**Dentist providing
SCD**

Community mental health teams

Doctors, GPs and hospital specialists

Community learning disability teams

Voluntary organisations

Scope of special care dentistry

Special care dentistry (SCD) is concerned with providing and enabling the delivery of oral care for individuals and groups of people with an impairment and/or disability (Box 114.1). This includes three groups of people who:

1 Experience disability due to oral function or structure
2 Have a condition that affects their oral health
3 Are disabled by their environment or society in a way which affects their oral health.

SCD is based on the ethos that all individuals have a right to:
- Equal standards of health care
- Autonomy in decision making
- The benefits of good oral health.

It is important to understand the different models of functioning, disability and health:
- **The medical model** of disability is a paternalistic model established by the WHO and focuses on the individual and his/ her impairment/ condition.
- **The social model** is preferred by disabled people and focuses on the impact of society on individuals with an impairment/ condition.
- **International Classification of Functioning, Disability and Health** (ICF) describes universal human experience in relation to a health condition, functioning and context, and is becoming the most acceptable classification globally (Figure 114.1).
- It is estimated that 1 in 4 adults in the UK will experience disability directly, or care for someone close to them who has a disability. Disability increases with age, with two-thirds of people with a disability being over 65. There is a spectrum of disability (mild – moderate – severe). Those with mild disabilities should be cared for in primary dental care services, with specialist services managing those with more severe disability (Figure 114.2).

Box 114.1 Definition of special care dentistry

Special care dentistry is the improvement of oral health of individuals and groups in society who have one or more commonly a number of these impairments or conditions:
- physical
- intellectual
- medical
- emotional
- sensory
- social
- mental

combination of any of these

Source: Joint Advisory Committee for Special Care Dentistry (2003). *A Case of Need – Proposal for a Speciality in SCD*. Royal College of Surgeons of England.

Access and barriers to oral health for people with disabilities

Disabled people experience barriers to good oral health (Table 114.1).

A patient-centred approach is needed to ensure the same level of choice, access and oral care services as other people. Recently, legislation has been introduced to help facilitate improvement in experience for disabled people (Box 114.2).

In dentistry this means providing appropriate:
- Access to buildings, e.g. ramps, signage, lighting
- Access to surgeries, e.g. width of doors, non-slip flooring, communication aids
- Access to the dental chair, e.g. hoists and transfer boards, wheelchair recliners

- Domiciliary care for patients unable to access care
- Training and education for staff to improve attitudes towards and knowledge of disability.

Whilst primary care practitioners need to consider all the above issues, specialist services will have access to more complex equipment, aids and expertise, and practitioners should know how to refer to appropriate services and provide appropriate information for patients for whom they are unable to provide care.

Table 114.1 Examples of barriers to oral health

User/ carer	Ability for self care Diet – need for food supplements, sugar-based medication Difficulty in communicating needs Fear and anxiety Poor standards of oral health Attitudes of carer to individual and to oral health
Dental service providers	Confidence in working with disabled people Attitudes to disability Training and experience NHS systems
Physical barriers	Physical access to dental services, e.g. transport for wheelchairs/ ambulance services Access to equipment, e.g. hoists

Box 114.2 Legislation

Disability Discrimination Act 1995 and 2004
↓
Equality Act 2010 (replaced all previous antidiscriminatory laws)
The Equality Act 2010 requires you to:
- Take reasonable steps to secure access to premises or make alternative provision
- Not refuse services on grounds of disability
- Not provide services which are different or not as good as those offered to others
- Encourage positive attitudes
- Promote equal opportunities

The all-encompassing Equality Act bans unfair treatment and helps achieve equal opportunities in the workplace and in wider society.

Communication skills for people requiring SCD

Good communication is the basis of good clinical care and for many people with disabilities our ability to communicate with them is compromised in some way. It is important to remember and make the most of the three elements of communication when we transmit or accept information:
- Words (7%)
- Vocal tone (33%)
- Facial expression and body language (60%).

Most common communication difficulties are found in people with:
- Sensory disability, e.g. hearing and visual impairment
- Neurological disability, e.g. stroke leading to aphasia and dysarthria, acquired brain injury
- Autistic spectrum conditions
- Learning disability.

Patients use many aids to communication (e.g. communication boards, computers, pictures and photos) and it is essential to find out how they manage communication every day (Box 114.3).

Box 114.3 Tips for good communication

- Face the patient
- Talk to the patient
- Be a good listener
- Speak clearly
- Do not shout
- Write things down
- Use gestures
- Allow time for patient to respond
- Reduce background noise
- Check hearing aids are on
- Check patients communication aids and use them, e.g. communication boards
- Employ help from carers
- Consider Sign Language, Makaton, British Sign Language, Signalong
- Use pictures and symbols, photographs and drawings

An essential consideration in SCD is obtaining consent from patients who may have communication, cognitive or sensory impairments. The capacity of the patient to provide consent is crucial to the process of gaining consent.

Impact of impairments and systemic conditions on oral health and functions

A good knowledge of human diseases is essential to practise SCD. There is growing evidence of the link between oral disease and medical conditions, for example diabetes, cardiovascular disease, arthritis, cancers, respiratory, disease and preterm and low weight births.

The impact of more common conditions on oral health are shown in Table 114.2.

Clinical management of patients requiring SCD

The care and treatment of patients should not be compromised because of impairment or disability but there are often complexities and additional issues to consider when treatment planning and managing clinical care.

- **Consent:** that is capacity of the patient to give consent
- **Good history taking:** this must include any medical, dental and social history that might affect care
- **Risk assessment:** this must take into account safety of the patient, staff and environment (especially in a domiciliary setting)
- **Treatment planning for prevention:** this is essential, particularly for those who have difficulty managing their own care; high-fluoride toothpastes are a useful adjunct for prevention of caries
- **Training for carers:** awareness of and ability to carry out good oral care is essential for those caring for disabled people
- **Behavioural management techniques:** there is a range of techniques available to facilitate oral care (Box 114.4)
- **Clinical holding:** it is occasionally necessary to support individuals by holding them to provide treatment; there should be appropriate protocols in place to facilitate this and staff should be adequately trained
- **Equipment and aids:** additional equipment and aids should be considered, e.g. modified toothbrushes for oral hygiene, hoists and manual handling aids to provide care that is safe for staff and patients (Figure 114.3)
- **Multiprofessional care and teamwork:** joint working with dentists and other dental-care professionals and liaison with other members of the medical and social team is essential to understand the patient and provide the best treatment (Figure 114.4).

Box 114.4 The range of management techniques

Behaviour modification techniques, for example:
- Tell, show, do
- Modelling
- Positive reinforcement

 Sedation: inhalation and intravenous General anaesthesia

Table 114.2 Common conditions and examples of possible impact on oral health

Condition	Impact on oral health				
Medical condition	Increased need for monitoring oral health/hygiene	Bleeding conditions	Increased risk of general infection	Drug Interactions	Cross-infection risks
Physical impairment	Access to surgery impaired	Involuntary movements	Inability to manage oral hygiene	Inability to open mouth for periods of time	With a degenerative disease a long-term treatment plan is important
Learning disability	Inability to understand care and/or communication difficulties	Inability to self-care	Reliance on carers to carry out care Training needs	Reduced ability to manage care and treatment	Diet Prescribed food supplements
Mental illness	Chaotic lifestyle	History of missed appointments and lack of oral care	Effects of medication	Possible affects of smoking/drug/alcohol abuse	Impaired/fluctuating understanding and communication
Effects of medication	May affect bleeding, e.g. after extraction	Bisphosphonate-induced osteonecrosis of the jaw (BIONJ)	Interactions with prescribed drugs	Allergies	Affect on periodontal condition and increase in caries, e.g. food supplements
Autistic spectrum disorder	Possible learning disability (see above)	Obsessive dietary habits	Low comprehension/concentration	Self injurious behaviour	Communication difficulties

115 Ethical care of patients

The 'ethics of health care' pervades the work of all healthcare professionals and healthcare workers. It has purported to do so for almost 2500 years, from the time of Hippocrates, hailed as the father of modern medicine.

The Hippocratic oath (*Attributed to Hippocrates c.460 c.377 BC, Greek philosopher and physician*): An oath to Apollo (the god of healing) and his daughters Hygeia (health) and Panacea (all healing) to convey basic ethical guidance to new physicians. Its most acclaimed injunction is 'First (above all), to do no harm'. Others include respecting teachers, maintaining knowledge and keeping patient's secrets.

There are varied types of ethical theory to enable justification of actions and acceptability of outcomes; the study of ethics is vast. This chapter explores the ethics of health care through four well established and accepted principles, originally devised by Tom Beauchamp and James Childress, and which have had a considerable influence in the field of medical ethics.

1 Autonomy
2 Non-maleficence
3 Beneficence
4 Justice.

Autonomy

The etymological derivation of autonomy is from Greek: *autos* meaning self and *nomos* meaning rule/governance. It embraces concepts of freewill, individual choice and the right of self-determination.

To be fully autonomous a person must be able to make decisions, and be able to act on those decisions, on the basis of rational thought and deliberation. Indeed, the delivery of health care itself promotes autonomy and enables a patient to lead as fully an autonomous life as possible.

In terms of health care respect for autonomy is about a patient's right to make decisions about their health and requires:
• Veracity/ truthfulness
• Fidelity/ trust
• Full explanations of the patient's presenting disease/illness or problem
• Full explanations of the available treatment options (including risks and benefits)

Both the above to be given in a manner that the patient can understand and, where required, given with assistance to enable the patient to understand.
• Respect for the patient's decisions – even if they do not accord with your own values
• Confidentiality.

Non-maleficence

The principle of non-maleficence imposes an obligation not to do harm, either intentionally or unintentionally. Importantly, it includes not exposing patients to the risks of harm. Generally within society, it is considered to be a negative obligation (that is, to fulfil it does not require action to be taken) and it is also considered to be a universal obligation, owed by all persons in society to each other irrespective of any extant relationship. Where there is a special relationship, however, this duty imposes positive obligations, which may require action to fulfil.

Beneficence

The principle of beneficence imposes an obligation to do good; to act for the benefit of others. It is a positive obligation, that is it requires action rather than abstention, and it includes the prevention of harm and the removal of risks of harm. It cannot be a universal obligation as it would be too onerous to be 'doing good' for others all the time.

However, within the context of health care, the obligation is engaged by the relationship of the state and its citizens, or the individual relationship between the healthcare provider and the patient.

Justice

The concept of justice, in the sense of fairness and not retribution or punishment, embraces the wider distribution of, and access to, health care within society, including the allocation of resources. It supports autonomy to the degree that every patient should receive equal consideration irrespective of sex, race, colour, age, wealth and social class.

Professional ethics

These four principles help to define what it is to be a professional person and a member of a profession subject to professional regulation as set out in a Position Statement by the UK Inter Professional Group, to which the GDC is a signatory.

Definition of a profession: A profession is an occupation in which an individual:
• uses intellectual skill based on
• an established body of knowledge and practice
• to provide a specialist service in a defined area
• exercising independent judgment in accordance with a code of ethics and in the public interest.

These principles also form the basis of the General Dental Council's guidelines set out in 'Standards for the Dental Team' 2013.

The core ethical principles of practice: there are nine principles registered dental professionals must keep to at all times. As a GDC registrant you must:
1 Put patients first
2 Communicate effectively with patients
3 Obtain valid consent
4 Maintain and protect patients' information
5 Have a clear and effective complaints procedure
6 Work with colleagues in a way that is in the patient's best interests
7 Maintain, develop and work within your professional knowledge and skills
8 Raise concern if patients are at risk
9 Make sure your personal behaviour maintains patients' confidence in you and the dental profession.

Ethics in action

The surgical removal of lower wisdom tooth, which has given rise to repeated bouts of pericoronitis and whose roots are in very close radiological proximity to the inferior alveolar nerve, provides a simple example of the competing principles.

There will be an obvious benefit from removal of the tooth but surgery will almost certainly cause postoperative pain and swelling and will also carry the risk of (perhaps) a significant nerve injury. The principles of non-maleficence and beneficence appear to be in clear conflict. How is such conflict resolved? Although it must be remembered that the principle of autonomy is not an overriding principle, in this scenario such conflict can easily be resolved by reference to it. A patient – fully and properly informed as to the risks and benefits of the treatment options (including no treatment) – will be empowered to make an 'informed choice' between running the risk of nerve injury and suffering further infective episodes.

Dentistry at a Glance. First Edition. Edited by Elizabeth Kay. © 2016 John Wiley & Sons, Ltd. Published 2016 by John Wiley & Sons, Ltd.
Companion website: www.ataglanceseries.com/dentistryseries/dentistry

116 Dentistry and the law

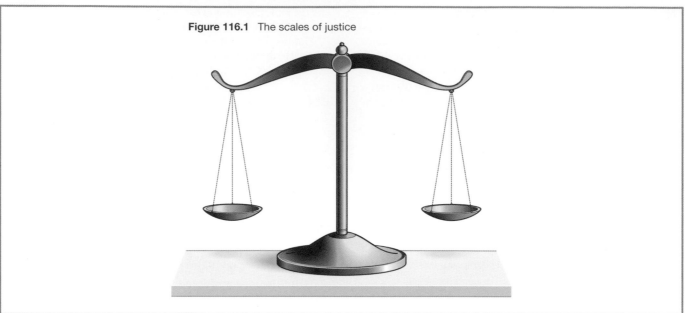

Figure 116.1 The scales of justice

The structure and principle of the law in England, Northern Ireland and Wales is that of a common law jurisdiction. The law of Scotland is a mixture of common law and of the civil law (Roman law) basis to the jurisdictions of continental Europe.

A common law system is one that operates through precedent of previously decided cases but which is also subject to the provisions of statute (Acts of Parliament) and statutory instruments (originating from the enabling Act) (Figure 116.1).

Both jurisdictions are subject to European Community law as applied by:

• Regulations, which have direct effect on all member states without the need for legislation to be passed

• Directives, requiring the member state to pass/amend legislation to achieve the result desired in the Directive; for example, the statutory instrument The Medical Devices Regulations 2002/618 (as amended) relating to standards and quality of crowns, dentures, removable orthodontic appliances etc., which is derived from the Medical Devices Directive 93/42/EC (again as amended)

• Decisions of the European Court of Justice.

Dentistry – the profession

The practice of dentistry in the United Kingdom is regulated by the Dentists Act 1984. Of that Act:

• Part I provides for the continuation of the General Dental Council, established in 1957, setting out the constitution and general rules and its committees.

• Part II deals with dental education, and its supervision, leading to the conferment of degrees and licenses.

• Part III deals with the dental profession and its individual members through the 'dental register' by reference to professional conduct, fitness to practice and continuing professional training and development.

• Part IV deals with the practice of dentistry defined as 'the performance of any such operation and the giving of any such treatment, advice or attendance as is usually given or performed by dentists' setting out the restrictions on those who can lawfully practice within the UK.

• Part V deals with dental auxiliaries.

Since 1984, there have been a number of amendments to the Act. For example, in 2005, the inclusion of professions complementary to dentistry at Part 3(A) of the 1984 Act.

Agreeing to treatment

The law upholds the principle of autonomy and a patient's right to make choices; the provision of treatment on a patient without their consent or without lawful authority would be a trespass to their person (a battery but commonly called an assault).

• Patients over the age of 16 years are presumed to have capacity to consent to treatment.

• The lawfulness of treatment for persons over the age of 16 years who lack capacity is governed by statute, and common law if below the age of 18 years (see below). In England and Wales, the Mental Capacity Act 2005 provides that treatment will be lawful if the person providing treatment reasonably believes that the patient lacks capacity and the treatment is in the patient's best interests; on the authority of a Lasting Power of Attorney; or on the declaration of a Court appointed Deputy; and the Court itself. In Scotland the relevant statute is the Adults with Incapacity (Scotland) Act 2000. The Mental Capacity Bill, which will provide similar legislation to the Mental Capacity Act 2005, is still making its way through the Northern Ireland Assembly.

• Children below the age of 16 years can have capacity depending on their level of maturity and understanding in respect of the proposed intervention (the concept of the 'Gillick competent child').

• For children below the age of 18 years who lack capacity, treatment would be lawful with consent from anyone with parental responsibility for that child or from a person who has care for the child and treatment would be in furtherance of that child's welfare.

• Consent for treatment for children below the age of 18 years who themselves will not give consent can be obtained from a parent or other person with parental responsibility or by the Court (even if the parents do not consent).

The latter three principles are derived from the common law.

By reference to the principle of autonomy for consent to be valid it should be an informed decision and should be given freely. The issue of an 'informed consent' and a patient's remedies in law are broadly divided into a lack of consent *per se* and a lack of information. For a consent to be valid in respect of a trespass the patient only needs to be advised of the 'nature and purpose' of the proposed procedure. A failure to provide the patient with sufficient information – the 'informed consent' – is embraced within the tort of negligence.

Providing treatment

Every dentist has a duty to provide treatment with reasonable skill and care, such a duty being imposed by common law in the tort of negligence, and by both common law and statute in contract (for private treatment only) when it will be an implied term. The law expects dentists to provide treatment (including advice) of a reasonable standard. It does not have to be of the highest possible standard.

Whether a dentist has
1 Provided appropriate treatment
2 Provided treatment of an adequate standard
is determined by reference to the professional standard test of 'accepted practice', often referred to as the 'Bolam test' from a case in 1957 in which the judge referred to

> 'a practice accepted as proper by a responsible body of medical men skilled in that particular art.......'

There is much evidence based research in the practice of dentistry and in consequence there are many 'guidelines' to formulate the determination of accepted practice. Remember that within this context 'common practice' is not the equivalent of accepted practice.

However, 'accepted practice' is not necessarily determinative in any claim. The Court remains the ultimate arbiter of the standard of care provided, for all aspects of care. In the face of competing views the Court would have to be satisfied that contrary opinions, for example supporting a particular treatment modality that was outside of mainstream dentistry in the UK, were reasonable, responsible, respectful and capable of withstanding logical scrutiny.

In terms of expected skill levels and expertise, the standard of care will be judged on a like for like basis. That is, a general practitioner will be judged by the expected standards of a general practitioner, a specialist by the expected standards of a specialist. A dental student under supervision or a vocational trainee will be judged by the standard of a qualified and reasonably competent dentist.

Until very recently, whether or not a dentist had provided a patient with sufficient and adequate information for the purposes of 'informed consent' would have also been determined by reference to the professional standard, the Bolam test. In March 2015, the Supreme Court departed from that standard and a dentist will now be:

> 'under a duty to take reasonable care that the patient is aware of any material risks involved in any recommended treatment, and of any reasonable alternative or variant treatments. The test of materiality is whether, in the circumstances of the particular case, a reasonable person in the patient's position would be likely to attach significance to the risk, or the doctor is or should reasonably be aware that the particular patient would be likely to attach significance to it.'

Perhaps this will become known as the 'Montgomery' test or the 'particular patient test'.

Where a dentist has failed to provide treatment with reasonable skill and care and that failure causes the patient more than minimal harm, the constituent elements of liability for a claim for negligence (or a breach of contract) are complete. This is in contrast to professional regulation where a failure to adhere to professional standards need not necessarily cause the patient any harm for the Professional Conduct Committee of the General Dental Council to make a determination that a dentist's fitness to practice was impaired, the exposure to a risk of harm being sufficient.

117 Risk management

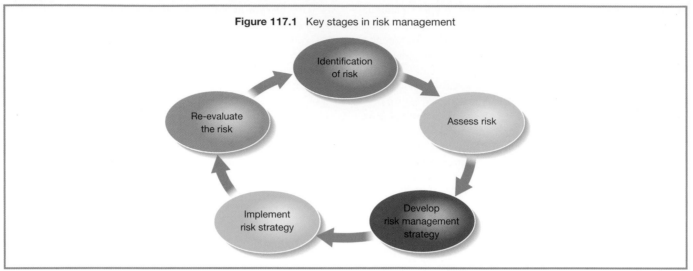

Figure 117.1 Key stages in risk management

Identification of risk

Assess risk

Develop risk management strategy

Implement risk strategy

Re-evaluate the risk

Introduction

Dentists have a duty of care to ensure that the health, safety and welfare of their staff and patients are maintained. This requires identification of any risks, with appropriate action taken to minimise the impact (Box 117.1).

Risk: The Health and Safety Executive defines 'risk' as 'likelihood that a hazard will actually cause its adverse effects, together with a measure of the effect'.

Risk management: NHS Scotland defines 'risk management' as 'the systematic identification and treatment of risk'.

Risk management in general dental practice includes a range of potential threats, which can involve every aspect of the practice. Box 117.1 highlights key areas that need to be considered when managing risk within a dental practice.

Box 117.1 Potential areas of risk in dental practice

Business
Professional liability
Health and safety
Legal and ethical
Clinical
Personal

Irrespective of the area of risk identified, the approach and strategy should be the same. The key stages of risk management are shown in Figure 117.1.

The first stage in risk management is **identification of risk.** This is about asking a series of questions around 'what could happen'? This approach is best undertaken as a group with team members fully engaged in the process. Once a risk has been identified it needs to be **assessed** and the nature and probability of the risk analysed. Consideration then needs to be given as to what measures can be **implemented** to minimise the risk. These actions are then implemented and the risks subsequently **re-evaluated**.

Clinical governance is a statutory requirement within the NHS and provides a quality assurance framework designed to deliver high standards of care aimed at continual improvement. A key aspect of the framework is to identify risks and manage them appropriately. **Clinical audit** plays an important role in improving quality and is a highly effective tool in managing clinical risk.

Areas of potential risk in dental practice

Business

Dental practices are businesses and as such are exposed to the same financial risks as any other business. Increased costs, reduced income, illness, competition, government regulations or economic climate can all have an adverse affect on a dental practice and severely compromise the business. These risks need to be identified and managed effectively through development of a sound business plan and sound financial management.

Professional liability

All GDC registrants are required to have appropriate professional indemnity insurance to mitigate against compensation claims by patients. This might be considered to be the ultimate **risk containment** strategy to allow a dentist to continue to practise, when other aspects of risk management had been ineffectual. The level of indemnity required for an individual practitioner is assessed by the dental defence organisation and this is based on risk.

Health and safety

Assessing risks within the work environment is central to Health and Safety legislation and the Health and Safety at Work Act 1974. Health and safety covers a wide range of risks for both staff and patients which may include fire safety, hazardous substances, pressure vessel regulations, physical environment, electrical appliances, computer equipment and stress. These risks need to be recognised and policies put in place to ameliorate the risks associated (Box 117.2).

Dentistry at a Glance. First Edition. Edited by Elizabeth Kay. © 2016 John Wiley & Sons, Ltd. Published 2016 by John Wiley & Sons, Ltd.
Companion website: www.ataglanceseries.com/dentistryseries/dentistry

Box 117.2 An example of risk management in dental practice

Exposure to nitrous oxide during inhalational sedation
Potential risk of overexposure identified
Risk assessed by measuring individual exposure to N_2O
Risk minimised by use of scavenging system and rotation of staff
Re-evaluated exposure following implementation of changes

Legal and ethical

Patients place a considerable degree of trust in their dentist, and with that trust comes responsibility. Patients understandably expect dental professionals to do their best for their patients and if this is not seen to be done, the trust is undermined. This can result in a complaint and, if pursued by the patient, may even escalate to a disciplinary hearing.

Prevention is better than cure, and communication is key in establishing a good relationship with patients. Good communication is also vital in ensuring that patients understand the treatment proposed and the potential risks and benefits, as this is a fundamental component of informed consent. Good clinical record keeping is of paramount importance in addressing a complaint or defending an accusation of poor practise. Irrespective of the validity of the complaint, poor note keeping will result in a poor defence, which is not a risk worth taking.

Clinical risk

Dentists are highly skilled professionals who are trained to improve oral health and aim to provide a standard of care that is non-maleficent. No treatment is one hundred percent successful and treatment failure can occur through no fault of the practitioner. However, the patient needs to be aware of the risks involved prior to consenting to treatment and all efforts must be made to minimise the risk.

All General Dental Council (GDC) registrants have a mandatory obligation to undertake continuing professional development; however, they must ensure that they work within their scope of practice and within their own level of competency. An example of this is highlighted in Box 117.3.

Box 117.3 An example of risk management in third molar removal

Recurrent pericoronitis affecting lower third molar necessitating removal
Recognised potential risk of damage to inferior dental nerve
Risk assessed by appropriate radiographs revealing close proximity to inferior dental
Patient aware of risks but in view of history, tooth removal required
Procedure deemed as beyond competency of individual practitioner resulting in specialist referral

Communicating with patients is a fundamental aspect of patient-centred care and has to be done effectively if shared decision making is the purpose of the consultation. Patients need to be aware of the risks of treatment and understand them fully.

Risk management of disease

Assessment of risk in managing disease has become increasingly important and this is highly relevant in dentistry. Within the NHS this has become particularly apposite in targeting time and resources at those most in need of prevention or treatment. In dentistry, assessment of caries risk will allow an individualised treatment plan to be developed which will determine the preventative regime, frequency of radiographs and indicate the appropriate recall interval. Such information is extremely useful and will ensure the appropriate treatment is being implemented and resources are being used effectively.

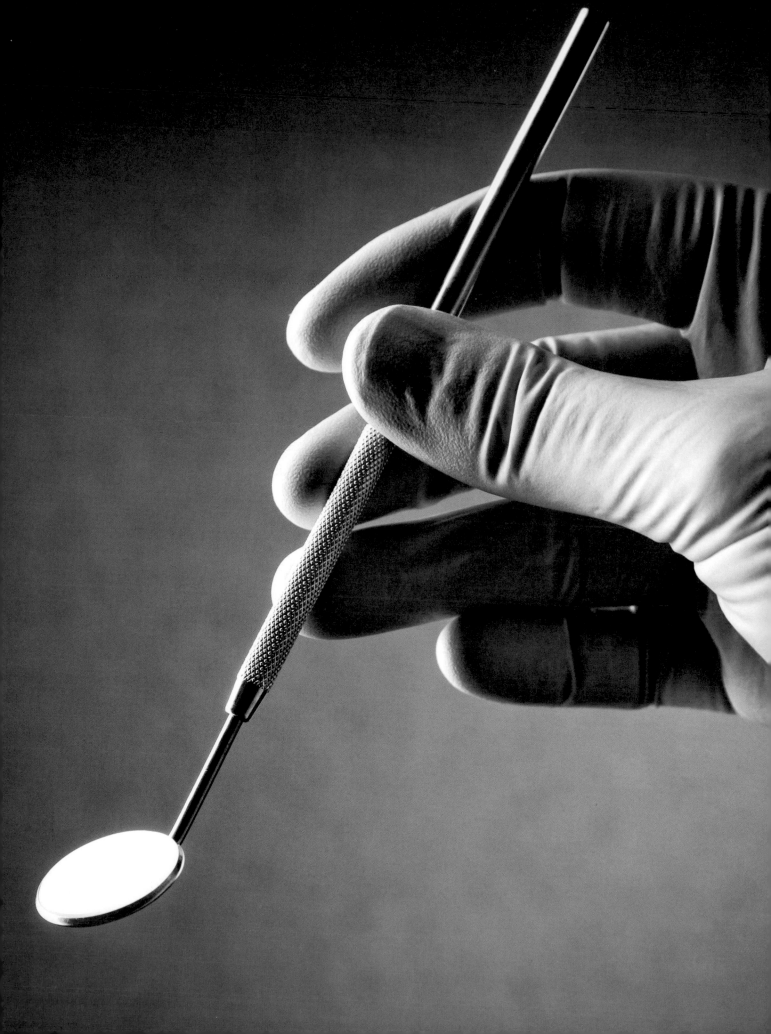

Running a dental practice

Chapters

118 Infection control

Dentistry at a Glance. First Edition. Edited by Elizabeth Kay. © 2016 John Wiley & Sons, Ltd. Published 2016 by John Wiley & Sons, Ltd.
Companion website: www.ataglanceseries.com/dentistryseries/dentistry

Figure 118.1 Infection control in practice

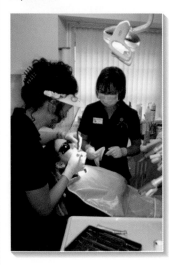

Box 118.1 Decontamination process

1 **Transportation:** Transfer of instruments from surgery to decontamination area safely and securely.
2 **Cleaning and decontamination:** Thorough cleaning of instruments with either:
   a Manual cleaning
   b Ultrasonic bath
   c Washer disinfector.
3 **Inspection:** Examination of instruments under magnification to ensure cleanliness.
4 **Sterilisation:** Instruments sterilised in autoclave, which is normally 134°C for 4 min.
5 **Storage:** Sterilised instruments are bagged and then returned to storage.

Box 118.2 Sharps injury policy

Every possible care should be taken to prevent sharps injuries. However, should a sharps injury occur the following protocol must be followed:
• Squeeze the wound to expel blood and continue to do so for several minutes with the wound under running water.
Do not suck the wound.
• Dry the wound and apply a waterproof antiseptic dressing.
• Immediately inform the dentist/ practice manager who will decide if you should seek the attention of a doctor.
• Dentist/ practice manager will contact GP/ occupational health.
• Keep the sharp item that caused the injury in a safe container and keep a record of the patient upon whom it was used.
• Check the patient's medical history with the dentist.
• Ensure the event is recorded in full in the accident book.

Figure 118.2 HTM 01-5 Decontamination in primary dental care practices

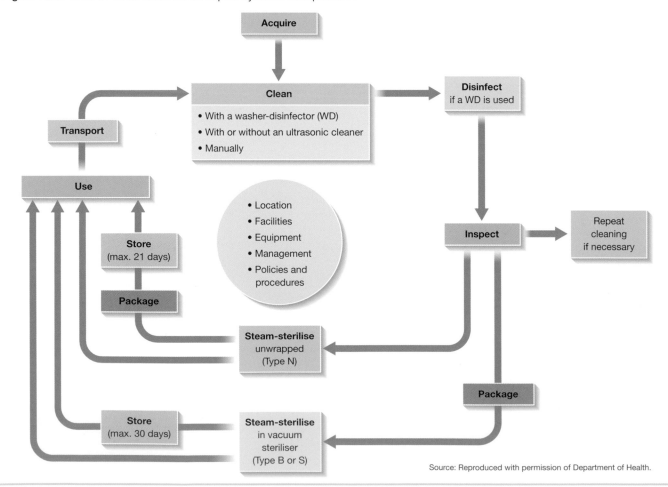

Source: Reproduced with permission of Department of Health.

Introduction

Infection control in health care is an area of extreme importance and this is reflected in the degree of training and investment made by dental practices to ensure that both staff and patients are protected. Effective infection control protocols and processes are ultimately the responsibility of the practice owner, but implementation of these procedures requires the full compliance of the whole dental team. Every practice must have a written infection control policy, which is tailored to the routines of the individual practice and regularly updated.

Infection control in dentistry
Standard precautions

The oral environment is host to a multitude of microorganisms, which can potentially be transmitted during dental procedures. Transmission can be via saliva, blood, aerosol or direct contact, with potentially serious consequences. Some patients may unknowingly be carriers of infective agents and despite thorough questioning may not be aware of the risk of infection which they pose during dental treatment. The same principle applies to dentists and other dental care professionals.

In view of this, it is vitally important that 'Standard Precautions' are applied universally within the dental practice. This ensures that a standard protocol is applied to all patients, which is robust and designed to minimise the risk of infection to staff and patients.

Medical history

A thorough medical history should be obtained for all patients at the first visit and updated regularly. The medical history should be retained as part of the patient's dental records and will provide valuable information on the patient's fitness to undergo dental treatment, the potential impact of systemic disease on the oral environment and potential risks or drug interactions. It may also allow a risk assessment to be made on the appropriateness of treatment, and indeed the scheduling of such treatment. The medical history and examination will not necessarily identify asymptomatic carriers of infectious disease and standard precautions must always be adopted.

Practice policies and staff training

Every practice must have a comprehensive written infection control policy, which is tailored to the routines of the individual practice and regularly updated. All staff must be familiar with the practice Infection Control Policy and aware of the procedures required to prevent the transmission of infection with regular training conducted.

Prevention of transmission of infection
Personal protection

All staff carrying out exposure-prone procedures should wear appropriate personal protection, including gloves, masks, visors and eye protection. Hands should be washed with water and antimicrobial soap at the beginning and end of each clinical session and if hands are visibly soiled following a procedure. Hands should be cleaned with a disinfectant gel between patients, and moisturiser applied regularly to maintain the integrity of the skin. Patients should be provided with protective glasses and a single-use protective bib, with rubber dam used wherever possible. All team members should wear personal protective clothing, which should be changed daily and machine washed at 60°C.

Immunisation

It is possible to confer a level of protection against certain transmissible diseases through immunisation and it is currently recommended that dental staff be vaccinated against:
- Diphtheria
- Hepatitis B
- *Bordetella pertussis*
- Poliomyelitis
- Rubella
- *Mycobacterium tuberculosis*
- Tetanus

Disinfection of surfaces, water lines and laboratory work

Work surfaces, water lines and laboratory items can potentially be a source of infection and need to be disinfected in line with the practice Infection Control Policy. Surgeries and local decontamination units should have 'zoning' in place, with clean and dirty areas clearly marked, which reduces the risk of contamination. Tubing in dental unit waterlines predisposes to build up of biofilms, which harbour potentially dangerous organisms, notably *Legionella* and *Pseudomonas*. No single process is currently available that will totally eliminate the build-up of biofilms; therefore, a combination of methods is applicable to reduce the risk of cross-infection. These include flushing of water lines at the beginning of each session, use of bottle water and antiretraction valves, and regular testing.

Waste disposal

Clinical waste needs to be separated and disposed of appropriately as it can potentially be a source of infection. Amalgam and sharps need to be dealt with responsibly and disposed of in the appropriate container.

Decontamination of instruments

Wherever possible single-use, disposable instruments should be used. This is not always practicable and an effective decontamination process needs to be in place to manage contaminated instruments (Box 118.1). In the UK, guidance is based on HTM 01-05: Decontamination in Primary Dental Care Practices (Department of Health) and 'best practice' stipulates the use of a dedicated Local Decontamination Unit, which is believed to provide a safer and more reliable process (Figure 118.1).

Inoculation injury

Inoculation injuries are the most likely route for transmission of blood-borne viral infections in dentistry. Prevention of such injuries is paramount and staff need to be fully aware of the risks and the need to minimise exposure. Should an inoculation injury occur, staff should act promptly and follow the appropriate policy. An example of this is shown in Box 118.2. A risk-based decision on whether to commence postexposure prophylaxis (PEP) with an antiretroviral may be indicated following evaluation of the patient record or discussion with the patient.

119 Regulatory bodies and best practice

Healthcare has become increasingly regulated over recent years, driven by a desire to raise standards, improve safety and ensure accountability. Over the last 20 years there have been significant changes in the UK within medicine and dentistry, partly as a consequence of a series of damning reports into patient care within the NHS. As dentists we have a duty of care to our patients, our staff and our profession to uphold the highest standards, comply with current regulation and deliver best practice.

Regulation in dentistry

Dentistry in the UK is highly regulated and dentists are obliged to comply with regulations and guidelines that have been put in place by various authorities. A selection of these are included in Boxes 119.1 and 119.2.

Box 119.1 UK dental regulations

- General Dental Council
- Care Quality Commission
- National Health Service
- Health and Safety Executive
- Employment Law
- Ionising Radiation Regulations
- Disability Discrimination Act
- Equal Opportunities Act

Box 119.2 Legislation specifically relevant to general dental practice

- Infection control
- Radiography
- Waste disposal
- Complaints handling
- Pressure vessel regulations
- Transportation of clinical materials
- Electricity at work
- Fire precautions
- First aid regulations
- Use of computers
- Accidents at work
- Data protection

General Dental Council

In the UK, the General Dental Council (GDC) is the regulator of dental professionals including dentists, dental nurses, dental technicians, clinical dental technicians, dental hygienists, dental therapists and orthodontic therapists. The primary role of the GDC is to protect the public and they do this by maintaining a register of dental professionals, setting standards, quality assuring dental education, recording Continuing Professional Development (CPD) and investigating complaints. It is illegal to carry out the practice of dentistry in the UK if you are not registered with the GDC (www.gdc-uk.org).

Care Quality Commission

The Care Quality Commission (CQC) was introduced in 2009 as the independent regulator of health and adult social care in England as a replacement for the Healthcare Commission. The role of the CQC is to ensure that health-care providers, including dentists, meet nationally agreed standards of quality and safety. The national standards cover all aspects of care and ensure that patients are treated with respect and dignity in a clean and safe environment. If a dental practice does not meet the agreed national standards registration with the CQC will be revoked and the practice will no longer be able to provide dental services (www.cqc.org.uk).

National Health Service (NHS) regulations

The majority of patients receiving dental care in the UK are seen under the NHS; 77% of patients who regularly attend a dentist in England have their care provided by the NHS. In monetary terms this equates to 58% of the dental market, which is valued at £3.3 billion (Source: Dentistry on Office of Fair Trading Market Study, 2012). Within the NHS, patients are still required to make a contribution to the cost unless they are exempt from charges. The General Dental Services Regulations provide a rigid framework for dentists providing NHS treatment under the Health and Social Care Act 2012. These regulations provide clear terms and conditions for the delivery of dental care within the NHS.

Health and Safety Executive

Dentists have a general duty under the Health and Safety at Work Act to ensure the health, safety and welfare of employees whilst at work. This duty of care also extends to patients. Employees also have a duty to cooperate with their employer to 'take reasonable care for their own and others' health and safety'. The Health and Safety Executive is responsible for enforcing the Health and Safety at Work Act 1974. HSE Inspectors can visit a practice at any time and examine and investigate all areas of the practice. The HSE has provided specific guidance on Control of Substances Hazardous to Health (COSHH). Under the specific guidance all dangerous substances supplied to practices must be sent with a safety data sheet when the product is first ordered. Safety data sheets provide information on chemical products that help users of those chemicals to make a risk assessment related to their storage, use and disposal.

The HSE are also responsible for ensuring that practices comply with the Pressure Equipment Regulations (1999/2001). Practices use pressurised vessels in the storage of oxygen and possibly nitrous oxide, and the use of compressors. Such equipment needs to be serviced regularly and comply with the current regulations.

Employment law

Dental practice owners have a duty of care to their staff and are bound by employment law to ensure that employees are treated fairly and equitably. Employees have rights that must be recognised, which include minimum wage, annual holidays, maternity leave and sickness pay. Employers also have a duty to ensure fair recruitment and treatment of staff under the Equal Opportunities Act 2010 and the Disability Discrimination Act 2005.

Radiation regulation

The use of ionising radiation in dentistry is governed by the Ionising Radiations Regulations 1999 (IRR99), which relate principally to the protection of workers and the public and the Ionising Radiation (Medical Exposure) Regulations 2000 (IR (ME) R2000), which relate to patient protection. The practice owner is responsible for the appointment of a Radiation Protection Advisor (RPA) such as the National Radiation Protection Board (NRPB) to ensure that the equipment is functioning safely and effectively. A set of local radiography rules is a requirement for each practice to ensure radiation safety and this is administered by a Radiation Protection Supervisor (RPS) who is normally a member of the dental team.

Disability and Discrimination Act

The Disability Discrimination Act was passed in 2005 to ensure that a disabled person is not treated less favourably for any reason relating to their disability. In dentistry this applies to staff and patients, and provision must be made to ensure inclusion is managed effectively.

Best practice

In the UK, a number of authorities provide guidance on standards in dentistry, including the General Dental Council, the British Dental Association, the National Institute for Clinical Excellence, the Royal College of Surgeons and the Faculty of General Dental Practice (FGDP). The FGDP has guidance on various aspects of general dental practice, including standards in dentistry, record keeping, radiography and prescribing (www.fgdp.org.uk).

120 Clinical record keeping

Figure 120.1 Digital radiograph

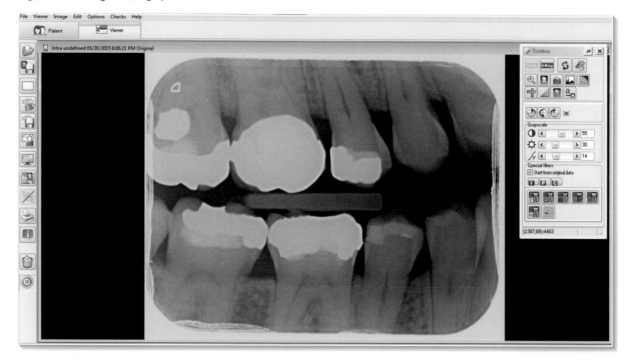

Figure 120.2 Clinical notes

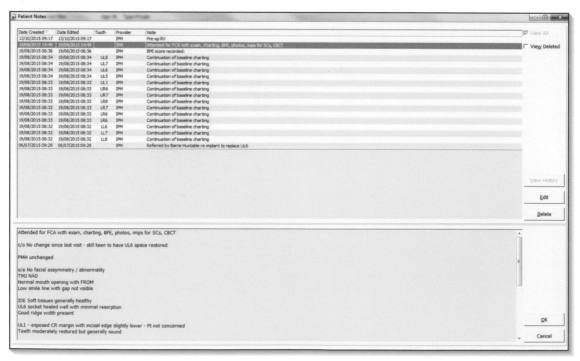

Introduction

The keeping of concise clinical records is a simple, yet important responsibility that every dental professional should take seriously (Box 120.1). The General Dental Council (UK) states that as dental professionals we have an obligation to maintain and record accurate clinical records for all treatment provided to patients under our care. This obligation is applicable to all patients, whether NHS or private. The importance of maintaining good clinical records is also recognised and advised by:

- Indemnity organisations such as Dental Protection, Medical and Dental Defence Union of Scotland
- Faculty of General Dental Practice – FGDP (UK)
- British Dental Association.

Box 120.1 Legislation that requires dentists to maintain clinical records

- Health and Social Care Act 2008
- Data protection Act 1998
- Consumer Protection Act 1987, under which an action could arise for a defective product
- Medical Devices Directive (Directive 93/42/EEC), which relates to custom-made devices
- Medicines Act 1968 and Misuse of Drugs Regulations 2001
- Freedom of Information Act 2000, primarily applicable to NHS practices

---

The **Health and Social Care Act (2008)** has led to the formation of the Care Quality Commission (CQC), and as of the 21st October 2010 all dental practices are required to register with the CQC. One of the requirements of registration, among many, is the appropriate recording and storage of patient records (Box 120.2).

Box 120.2 Health and Social Care Act 2008

Regulation 20 of the Health and Social Care Act 2008 states that providers will:
- Keep accurate personalised care, treatment and support records secure and confidential for each person who uses the service.
- Keep those records for the correct amount of time.
- Keep any other records the Care Quality Commission asks them to in relation to the management of the regulated activity.
- Store records in a secure, accessible way that allows them to be located quickly.
- Securely destroy records taking into account any relevant retention schedules.

In addition to complying with legislation, the maintenance of accurate and contemporaneous records provides a number of benefits for dental practitioners. Dental records provide dentists and patients with a concise history of previous findings, discussions and treatments. Recording notes and findings also allows a dentist to monitor any changes in a patient's oral health. If appropriate, this information can also be shared with other dental professionals to give an understanding of treatment previously provided, and any other relevant information to continue treatment.

Clinical records

Clinical records may include written or digital clinical notes, all correspondence, reports, estimates, consent, medical history forms, radiographs, study casts and laboratory sheets (Figures 120.1 and 120.2). All information within the clinical record needs to be detailed, accurate and contemporaneous. All entries must be complete entries and made at the time of the clinical visit. Any subsequent alterations or adjustments should be clearly indicated and signed and dated.

Storage of clinical records

Clinical records should be stored securely in compliance with the **Data Protection Act 1998** (DPA). Electronic data needs to be safe and secure with appropriate password protection and regular data back-up scheduled to prevent catastrophic loss of information.

The DPA (1998) states that patient records should be should be retained 'no longer than necessary'. The Department of Health advises in the Code of Practice on Retention/ Disposal of Records that practitioners should store adult records for a minimum period of **11 years** and for children up to the age of **25 years** or for a period of 11 years (whichever is longer).

Confidentiality

Dental staff have access to patient information, which may be of a personal and confidential nature. Staff must be cognisant of this fact and ensure that they take this responsibility seriously. Patient confidentiality is extremely important and any breach of trust can result in disciplinary action. The General Dental Council (UK) has clear guidance on patient confidentiality and failure to comply may be viewed as professional misconduct.

Patient access to records

In accordance with the DPA (1998) and the **Freedom of Information Act 2000** (FOIA), patients are allowed access to their own clinical records. The DPA (1998) allows patients the right to access any personal information held by the practice. The FOIA (2000) on the other hand relates to government information. As many dental practices in the UK receive government funding through the National Health Service (NHS), they are also covered by the FOIA. Third parties can only have access upon the explicit written consent from the patient unless requested otherwise by law or court order.

Should a patient wish to see their dental records, this should be requested in writing and the dentist must respond within 40 days. The identity of the person, to whom the disclosure is to be made, must be checked and if another individual is mentioned in the records their permission must be obtained. Patients have the right to have their records amended if they feel they are not correct. Records may only be withheld if the patient is deceased or if the record holder feels disclosure would cause serious harm to the patient or identify another person.

Disclosure of clinical records

Patient's records and information can only be disclosed in specified situations. These include;
- Disclosure of information to a different health-care professional (permission should still be sought)
- Disclosure in the public interest, e.g. potential for harm if a patient ignores post-IV sedation instructions
- Disclosure required by law (a warrant is necessary)
- Disclosure if necessary for a legal case against a patient (a court subpoena is required).

Accurate and contemporaneous notes, which can be easily and reliably accessed, are a fundamental aspect of managing a modern dental practice. Computerised record keeping and practice management software are already an integral part of delivering quality health care, and we are likely to become even more dependent on information technology in the future.

121 Team management

Figure 121.1 The dental nurse team

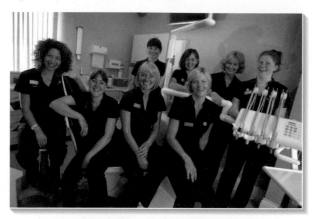

Figure 121.3 Teamwork in a clinical setting

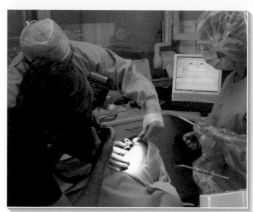

Figure 121.2 The dental team

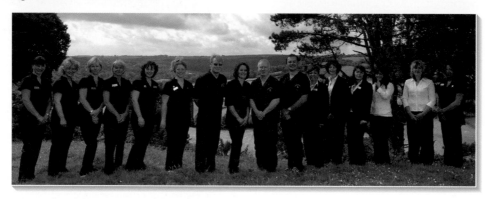

Figure 121.4 Extracurricular team bonding

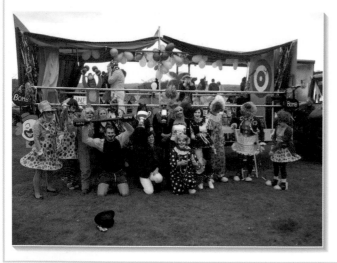

Figure 121.5 Team-building activities

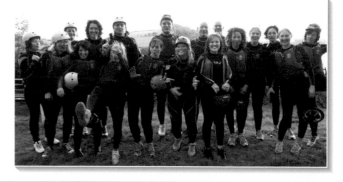

Introduction

The concept of **teamwork** is an extremely important aspect in the performance of any team, whether this is in sport, business or dentistry. The delivery of quality dental care cannot be provided in isolation and dentists operate within a team of dental care pro-fessionals (DCPs), including receptionists, practice managers, dental nurses, hygienists, therapists and dental technicians (Figures 121.1 and 121.2). The quality of care provided to the patient will be largely dependent on the effectiveness of the dental team and its individual members (Figure 121.3).

Dentistry at a Glance. First Edition. Edited by Elizabeth Kay. © 2016 John Wiley & Sons, Ltd. Published 2016 by John Wiley & Sons, Ltd.
Companion website: www.ataglanceseries.com/dentistryseries/dentistry

Teamwork

Teamwork can be defined as 'collaborative working within a group of individuals in order to achieve a goal'. A key aspect of teamwork is creation of a clear vision with appropriate goal setting. Each member of the team should be involved in creating the vision and setting the goals to ensure 'buy-in' and 'ownership' of the team strategy. This can be done through creating a 'mission statement' and 'team charter' to ensure that each individual is clear about their own role and the role of others in achieving the team aims and objectives. An example of a vision for a dental practice is shown Box 121.1.

> ### Box 121.1 Vision for a dental practice
>
> Our aim is to provide high quality dental care in a pleasant and friendly environment, working with our patients and the local community to improve oral health. We are committed to continual development to reflect our patients' needs, and the aspirations of the dental team to allow us to deliver the highest standard of care.

In the UK, the General Dental Council (GDC) recognises the importance of teamwork and has produced a document *Principles of Dental Team Working* to support a team approach. Within this document they state that 'the quality of teamwork is closely linked to the quality of care the team provides'.

External teamwork is also important in developing services for patients through relationships with secondary care providers, commissioners of dental services or other health-care professionals. Patient-centred care is an important aspect of providing high-quality health care and co-ordination of that care through effective teamwork between professionals is recognised as key.

Benefits of teamwork

It is widely recognised that we can generally achieve more collectively than we can individually. A group of individuals will often have different skills and talents, which can complement each other, and considerable research has been undertaken into the different roles that are important within a team. Dr Meredith Belbin identified specific roles within a team, which when present are most likely to succeed. These various roles are shown in Box 121.2, and highlight the importance of diversity and the value that individual members can bring to the success of a team.

> ### Box 121.2 Belbin's team roles
>
> - The Co-ordinator
> - The Plant
> - The Implementer
> - The Team Worker
> - The Shaper
> - The Monitor–Evaluator
> - The Resource Investigator
> - The Finisher

There are many other benefits to working as a team, including increased efficiency, creativity, morale support, work satisfaction, camaraderie and the opportunity to our share our successes and failures.

Developing a team philosophy

Placing a group of individuals together will not necessary provide a successful team. Suitable individuals need to be recruited who share the same values as the existing team members and are willing to 'buy into' the team vision. In addition to appropriate recruitment, team members need to understand and appreciate the practice vision, undergo regular training and above all feel valued. Leadership is an important aspect of any team. Many different styles of leadership have been described but each have the common features of a sense of purpose, a clear vision and respect of their team.

Team training

In sport, a successful team trains regularly and to a high standard. A dental team is no different. The more often they train and work together, the better they will perform. Whether this is welcoming a new patient, perfecting four-handed dentistry or dealing with a medical emergency; the result will depend on each individual playing their part with an appreciation of the importance of their role and the responsibility they have within the team. This needs to be learned and can only be achieved with regular training.

Such training can be specific to the task, such as medical emergency training: knowing how to manage a collapse, what to do in such an event and understanding the various roles in the team. The GDC has clear requirements for Continuing Professional Development (CPD) for all DCPs and core training is mandatory for radiology, infection control and medical emergencies. Each DCP should have a Personal Development Plan (PDP) to identify further areas of educational development and all training should be recorded in a training log.

Team training is also invaluable and this can be undertaken in a variety of ways. Specific training, such as fire drills or medical emergencies, is vital as it ensures that each individual can operate effectively within the team. More prosaic approaches to developing team work can be undertaken by team-building exercises. These may be completely unrelated to the 'day job' but often deliver huge benefits in creating a strong team spirit (Figures 121.4 and 121.5).

Communication and appraisal

In any successful team, communication is a key factor in success. Regular practice meetings are an extremely important part of running a successful dental practice, and additional team meetings may be beneficial, depending on the size of the practice.

In addition to team meetings, it is important that team members have the opportunity to meet and discuss their own individual needs with the management. Annual appraisal provides an ideal opportunity for staff to feedback any issues or concerns that they may have, and also provide the management with the chance of communicating with the employee about aspects of their performance. More importantly, appraisal is an opportunity to look at personal development, career planning and future training opportunities, with consideration given as to how this will fit into the strategic business plan of the practice.

An annual appraisal is insufficient and more frequent 'job chats' or '1-2-1s' need to be timetabled to allow staff to be fully engaged. It is important that dentists also have the opportunity for appraisal and an effective approach is through 360° feedback, with staff encouraged to express opinions on a clinician's performance. This provides good lines of communication and supports an open and transparent culture where staff feel able to raise concerns, should they arise.

Awards

Teamwork is a vital aspect of a developing a successful dental practice and this is recognised by various institutions. Many practices in the UK have been accredited by **Investors in People** and **BDA Good Practice**, which recognises a high level of teamwork. Such awards are a useful marker of Quality Assurance, but also provide an excellent way of acknowledging the hard work of successful dental teams.

122 Intrateam communication

Figure 122.1 Verbal messages need to be brief and succinct

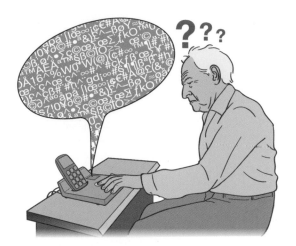

Figure 122.2 Business plan

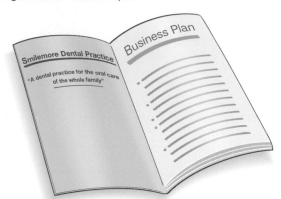

Figure 122.3 (a) Written policies and procedures need to be regularly reviewed. (b) Team meetings are essential

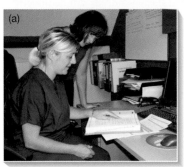

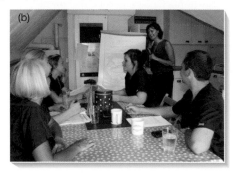

Figure 122.4 (a) A forward lean tells other person you are interested. (b) An open stance and a smile are welcoming. (c) Beware the cold shoulder, (d) Facial and postural messages are powerful, and (e) Folder arms signify defensiveness

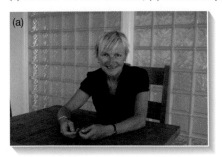

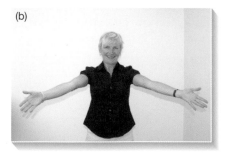

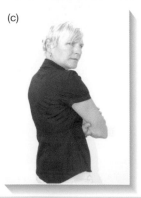

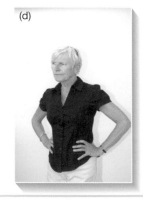

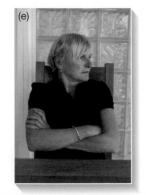

The most important questions to ask before considering any communication at all to anyone are:

- What do you want to convey?
- Why do you want to convey it?

This may seem so obvious that it is not worth mentioning but although it is supremely important it is overlooked, confused or mismanaged countless times, leading to many of the problems in dentistry, as in life.

One example with which we are all familiar is the rambling voicemail message (Figure 122.1). Basically, you are unavailable and the caller needs to leave a succinct summary of why they want to speak to you and what they want to tell you. Yet many people seem incapable of this because they are not clear from the outset (or when they hear that you are not available) what it is they want to say or why. I am sure you have many examples of your own but put simply: 'Hi, it's Stephen, calling to arrange a meeting about the implant course. Please call me back on my mobile number when you get a chance. Cheers for now.' Job done.

Business plan and objectives

In order to help formulate what it is we want to communicate and why, we all need guidance as to the situation. Most importantly, the practice, department or clinic needs a clear business plan and/or set of objectives (Figure 122.2). For example, what is it that the practice does? 'Smilemore is a dental practice for the oral care of the whole family' or 'Going Straight is a practice dedicated to orthodontics'. Everyone is clear.

From this will flow all your internal and external communications. Does asking a team member to order orthodontic brackets fall into the remit of Going Straight? Almost certainly. Would it be appropriate for a Smilemore team member? Probably not as the practice is more likely to refer patients to an orthodontist. But this will form an important part of external communications (see Chapter 123).

Written communication

A good deal of important information for the team will be written and be available either as hard copy or electronically, or both. Such documents will include instructions for procedures and use of equipment, practice policies on a variety of issues, health and safety information, induction packs for new team members. These should be collated and regularly reviewed and updated by the practice manager or the team member designated to the task (Figure 122.3a).

Verbal communication
Instructions and discussion

A happy and successful dental team will spend a lot of time talking to one another, whether this is directly involved in clinical work or the running of the practice or in 'social' conversation on day-to-day life in general. Good teams in any walk of life have

fun and, conversely, team that have fun are usually very good at what they do. People who have job satisfaction invariably report that they have fun at work without in any way lessening the seriousness of what they do.

Patients sense happy atmospheres and this leads to a general upward spiral of good communication and clear understanding.

Once again, the need for clarity is paramount. If a dentist says, 'pass me that curvy looking thing', the nurse may have a range of instruments to choose from, and may pass the wrong one. This will require another request 'not that one, (points) that one' (raised eyebrows, irritated tone of voice, two upset people). If instead the dentist had said 'can you pass me the Hollenbach carver so that I can finish this amalgam' everyone would be clear.

In this example, after working together for a time the nurse will probably be able to anticipate what the dentist needs and when; a simple nod may be then enough to transact the communication.

Team meetings

Team meetings can be tedious nightmares or great opportunities for all team members to communicate and contribute to the success of a task or project (Figure 122.3b).

Once again, the key is to be sure why the meeting is being held and what is to be achieved. An agenda or list of topics to be discussed or described is essential so that everyone is clear of the purpose. Allowing everyone to contribute will ensure that all team members feel part of the discussion and the project under consideration, and the practice. It will also ensure that no one harbours grudges or feels that 'no one listens to me anyway, so what's the point?'

Written notes, reports or minutes of the team meeting help as reminders on action points as well as refreshing individuals' memories of what was said and agreed. These can also provide a useful reference point as well as a measure of progress on particular issues; for example, from an initial idea in January through to a report of a successful practice open day in September.

Non-verbal communication (body language)

This is a huge subject and readers are encouraged to investigate this more fully as it is so often the key to successful communication.

We are all aware of the extremes of negative and positive body language (Figure 122.3). Turning your back on someone or welcoming them with open arms are obvious examples. But there are countless stances in between these limits invariably augmented by facial expressions to support the emotion being conveyed: angry, smiling, confused, listening and so forth.

An important element is awareness. Be aware of your own body position and what it is 'saying' as well as observing others and what they are 'telling' you without speaking. Picking up on these clues will help you modify your own body language to enable you to convey what you want to communicate and why.

123 External communication

Figure 123.1 All your practice's external contacts should be documented

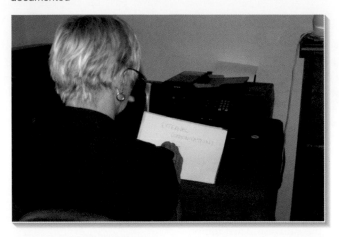

Figure 123.2 (a, b) Use the appropriate medium for a given recipient

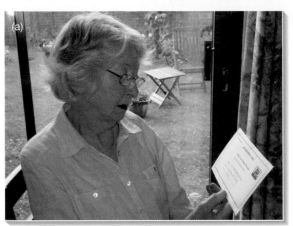

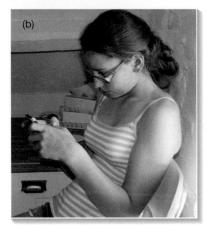

Figure 123.3 Write prescriptions clearly

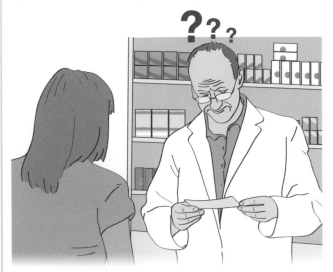

As with intrateam communication (see Chapter 122), the key questions to ask before considering any external communication are:

- What do you want to convey?
- Why do you want to convey it?

This bears repetition as it is central to achieving successful communication.

Who is external?

Firstly, it is valuable to list all the external people with whom you, or the practice, communicate (Figure 123.1). When you sit down and make a list, which you should, you'll be surprised at how long it is: patients, dental suppliers, suppliers of other goods and services, referral practices, hospitals, pharmacies, newspapers, advertising agencies, government agencies and departments to name only some. The contacts will be very diverse, from professional to lay, and will each need careful consideration as to the most appropriate form of communication to employ.

What form of communication is appropriate?

There are many ways in which we can convey our messages, or receive responses, including written, verbal, electronic, internet and social media. Often the reason for the communication and the context will dictate the means. For example, if you need to order goods quickly then the internet or a phone call will be preferable to a postal route. A reminder to call for a check-up appointment may, however, be best sent by conventional mail.

However, careful consideration is needed (Figure 123.2). Would your patients prefer to be contacted by email or text? Would they regard your practice as being up-to-date and efficient or would they consider this a nuisance?

Advertising

In former times, the General Dental Council (GDC) (the regulatory body appointed to regulate dental professionals and protect the public) had very strict rules about dentists and dental practices advertising. Although these were relaxed some years ago, the GDC does still have guidelines as to appropriate advertising and it is important to check these (www.gdc-uk.org).

Advertising can be for a variety of purposes. It may be for team recruitment, in which case a professional journal, such as the *British Dental Journal*, may be appropriate if the team member might be attracted from outside the immediate locality of the practice. Alternatively, if the applicants are likely to be from the surrounding area a local newspaper or online jobsite may be better.

In either case, the usual rules of advertising content 'decent, honest, legal and truthful' should be followed as well as avoiding discrimination. The publication or website owner will be able to give guidance on this. Additionally, this provides the opportunity to promote the practice in a positive light. 'Nurse wanted for dental practice' might sum up the actual requirement but some elaboration can make the prospect seem more attractive, even if the reader is not specifically interested in the position.

'Smilemore, a happy family dental practice in Gleamtown seeks an enthusiastic dental nurse to join a dedicated and expanding team' still conveys the requirement but adds extra value and encouragement as well as clearly setting down the practice philosophy and outlook.

Prescription writing

This form of communication is necessarily very specific and involves two important external 'customers', the patient and the pharmacist. The standard joke is of illegible prescriptions written by busy doctors but taking heed of this cliché provides a valuable lesson. In dentistry it is unusual for prescriptions to be long or over-complicated. It is therefore a straightforward matter to ensure that they are written or typed clearly and without any obvious confusion (Figure 123.3).

It is also important to tell the patient the details of the drugs or medicines and their purpose. This will include the number of times a day that they are to be taken, and when (e.g. before or after meals) and for how long. Patients often do not take in such details in the surgery and will ask other team members in reception or the waiting room. Therefore, making team members aware of what constitutes a prescription and the specific details of interpretation is an important element of internal communication, even if the instruction is to refer back to the prescription writer if in doubt.

Referral letters

One of the most important pieces of written communication from a practice, whether in hard copy and/or electronic form, is the referral letter. By its nature it is a request for further expertise or knowledge from a fellow professional and it is thus in the interests of the referring professional, the receiving professional and, most importantly, the patient that the content is clear, complete and concise.

Complete: The letter should be on headed practice paper and contain all the anticipated information that will be necessary for the receiving professional to:

- Take action in contacting the patient to make an appointment (patient's name, address, phone number, email address)
- Assess the need for an appointment appropriate to the patient's likely needs (consultation, active treatment session etc.)
- Contact you in the event of further immediate queries (your contact address, phone numbers and email)
- Understand the background to the referral, including relevant medical, dental and social history of the patient.

Clear: The letter should clearly state the reason for the referral and the urgency for requested action on the part of the receiving professional.

Concise: Being concise is in everyone's interests in that it will enable the important information to be communicated swiftly and without unnecessary confusion of detail or extraneous information. Speed is often of the essence in such circumstances but taking time to compose, write and review a referral letter can pay dividends in terms of patient care and organisational efficiency. To be extra sure, and if time permits, ask a colleague to read the letter before sending it so that any missing detail can be added or unneeded text can be removed.

124 Being part of the profession

Figure 124.1 The Royal College of Surgeons of England, Lincolns Inn Fields, London
Source: Reproduced from RCSEng photo archives with permission of the Royal College of Surgeons of England.

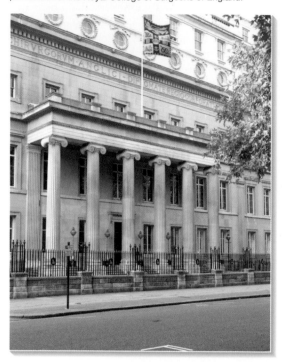

Figure 124.2 The Guy-Whittle Auditorium at the Royal Society of Medicine, London
Source: Reproduced with permission of the Royal Society of Medicine, London.

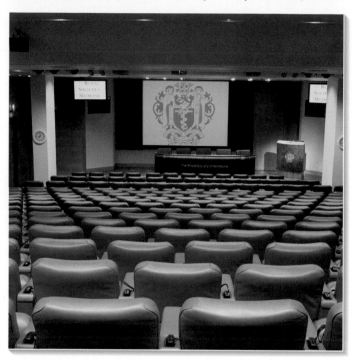

Figure 124.3 The Atrium at the British Dental Association Building in Wimpole Street, London
Source: Reproduced with permission of the British Dental Association.

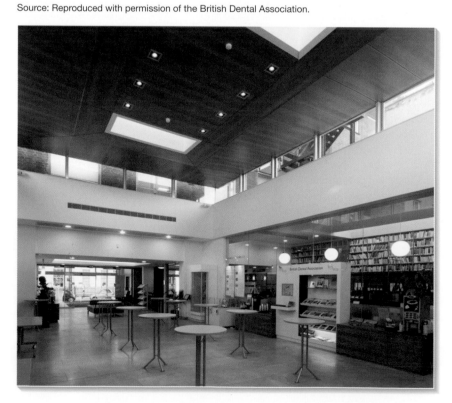

Being part of a profession is a matter of privilege and pride. Just having a qualification or skill is not sufficient, as a professional person has to follow a code of ethics, attitudes, behaviours and values set by peers, in addition to obeying the laws of the land and the community.

On qualification, the first requirement is to register with the General Dental Council (GDC), the regulatory body whose key function is patient protection. On paying an annual retention fee, registrants are required to follow a set of standards and additional guidelines, plus keep up to date by maintaining Continuing Professional Development (CPD). In case patients make a claim, the registrant is also required to have indemnity cover from a dental defence organisation, an insurance company or be covered by NHS/ Crown indemnity.

The hallmark of a professional person is their eagerness and enthusiasm to learn and continue to do so for life. After graduation, most dentists will undertake Foundation Training (FT) organised by their local Deaneries, which are co-ordinated by the UK Committee for Postgraduate Deans and Directors (COPDEND).

The Faculty of Dental Surgery and the Faculty of General Dental Practice are the two Dental Faculties of the Royal College of Surgeons of England, which dates back to the Guild of Barber Surgeons in the 14th Century (Figure 124.1). These two Faculties exercise the crucial roles of overseeing standards of practice and standards of training to ensure the best oral health for patients and to promote professional excellence in all aspects of dentistry.

The Faculties fulfil these roles in setting and monitoring standards for both generalist and specialist practice, including the dental team, by setting the curricula for and conducting examinations and awarding diplomas in the full range of dental surgical practice, offering a benchmark for dentistry.

Playing a wider role in the promotion of standards in practice, they liaise with other bodies involved with health care at the highest level, providing input to national consultations on changes to the health service, programmes of postgraduate education, continuing professional development, revalidation, promotion of clinical audit and research, and publications on clinical guidelines and standards

The Faculties accomplish all of these things through the active engagement and work of their Members and Fellows. That, ultimately, is what the Royal College Faculties are – highly committed professionals working together for the safety of patients and the further enhancement of dentistry. In the UK, the Scottish Royal Colleges in Glasgow and Edinburgh also carry out similar activities.

The Royal Society of Medicine (RSM) is another major provider of postgraduate medical education and has one of the largest postgraduate medical libraries in the world (Figure 124.2). All members, including students, can use this library, which also has several hundred ejournals, ebooks and an extensive collection of online lectures.

The Odontology Section provides a forum for the continuing professional development for all those working in the field of oral and dental healthcare sciences by organising a broad range of educational activities throughout the year. The Oral and Maxillofacial Section provides education aimed at consultant level to keep members updated on the constantly evolving innovations in the specialty.

The RSM is located in the heart of London's West End, with club facilities available to all members including restaurant, bar and hotel accommodation.

Dentistry is not just a job; it isn't even just a vocation; it's a profession. So in qualifying as a dentist one joins a proud history and community. In seeking to advance their profession, dentists have always acted proactively, sharing best practice, advancing the science of their work and seeking to provide the best care they can for their patients. From that philosophy was born the British Dental Association (BDA), which is the leading professional association for dentists (Figure 124.3). This not-for-profit organisation is run by dentists for dentists. It has nearly 23 000 members and has been supporting dentists for over 132 years.

As a trade union the BDA is responsible for negotiating with external organisations, and lobbying on all issues that affect dentists and dental students. It also represents individuals who may have a problem at dental school or work. It supports students at each stage in their career and continues to protect them throughout their careers.

Local Dental Committees (LDCs) are the statutory bodies recognised by successive NHS Acts as the professional organisations representing general dental practitioners. They are independent self-funding bodies, not trade unions. They advise on contracts, terms of service, complaints, disciplinary matters and clinical governance. They are local and it is this local knowledge and insight into practice activity that make each LDC very important. They allow practitioners to be part of a network.

During a period of considerable change, it is these LDCs that retain the greatest knowledge of the services in their particular areas. This vital resource is invaluable in supporting transitions to new commissioning structures. LDCs therefore have an important part to play in providing advice to Health and Wellbeing Boards when devising strategic needs assessments and health and wellbeing strategies.

As a professional person, the dentist always puts the patients interests first, constantly respecting their rights, dignity and autonomy. As their career advances, the dentist will begin to realise the value of being part of the professional network provided by their peers and support organisations. An integral part of being a fulfilled professional person is the 'giving back' to the profession. By contributing at all levels from teaching, mentoring and advising other colleagues to examining, representing and ultimately leading local or national professional bodies, a career-long sense of satisfaction, pride and achievement can be gained. Most successful personalities will agree that they gained much more from their profession than they gave to it.

Index

Dentistry at a Glance. First Edition. Edited by Elizabeth Kay. © 2016 John Wiley & Sons, Ltd. Published 2016 by John Wiley & Sons, Ltd.
Companion website: www.ataglanceseries.com/dentistryseries/dentistry